MEDICAL CHOICES, MEDICAL CHANCES

MEDICAL CHOICES, MEDICAL CHANCES

How Patients, Families, and Physicians Can Cope with Uncertainty

HAROLD BURSZTAJN, M.D.   RICHARD I. FEINBLOOM, M.D.
ROBERT M. HAMM, PH.D.   ARCHIE BRODSKY

A Merloyd Lawrence Book
DELACORTE PRESS/SEYMOUR LAWRENCE

A MERLOYD LAWRENCE BOOK
Published by
Delacorte Press/Seymour Lawrence
1 Dag Hammarskjold Plaza
New York, N.Y. 10017

Photographs by Michael Lutch
Courtesy of Beth Israel Hospital, Boston, Massachusetts
Permission to publish elsewhere may be granted by Beth
Israel Public relations.

Photograph accompanying Chapter 8
Courtesy of A. Stone Freedberg, M.D.

Photograph accompanying Chapter 13
Courtesy of Diana, Don, and baby Maxwell Jillie.

Manufactured in the United States of America

First printing

Designed by Laura Bernay

Library of Congress Cataloging in Publication Data
Main entry under title:
Medical choices, medical chances.
"A Merloyd Lawrence book."
Bibliography: p.
Includes index.
1. Medicine—Philosophy.   2. Medical logic.
3. Medicine—Decision-making.   4. Probabilities.
5. Uncertainty.   6. Physician and patient.
I. Bursztajn, Harold.
R723.M36   610'.1'9   80–22631
ISBN: 0–440–05750–7

To
A. Stone Freedberg
a model of wisdom in clinical practice
and
Stanley Sagov
a model family physician

CONTENTS

CONTENTS

ACKNOWLEDGMENTS

We wish to acknowledge some of the people who have contributed to this book and to our lives and works. They range from patients to philosophers, doctors to typists—and, of course, loved ones and friends. They are: Joel Alpert, M.D., William Bayer, M.D., William Berenberg, M.D., Judy Bevis, Sissela Bok, Lilly Bursztajn, Sherry Bursztajn, Buzzy Chanowitz, Sey Chassler, André Churchwell, M.D., Max Day, M.D., John Drimmer, Robert Ebert, M.D., Werner Erhard, Peter Farquhar, Betty Forman, Thomas Gates, M.D., Donna Gertler, David Gordon, M.D., Robert Haggerty, M.D., Michael Harris, Reid Hastie, Leston Havens, M.D., Harvey Jackins, Charles Janeway, M.D., Frances Judkins, Arthur Krieger, M.D., Robert Lawrence, M.D., Duncan Luce, James Lyons, M.D., Peter McFarren, Melissa Mahaney, Matthew Movsesian, M.D., Alexander Nadas, M.D., Thomas Nagel, Norman Paul, M.D., Eric Proctor, Hilary Putnam, Howard Raiffa, Julius Richmond, M.D., Klaus Riegel, Kim Ruth, Paul Schrecker, Miles Shore, M.D., Harold Solomon, M.D., John Stoeckle, M.D., Michael Sukale, Joanne Sullivan, and Daniel Tosteson, M.D. We also thank the staffs of the Family Practice Group of Cambridge, Massachusetts, and the Ambulatory Screening Clinic at Massachusetts General Hospital.

We are deeply grateful to the many patients and families who have worked with us in developing our ideas in practice. The experiences we have shared with them form the basis of the accounts in this book. In the course of preparing these case studies a number of families have given freely of their time to review experiences that were sometimes painful in order that others might benefit. In so doing they have made this their book as well as ours. The same is true of Merloyd Lawrence, a gifted editor whose critical readings have helped to clarify and at times inspire our ideas. This book would not have been possible without her support. Nor would it have been possible without the warmth and wisdom of the families in which our education began.

H.B.
R.I.F.
R.M.H.
A.B.

INTRODUCTION

When we deal with questions of health and illness, as patients or concerned family members, as doctors or other health professionals, each of us has some notion of what is true and what is good. We are all guided by some implicit philosophy of science. That philosophy, whatever it may be, has a lot to do with how we feel about the pain, fear, and risks associated with illness, how we think about the decisions that are to be made, and what actions we take on our own behalf or that of someone else who is ill.

Of course, most of us don't think in terms of an *explicit* philosophy of science when we are confronted with illness. But we do have some idea of what we know, how we know it, and how sure we are about it. That is our implicit philosophy of science. Even if we don't think of ourselves as scientists, we do think of medicine as a science. We have some idea of what science is and of what constitutes good science and bad science. One question we need to ask ourselves is whether our ideas about science correspond to what scientists today understand science to be. Another is whether these ideas can help us make the best possible decisions about illness and health.

When a number of writers, dissatisfied with medicine as it is generally practiced by physicians, address these questions, they argue that medicine should not be thought of as a science at all (Carlson, 1976; cf. Cousins, 1979). Science cannot be an adequate basis for medicine, they claim, because medicine deals with human life and human feelings. The logic behind this critique is as follows: Science is "exact"; human beings cannot be understood exactly; therefore human beings cannot be understood by means of science.

But science is not what these critics of medicine seem to think it is. By their definition not only medicine but all of the biological and social sciences (at least in the twentieth century) fail to qualify. Although the sciences that deal with living beings cannot claim one hundred percent predictability, it still is useful to characterize particular ways of understanding living beings as scientific.

What the critics really seem to be saying, then, is that medicine cannot be a science because it is not like physics. But physics, too, has changed during this century from a *science of certainty* to a *science of probability*. Most of us have at least heard of the Heisenberg Uncertainty Principle. We are aware that the physics of Einstein and his successors is not the physics we learned in high school, where cause-and-effect relationships could be known with precision and predicted with certainty through the use of Newton's laws. But we haven't thought systematically about what it means to "know" in the age of quantum physics, because we haven't tried to apply the new science to everyday thought, feeling, and action. We still think we can "know" in the old, mechanistic way.

Physicists have realized that the new way of thinking has revolutionary implications. Indeed it represents what T. S. Kuhn (in *The Structure of Scientific Revolutions,* 1962) calls a "paradigm shift"—i.e., a change in the fundamental assumptions and procedures of science. As long as scientists work within a familiar, agreed-upon paradigm, the philosophy that guides their work can be left implicit. During the period of a paradigm shift, however, this implicit philosophy becomes a matter of explicit discussion. After a period of questioning, debate, theorizing, and experimentation, it is replaced by a new philosophy which, once articulated, agreed upon, and learned, can itself become implicit as the new paradigm that guides scientific investigation.

Paradigm shifts tend to occur when an existing paradigm isn't working— when scientists can no longer use it to solve the problems they set out to solve. Such a crisis of confidence exists today in the science of medicine. Amid malpractice suits, the holistic medicine and "patient's rights" movements, and a growing concern over the cost of medical care, we need to make explicit the assumptions that guide our thinking in medicine. In making these assumptions explicit, we have the opportunity to change them. In this book we will show that medical questions can continue to be approached scientifically if the science of medicine partakes of the standards of twentieth-century physics. It took two hundred years for medicine to incorporate the insights of classical physics, the physics of Newton. More than fifty years after the "quantum revolution" in modern physics, medicine has yet to incorporate its standards.

It may be natural to think that medicine always was and always will be what it is today, but in fact, what we know as "modern medicine" is less than a century old. In the latter part of the nineteenth century the French physiologist Claude Bernard introduced principles adapted from classical physics into experimental medicine, thereby revolutionizing all of medical practice, experimental and clinical. With medicine now in search of a new science we can once again turn to physics as a model. We will refer to the Newtonian paradigm of science as the Mechanistic Paradigm, and to the paradigm that guides the work of modern physicists as the Probabilistic Paradigm. The new science of the Probabilistic Paradigm is one that accepts a degree of uncertainty as an inherent part of reality. It questions whether causation can be specified with certainty, whether there is such a thing as a conclusive experiment, and whether subjective knowledge can be entirely separated from objective knowledge.

Under the Probabilistic Paradigm, a set of probable causes in constantly changing configurations replaces the concept of a definite cause or causes for a given effect. Experimentation, rather than linking cause and effect in a relationship of certainty, becomes a way of exploring what probabilities may obtain. Instead of an "objective" reality that exists independently of the observer, there is a many-sided reality that includes the effect of the way one observes on what one observes. Instead of a strict distinction between facts that are "value-neutral" and values that have no basis in fact, there is a recognition of the subjective component of factual knowledge and the objective, rationally discussable aspect of values and feelings.

All of these distinctions have vast implications for medical practice. Of particular significance for medicine is the fact that the Probabilistic Paradigm recognizes values and feelings to be an inescapable concern of science. A paradigm of science is a paradigm of thought and action. The Probabilistic Paradigm, as distinct from the Mechanistic, incorporates the realization that thought and action take place in the context of feeling. Under the new paradigm the scope of thought and action in medicine is enlarged to take into account the feelings that affect people's health and well-being.

We are all, to some degree or other, afraid of uncertainty. Because our conception of rationality is grounded in the Mechanistic Paradigm, which has no place for uncertainty, we find it difficult to be rational about uncertainty. Instead, when faced with uncertainty, we become anxious—most of all when our lives are on the line. When we are sick or are in the presence of illness (as family members or medical personnel), pain and fear make it hard to be as rational as we would like to be. We are tempted to retreat into a false sense of certainty, which affects our capacity to make decisions. For when uncertainty is too painful to face directly, we block it out. But we cannot make wise decisions when we deny ourselves the benefits of conscious awareness of uncertainty.

Not only patients and their families are prey to anxiety. While a patient may have reason to fear imminent death, a doctor may dread the intimations of mortality that come when the limits of knowledge and power are revealed. Just as a patient may seek to evade the unknown future consequences of an illness by simply failing to acknowledge them, so a doctor may do anything to avoid being exposed as uncertain or in error—in his or her own eyes, in the eyes of colleagues, in the eyes of patients and families who have been taught to expect "scientific" accuracy from medicine, and perhaps even before a court of law. A woman who fails to perform regular breast self-examinations and a doctor who relies on laboratory readings in place of clinical judgment may both be fleeing from the responsibility of making choices in an uncertain world.

One way to avoid the anxiety that accompanies uncertainty is to bury one's head in the sand. Another way is to seek assurance from technology. While much is said about overtreatment in critical commentaries on contemporary medicine, the damaging influence of the Mechanistic Paradigm can also be felt in overdiagnosis. In practically any teaching hospital conscientious interns and residents daily bring to bear every available piece of diagnostic machinery on difficult cases in an effort "not to take any chances" and "to find out for sure." Trained to seek certainty, they may not realize that they *are* taking chances, not only with time and money, but with the health of patients who are already in a weakened condition. Putting needles or tubes into a person's body and drawing blood (or whatever) drains the patient's strength and increases the risk of infection —often in a search for esoteric conditions that are unlikely to be found and would be untreatable if diagnosed. Mechanistic medical science all too frequently loses sight of the goal (treatment) in the exaltation of the means (increasingly refined diagnosis). The aim of medicine traditionally has been, and should still remain, that of making people who are ill feel better, not that of making doctors feel better about the state of their knowledge.

We are thus in agreement with those who criticize physicians for often being too hasty in turning to technological intervention instead of observing the natural course of illness, being emotionally supportive, and providing treatment in the context of a patient's life. But we come to this conclusion from a different perspective. Rather than question the value of reason as a tool for solving medical problems, we would suggest that reason is often abandoned in "establishment" medical practice. Technical procedures, valuable as they are when there is a rational basis for using them, are invoked mindlessly and automatically, as rituals to reassure anxious physicians. Precise laboratory measurement is accepted as a substitute for a complex, elusive reality that may be understood only with patience and sensitivity. Indeed, future anthropologists may look at our medical rituals the way we look at, say, the savage ritual of offering sacrifices to bring rain. We take the healing rain that eventually comes as conclusive evidence that we have finally chosen the right sacrifice.

The Probabilistic Paradigm offers both patients and doctors a way to make peace with uncertainty without paying the high costs involved in denying uncertainty altogether. Once it is understood that science accepts uncertainty, it should be easier for people to accept uncertainty. By using the new science of probability, people can support each other in uncertain situations by sharing the risks and helping each other cope with them consciously and rationally. The acknowledgment of uncertainty removes a large barrier to trust (whether between family members or between doctor and patient), since people can trust one another more readily when the unreasonable expectation of certainty is removed. At the same time, the realization that uncertainty is inescapably a part of reality motivates people to work at creating the trusting relationships and mutual support necessary in a world where no one can have a sure or final answer. Thus, along with its other benefits, the new science of medicine offers patients and doctors the opportunity to deal with each other as *allies* instead of *adversaries,* which is too often the case today.

An understanding of probabilities also enables patients and doctors to exert all possible influence over the outcome of an illness and to gain the satisfaction and the sense of control that comes from doing so. Although shielding ourselves from uncertainty may reduce anxiety in the short run, it does not help us achieve better outcomes in the long run. By giving up the dream of total certainty and sharing the uncertainty that does exist, we can realistically make decisions that in effect reduce uncertainty. We can better predict how things will turn out, do something about making them turn out for the better, and (when that is not possible) live with disappointment. It is only when we face the fact that we are taking chances that we can begin to make choices.

* * *

Medicine provides a natural focus for bringing the perspectives of twentieth-century science into our lives. Some of our most powerful fantasies about ourselves are nurtured and expressed (or left unexpressed) in our relationship to medicine: the fantasy of omniscience and omnipotence, as embodied in the doctor who commands the wondrous apparatus of modern science; the fantasy of ignorance and weakness, as embodied in the uncertain, dependent patient. Medicine is where our very existence may be at stake in the choices we make. It is one of the places where we learn early in life about certainty and uncertainty, trust and mistrust. If in the past medicine has contributed to teaching us mechanistic habits of thought, feeling, and action, perhaps we can now change medicine so that it can teach those who come after us different habits, habits that are more useful and more humane.

The new approach to medicine we propose here contains some ingredients that in themselves may seem familiar. The language of probability is already used a great deal in medicine. For example, doctors may obtain informed consent from patients by specifying the odds for success of various treatment outcomes. In addition, many recent developments in medical practice, emanating from the public as well as the profession, are aimed at breaking down both the intellectual rigidity of mechanistic medical science and the authoritarian doctor-patient relationship that coexists with it. They include self-care, holistic medicine, family medicine, patient's rights, patient advocacy, and patient education. Supporters of these changes may find much in these pages that strikes a sympathetic chord.

From a scientific perspective, however, the current efforts to humanize medical practice (admirable as they are) are a probabilistic icing on a mechanistic cake. When an outmoded paradigm breaks down, scientists naturally try to patch it up before giving up on it completely. This is what is happening in medicine today. While the patchwork repairs now being attempted may be moves in the right direction, they are not likely to have much effect in the absence of a systematic change in our habits of thought, feeling, and action. Until we learn to think about medical decision-making in a new way, the old way of thinking will continue to shape the questions we ask and the ways in which we answer them.

This is why we propose to use the Probabilistic Paradigm, originally developed in physics, in the applied science of medicine. We wish to explore this theme in a useful and not unnecessarily forbidding manner, since we believe that philosophy has meaning only insofar as it is consciously applied in everyday life—in this case by patients, doctors, and all who are concerned with medicine. We have therefore written this book as an episodic tale of how a doctor and his patients attempt to learn and practice the new paradigm. As our fictional Dr. S. makes a pilgrim's progress that loosely reflects the experiences (including the mistakes) of the two of us who are physicians, his thinking and personal reactions reflect those of all four authors. In keeping with the Probabilistic Paradigm, S. is committed to helping patients and their families to make their own choices and work out their own medical destinies. At the same time, as a physician he sees himself as having knowledge and skill to contribute and comfort and caring to offer.

At the beginning of our story, S., as a hospital intern, witnesses a case of overdiagnosing and under-caring—a case that haunts him throughout his practice—that dramatizes the devastating impact mechanistic thinking can have, even in the hands of well-meaning people. It is then that S. begins to articulate the principles of the Probabilistic Paradigm. The remainder of Part I ("A New Science of Medicine") lays out these principles and shows how they depart from those of the Mechanistic Paradigm—first in scientific theory and research (with emphasis on physics), then in medical practice, and finally in everyday life. For after S. and his patients realize the advantages of the new paradigm, they must come to terms with the fact that life in our society—in the family, on the job, in the consumer marketplace, and in the doctor's office—continues to reinforce the use of the old paradigm that has shaped our society in the first place. The bulk of our social institutions, including our profit-oriented economic system, have not been set up to encourage independent critical thinking. It will be far from easy for patients and doctors to think probabilistically in their medical encounters when they are accustomed to thinking mechanistically in other areas of their lives.

In Part II ("Chance and Choice") S. seeks to translate the Probabilistic Paradigm into tools for decision-making that he and his patients together can use. First he tries the formal procedure called decision analysis, which has recently been introduced into medicine after having been developed in business and public policy planning. Although he finds it useful to learn decision analysis as a way of teaching himself what to keep in mind when making decisions probabilistically, he and his patients conclude that guiding their actions with decision analysis creates as many problems as it resolves. Even with decision analysis, they are still faced with large questions of judgment at every step of the way.

Realizing that they cannot avoid making judgments, they turn to a more practical, informal approach, one that treats every decision (in medicine and in life) as a gamble and attempts to distinguish between good and bad gambles according to the contexts in which they occur. The word *gambling* here does not have its usual connotations: a trivial recreation, a highly profitable business activity, or a form of compulsive, self-destructive behavior. Instead, the gambling we speak of here is guided by the principles of scientific experimentation under the Probabilistic Paradigm. On the one hand, it requires critical judgment, i.e., the capacity to doubt. On the other, it requires trust, i.e., the capacity to believe. Actually people gamble all the time, in everything they do. Because they don't always like to admit it, they gamble unconsciously. By gambling consciously together, S. and the families with whom he works are able to gamble in a way that is both reasonable and effective.

To do so, however, they have to learn to trust one another, and that is not always easy in a world that is full of mistrust. In Part III ("Relationships") S. and his patients confront the fact that decision-making takes place in the context of relationships among people (in the family, in the workplace, between doctor and patient, and so forth) and the feelings those relationships engender. When there is little trust in a family (as, for example, in the case that begins Part III), the family members are not likely to have the emotional security needed to gamble consciously. By working to achieve greater trust and mutual concern, S. and his patients become better able to gamble together. Conversely, through the experience of gambling together, they develop trust and concern. In this process of discovery and growth S. learns from his patients just as they learn from him.

Although S. is portrayed as a family doctor, a doctor who works not only with individual patients, but with families, one does not need to be or to have a family doctor in order to make decisions as S. and his patients do; any doctor or patient can do so. On the other hand, probabilistic thinking lends itself particularly well to situations in which a doctor, patient, and family work together.

Part IV ("Family Decisions") shows how families can make medical decisions in keeping with the Probabilistic Paradigm when an atmosphere of trust and caring is present. Here, with guidance and support from S., families create their own ways of coping with illness, death, and birth, even as they go through the range of emotions attendant upon these events. The cases in this section, which include a birth and a death in the home, center around the decision to use the home or the hospital as a site for care. They show how families can exercise varying degrees of control in different settings. They also show that it is much easier for patients to exercise critical thinking under conditions of uncertainty when there is a family to support them in facing uncertainty.

From the doctor's point of view we see how S. shares his understanding of the new paradigm with patients and their families. By working with families he can observe and point out the complex contexts of causation that affect the course of an illness, showing that each individual cause has effects that vary with time and cannot be precisely specified. He and his patients soon realize that the family itself can simultaneously be both a factor contributing to illness and a source of recuperative strength.

Like physicists who unintentionally influence the movement of electrons merely by turning on a light to observe them, the patient, family, and doctor cannot be detached observers. They are all involved observers affecting and being affected by the observed situation in countless ways that no laboratory test can measure. With regard to the doctor's observations, every form of diagnosis, from a kindly gaze to a complex X-ray procedure, has an impact, great or small, on what it is designed to reveal. By the same token, the patient's and family's understanding of symptoms can have a significant impact on the course of illness.

A doctor who maintains contact with families, rather than just individuals, can also more easily understand the many different ways in which people think, feel, and act, and the importance of values in medical decision-making. Does a lonely, disabled, elderly man want to prolong his life at the cost of having a painful, risky, and perhaps further disabling operation? Does a woman about to give birth want to go through an uncomplicated labor under anesthesia and pain medication or with coaching from her family? Does a single mother with severe high blood pressure want to try to live out a normal life span by taking pills that make her too drowsy to earn a living and care for her young children? Do a father and mother want to authorize surgery to save the life of a three-day-old baby with a heart condition who may also have Down's syndrome ("mongolism")? These are questions of value, and in the new science of medicine values are considered along with probabilities in reaching decisions. In this new science any doctor, regardless of specialty, needs to be a bit of a family doctor as well; and any patient, however isolated, needs to be in contact with the source of his or her values, i.e., the family, even if it is accessible only through memory.

Finally, as indicated in Part V ("Contexts"), even the most fully aware and committed doctors and patients will be practicing the new science in a world that is not yet hospitable to probabilistic thinking or to the spirit of trust and cooperation in which probabilistic thinking can most readily take place. Inevitably there will be obstacles, both in the immediate contexts of practice, where the setting (be it home or hospital) influences medical choices, and in the larger contexts—economic, legal, political—where further barriers of misunderstanding are raised. If one patient, doctor, or family learns to make decisions under conditions of uncertainty by thinking critically, it will not change the character of the social relations that limit everyone's freedom to make decisions, but it will mean more freedom and control for that one patient, doctor, or family. If we can all begin to think critically and to work together, then perhaps basic change will be possible.

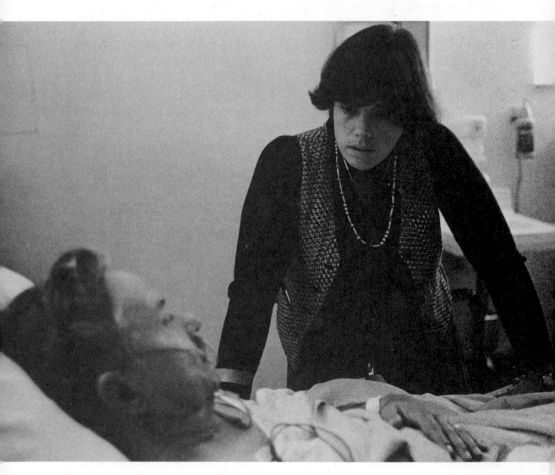

PART I

A NEW SCIENCE
OF MEDICINE

1

A CASE OF
UNCERTAINTY

In a large city with several renowned medical schools there is a leading teaching hospital which enjoys a well-deserved reputation (as hospitals go) for being efficient and humane at the same time. The pediatric facility of this hospital benefits from close association with the practitioners of adult medicine in an enlightened medical community. Yet its staff almost always has time to give a child a smile.

Not long ago the hospital admitted a twenty-one-month-old boy. It is difficult even now to write about him, using his full name. It is easier just to call him K.

What was wrong with him? Nearly everything. In addition to the ear infection that brought him to the hospital in the first place, he was emaciated, pale, and withdrawn. Though obviously starving, he refused to eat. What was *right* with him? It was hard to tell. He could not communicate verbally, and his capacity to experience and express love was not very well developed.

While K. was in the hospital, he came under the care of two groups of physicians who took very different approaches to diagnosis and treatment. His case enables us, therefore, to com-

9780873944009

pare two ways of thinking and two strategies for making choices.

K. lived in a working-class neighborhood far from the hospital-medical school complex. He was the only child of a young mother who claimed that the anesthesia used during childbirth had left her in a daze for two weeks. As a result, she said, when she was finally able to start taking care of the child, he refused to accept food from her. Under these circumstances her husband took charge of the boy's feeding.

When K. was seven months old, his father lost his job as a warehouse loader and subsequently moved out of the house, leaving K. in his mother's care. The mother, who was often out "partying," sometimes missed feeding him altogether. When she did feed him, it was on an inadequate diet consisting of jar baby food, skim milk, and potato chips. When he refused these feedings, as he usually did, she would force the food down his throat with a spoon and hold his mouth closed until he swallowed. More often than not he would spit the food up again.

At the time his father left home, K. was at the fiftieth percentile (i.e., average) in height and weight for boys his age. Within a few months he began to decline. In a classic picture of malnutrition he first stopped gaining weight, then stopped growing. By the time he came to the hospital, he was about thirty inches tall and weighed less than eighteen pounds. Fewer than three percent of all boys his age are shorter and lighter than this.

Meanwhile he kept getting middle ear infections (otitis media). According to his records he had twenty-six such episodes before coming to the hospital. These recurrent infections were, in fact, what brought him to the hospital. The neighborhood doctor who had been seeing him felt, quite properly, that he needed more specialized attention. But this physician, who did not himself have privileges at the hospital and was not well acquainted with its staff, did not make the referral in the spirit of a family doctor actively supervising his patient's care. He did not refer K. to a particular individual at the hospital; nor did he write a referral letter detailing his condition. Instead he simply told K.'s mother that the pediatric ward of this hospital was *the* place for a sick child. In the jargon of the trade this is called *dumping.* The doctor had had enough of this frustrating case.

K. was seen in the infectious-disease clinic. There was no effective provision at the hospital for a general evaluation of the child's health before the specialty consultation. The clinic staff found no apparent reason for the recurrent ear infections, and K. was sent home, with an appointment for a follow-up visit three months later. No one noticed that he was starving.

A few months later, when he showed up again, someone did notice. K. was then admitted to the hospital for failure to thrive, feeding problems, developmental delay, and recurrent otitis media. First seen by house officers (interns and residents) on the infectious-disease rotation, he was referred to Dr. S., a new intern on the acute-care ward. Having just come through four weeks of drawing blood, starting IV's, and other intensive-care procedures on this difficult rotation, Dr. S. felt confident enough to take charge of a case in the manner of the family doctor he aspired to be. And K. was a peculiarly appropriate patient for him to have. On the telephone the house officer referring K. had said of him, "He looks like one of those concentration camp survivors you see in films." And indeed he did, with his sunken eyes, his long eyelashes, his wasted arms and legs, and his distended stomach and protruding ribs. From the beginning, the resemblance made Dr. S., who had had relatives die in Auschwitz, take a special interest in K.

Under Dr. S.'s supervision the admission lab workup was kept to a minimum. Aside from minor metabolic abnormalities, all the test results were normal except for an elevated red blood cell sedimentation rate (indicating chronic infections and inflammations), a low white blood cell count (in particular, a low count of one kind of white blood cell that is crucial in fighting infections), and a slightly abnormal liver function (consistent with malnutrition). The tests, in other words, confirmed what the initial physical exam had already revealed.

At this point what were the options? Any doctor might have been uncertain. Dr. S. knew that he was, as were the other physicians with whom he consulted. But he was able to reach three conclusions:

First, whatever else was wrong with the child, he was

severely malnourished. He was also suffering from an immune deficiency, i.e., an inability to fight off infections. But the lab tests had failed to establish primary (genetic or constitutional) immune deficiency, as opposed to secondary (environmentally caused) immune deficiency. Malnutrition itself is a major environmental cause of immune deficiency. The tests had, moreover, ruled out most of the clearly treatable conditions that could contribute to immune deficiency. Thus it was unlikely that K.'s lack of resistance to infection could be specifically diagnosed or directly treated. But one *could* treat his malnutrition, and perhaps in so doing build up his immune defenses as well.

Second, K. would starve to death if he wasn't fed.

Third, K. was very brittle. While performing the initial lab workup, Dr. S. felt very uncomfortable having to draw blood from this emaciated child. Noticing even then that K. refused to eat after being poked with needles, Dr. S. resolved to limit any further invasive testing to the necessary minimum. "God knows," he thought, "he's had enough invasive things done to him with a spoon, let alone needles." He realized that he was thinking of the child, at least sometimes, as a survivor of a kind of concentration camp. He might have dismissed these feelings as mere "projections," but he did not.

Dr. S.'s treatment plan evolved from these perceptions. He decided to forgo the more powerful diagnostic tests, since these had not proved very powerful anyway, and since they were likely to harm the child (by weakening him physically, by increasing his resistance to food, and by alienating him further from those caring for him). Dr. S.'s aim was to treat what could be treated, and to diagnose by continuing to observe how well the child thrived under treatment. Here was a child whose response to food—and to people—took the form of an extreme reaction to real and expected abuse. The first priority was to build up his strength by seeing that he was fed in a loving atmosphere. Since it was likely that K.'s malnutrition was exacerbating, if not causing, his immune deficiency, the extent of this effect could be assessed by seeing whether he became more resistant to infection once he was better nourished. If he did not, invasive testing would be resumed, since in that case more precise information would clearly be required. But by then K. would also be stronger and better able to withstand the testing.

To help set up K.'s feeding program, Dr. S. brought in the hospital's one-man volunteer "feeding team," a genial man who inspired trust in children by speaking to them patiently until they were ready to eat. This "specialist" noticed that even though K. would not eat, he liked to suck on empty bottles. So he and Dr. S. set up a positive-reinforcement schedule for K. When he ate, they let him suck on a bottle. When he spat up food, they did not give him this reward, but they also did not punish him. They just let it pass. Previously the only emotion K. had been able to elicit from his mother was the anger she displayed when he spat up food. Now he was getting love when he ate. To make sure he would get it consistently, Dr. S. put one nurse in charge of K. Together they recognized that this was an emergency, and that love was needed on an emergency basis.

Meanwhile K. continued to run fevers. Instead of always trying to specify the nature and cause of these infections by testing, which involved restraining the child for up to fifteen minutes while fishing for a still-functioning vein in his neck, Dr. S. made educated guesses and treated the infections empirically. That is, he tried a particular antibiotic, which worked, and kept using it as long as it continued to work. As long as K.'s infections could be brought under control in this way and he continued to thrive, the infections would not interfere with his overall therapy. Therefore Dr. S. felt no need to investigate them more closely. He was more interested in watching K. eat and begin to gain weight. One test was taken during this period —a liver function, which was now normal.

K. progressed for about ten days. Then he developed a fever while Dr. S. was off duty. Dr. S. had left instructions that if this happened, K. was not to be given a septic workup (which includes a blood culture and a spinal tap) to determine the source of infection, but was to be treated empirically as before. When he came back on the floor, Dr. S. found that K. had had a complete septic workup, with "a tube in every orifice, and a needle wherever there wasn't an orifice." Two medications dripped into K.'s arm through an intravenous needle. The house officer in charge explained to Dr. S., "If we hadn't done this and he had gotten worse, it would have been my head!"

The septic workup revealed nothing—which was exactly how much K. ate for the next three days. After his trust was regained, he resumed eating and again gained weight.

In his effort to play the role of a family doctor for K., Dr. S. went beyond his duties on the hospital floor. By now the parents were back together (as often happens when a child becomes seriously ill), and Dr. S. tried to get to know them. He succeeded in establishing a relationship with the father, but found that he could only maintain contact with the mother by referring her to a psychiatric social worker. He could not help but notice the lack of emotion she showed on her occasional visits to her child in the hospital.

Dr. S.'s superiors in the hospital did not encourage him in these efforts. And on the acute-care ward the prevailing attitude toward his spending time with K. in order to feed and communicate with him was a patronizing one. "That's nice," thought his colleagues. "Dr. S. is playing with this feeding therapy. Now let's get back to what's important." What was important to them was diagnosing K.'s infections. Like K.'s original physician, the hospital staff was more concerned with his ear infections than with his diet.

As Dr. S. neared the end of his six-week rotation on the acute-care ward, he realized that his treatment plan for K. would not be followed on that ward once he was no longer there to assume responsibility for it. When it comes to providing continuity of care, an intern, whose patients disappear from his life every six weeks, cannot be a family doctor. Recognizing this, Dr. S. sought to have K. transferred to the psychiatric ward for children, where he would be given nurturant attention and would be less likely to be subjected to invasive testing.

Dr. S. persuaded a sympathetic senior physician (a child-development specialist) to support the transfer by offering this rationale: K., whose primary "medical" problem was susceptibility to infection, ran a high risk of infection on a hospital ward where he was exposed to "big bad bugs." This is a term used by hospital personnel to describe the virulent strains of infectious organisms that develop through natural selection in the hospital environment. Some say that these organisms thrive even on antibiotics as a culture medium. As one house officer put it, "They suck on gentamycin Popsicles for breakfast and eat chloramphenicol pies for lunch." K.'s lack of resistance to infection left him easy prey for these bugs, and his chances of infection were only increased when his skin was broken in drawing blood for tests. Thus, in what Dr. S. and the physician he consulted saw as a destructive cycle, infections led to more testing, and the testing led to more infections.

So K. went over to the psychiatric ward. Urging the psychiatrists to get in touch with him if any problems developed, Dr. S. briefed them on K.'s frequent infections and left instructions for these to be treated empirically. He also visited the child regularly during his off-duty hours. In this unofficial, almost subversive way, hollowing out a place for himself "between the lines" of authority in the hospital, Dr. S. continued to treat K. as his personal responsibility and to act as his physician. He was still serving as K.'s "advocate," though now without the authority to back up his recommendations.

K. thrived nicely on the psychiatric ward for about ten days before he developed his first—and last—fever there. The psychiatrists, feeling that they couldn't take the risk of leaving an organic condition undiagnosed and untreated, transferred him back to acute care for evaluation. Psychiatrists are often sensitive to the accusation of ignoring organic causes of illness. In this case they did not see it as taking a risk to transfer K. back to a ward full of big bad bugs and big bad house officers. They saw it simply as the right thing for them to do—even though K. had had a complete set of lab cultures and had responded consistently to empirical therapy for infection.

Back on the acute-care ward the diagnostic machine, no longer impeded by Dr. S.'s iconoclastic presence, went into full and impressive (albeit misguided) operation, with the house officers showing complete unanimity of purpose. They, too, felt that they couldn't take chances; or as a colleague put it, "If he dies without a diagnosis, then we have failed." By their conception of scientific medicine one had to find a cause before one could treat. Each of K.'s increasingly frequent, increasingly generalized infections brought on a new round of tests to determine its cause. In addition K. was the object of intensive and extended evaluation to determine the basic cause of his immune deficiency and his failure to thrive.

A host of distinguished specialists descended on K. The responsibility for K.'s care, to the extent that it had ever been fixed in Dr. S.'s hands, had by now been diffused among a coterie of specialists, each interested in applying a particular diagnostic technology to a particular part of K.'s anatomy. It had become "medicine by committee." No one doctor could be held accountable. After all, no one doctor could possess all the knowledge thought to be relevant to K.'s problems.

Over the next nine weeks K. underwent the following procedures: CT scan; barium swallow; upper GI; abdominal ultrasound; gastric biopsy; small-bowel biopsy; esophagoscopy; a second bone marrow biopsy; numerous cultures of blood, urine, stool, and throat; six lumbar punctures; serial blood gases; a prednisone stimulation test; screens for adenosine deaminase and nucleoside phosphorylase deficiency; urine assay for vanillylmandelic acid; and repeated b-cell and t-cell function tests. Most readers will not know what each of these tests is. Nor can we know what it must have been like for a two-year-old child (one who could not communicate in words) to be subjected to all these procedures.

What did the tests reveal? Nothing decisive. There were persistent abnormalities of white blood cell function, as before, indicating a compromised immune system. But there were still no grounds for distinguishing between a primary immune deficiency and an immune deficiency secondary to severe malnutrition.

The malnutrition, meanwhile, was becoming more severe, since under the barrage of testing K. stopped eating again. The staff compensated for this by putting in a hyperalimentation line—an intravenous line passed from a vein in the arm to the large vein that empties into the heart—through which K. was given all the nutrients needed to survive. But the hyperalimentation line carried only calories, not love, and by this point K. had been badly weakened by the combined effects of constant infection, starvation, and testing—so much so that he had to have infusions of blood to make up for iatrogenic blood loss from all the tests. (The word *iatrogenic* refers to complications brought on by the medical process itself.)

K.'s next scheduled test was a biopsy of the thymus gland. Whether he sought to avoid this—in the only way now left to him—is not known. In any case he had had enough. Two days before the scheduled test his breathing became very rapid, and he began to lose what little color he had. First his mouth turned blue, then his hands and feet, then his entire body. A vigorous two-and-one-half-hour resuscitation attempt was unsuccessful.

Shortly afterward, the man known as the "feeding team" walked up to Dr. S. in the outpatient clinic, to which he had now rotated, and laid a hand on his shoulder. "Do you know?" he said. "K. died today."

"God damn it!" said Dr. S. "God damn it!"

Other reactions to K.'s death were equally in character. His mother didn't show much response, and the senior resident wondered why. Both parents, saying that they wanted to know whether they should have any more children, asked an intern—and she took the question seriously—whether K.'s disease could be "inherited." The physicians involved, having failed to find a precise cause for K.'s disorder in all their testing, tried again at the autopsy, hoping to find one cause (perhaps an incurable underlying condition such as a cancer) that would explain what had happened to K. They tried again two months later at the clinico-pathological conference on the case. Again no luck.

One of the residents, commiserating with Dr. S., exclaimed that she had never seen such a valiant resuscitation effort. "Why, at one time he had three IV drips going at once! He was spared no test to find out what was really going on. He died in spite of everything we did!"

("In spite—or *to* spite?" thought Dr. S.)

"Nothing could have been done to save him," she went on, "because everything that could have been done *was* done."

("Yes," thought Dr. S., "nothing could have been done—which might have saved him!")

In the pediatric section of the hospital where these events took place numerous well-planned playrooms and multicolored walls hung with engaging designs present a bright, open face to child patients, as do the staff, who are trained to be friendly and reassuring to the children. There is even an "attending" physician assigned to patients like K. who do not have their own private physicians. Yet Dr. S. had seen children who did have private physicians, and whose families were better off financially than K.'s, get the same kind of treatment that K. did.

All this made the case that much more disquieting. No one in the hospital was evil. Everyone was trying to do the right thing, scientifically and morally. In spite of everything they did, or because of it, or for unrelated reasons, the patient died.

The people who "attacked" K. with needles were not sadistic. Nor were they thinking of the income that their procedures would generate for the hospital. They saw and felt the suffering they caused the child, and were distressed by it. They were quite capable of empathy, yet their "scientific" consciences, as distinct from their "personal" consciences, would not allow them to let up on the testing. But what if their "scientific" conceptions turned out actually to be *un*scientific?

No one can say for sure that they were. Yet it is worth noting that while every drug used in K.'s treatment has been thoroughly studied for its side effects, there is one "drug" which has not been subjected to the same scrutiny. It is the most potent, widely used drug in medicine: clinical reasoning. If there is any drug which, when used inappropriately, can kill a patient, it is the reflex reasoning done in the name of diagnosis and treatment. We don't know if it killed this particular patient. But we can look closely at how Dr. S. went about handling K.'s case and how his method differed from that of the physicians who succeeded him on the acute-care ward. When we articulate the assumptions, the thought processes, the clinical strategies that guided the two approaches to this case, we may find ourselves revising our notion of what constitutes scientific practice in medicine.

In general, the two approaches valued different kinds of information and went about getting that information in different ways. These preferences are linked, of course, since a given mode of investigation tends to yield a particular kind of information. Most of the physicians involved in K.'s case were looking for "hard," "scientific," "objective" biological data. They sought these data through precise measurements of organic processes. For example, a genetically based immune deficiency might be discovered by taking a bone marrow biopsy. On the other hand, Dr. S. and his collaborators (such as the child-development specialist and the "feeding team" specialist) took seriously the causal role of subjective psychological factors as well—the child's emotional state, his relationships with the people around him, and his reactions to medical procedures. They realized that their own actions toward K. would be interpreted by him in the context of his family's past actions. These factors do not lend themselves to precise laboratory measurement. Consequently Dr. S.'s diagnostic tools included observation over time and subjective judgment.

These psychological variables are also not easy to isolate from one another, or from other causes. Working on the assumption that K.'s immune deficiency may well have had both genetic and environmental causes, Dr. S. knew that he probably would not be able to tell just how much each was responsible for K.'s condition. But he was comfortable with this uncertainty, because he felt that ongoing treatment and observation would reveal to what extent he could successfully treat K.'s lowered resistance as a complication of malnutrition, and to what extent he would need to investigate its causes further. Dr. S.'s approach assumed that a patient's condition might have many causes, that the relative influence of these causes might change with time, and that the various causes together might act in a way that none would separately. Thus he took into account genetic, nutritional, and psychological factors, even though each of these alone might not be sufficient to account for K.'s illness.

To the other physicians, however, every effect ideally could be traced to a single cause. They seemed to work on the principles that once one cause has been found, it is not necessary to look for other causes, and that the sort of cause worth looking for is one that can account for all that is happening to a patient. For every condition that K. developed, whether acute (a particular fever or ear infection) or chronic (his immune deficiency and failure to thrive), they tried to find one causative factor that would explain how that condition came about. They did so by conducting tests that isolated and measured one hypothesized cause at a time while holding other factors constant or ignoring them entirely. Even when psychological causation *was* considered, the one-cause model was adhered to. K.'s running a fever on the psychiatric ward was taken to "disprove" the psychological hypothesis, and he was immediately sent back for medical examination. The psychiatrists and acute-care physicians did not seriously consider that psychological and physiological causes might both be present, or that causes might come and go with time.

As these other physicians saw it, treatment could not be undertaken scientifically without first having a definite diagnosis, while to Dr. S. the primary purpose of diagnosis was to enable one to treat. He attached less value to the diagnosis of incurable conditions. By the same token, he was quite prepared to treat experimentally without having a very sure diagnosis, on the grounds that treatment could be a form of diagnosis, a way of obtaining information while helping the patient. Dr. S. and the other physicians undoubtedly would have agreed in the abstract that diagnosis is not an end in itself, but a means of discovering the appropriate treatment. In fact, though, the acute-care milieu placed primary emphasis on establishing a diagnosis, while Dr. S., having a more pragmatic disposition, kept treatment foremost in mind.

These divergent biases shaped the course of K.'s treatment under the two medical regimens. Dr. S., by emphasizing the feeding and nurturing of the child, tried to bring about a gradual, day-by-day improvement in his condition. In curtailing diagnostic tests he accepted a small risk of failing to discover a serious condition that might cause a large negative outcome, perhaps a fatal one. This risk was unacceptable to the house officers who took over K.'s care from Dr. S. In their zeal to avoid it by testing for every remotely relevant disease, they undertook stressful procedures which brought about a gradual, day-by-day deterioration in the boy's condition. To the extent that they noticed this downward progress, they considered it an unavoidable consequence of their efforts to achieve a large (though unlikely) positive outcome, i.e., a definitive diagnosis which, if the condition diagnosed was treatable, could lead to an instant cure. However, the progressive weakening of K.'s condition led in the end to the very outcome they were so concerned to prevent.

Several observations can be made about the clinical reasoning of this latter group of physicians:

First, in focusing on extreme outcomes, they disregarded incremental effects. Preoccupied with large gains and large losses, they didn't see that a succession of small losses can add up to a total loss. Dr. S. was sensitively attuned to incremental changes—the small gains from feeding, the small losses from drawing blood. Therefore he tried to put K.'s condition on a gradual upward course. Since his treatment program was interrupted, however, we cannot say whether small gains ultimately would have added up to a large gain for this patient.

Second, they failed to take into account the effects of their own actions. Working from the assumption that K.'s illness had only one cause—the one they were looking for—they naturally saw themselves as observers—*only* as observers. To them *the* cause lay somewhere in K.'s body, so they had no reason to consider whether their own procedures might also influence his condition, perhaps decisively. As human beings they could share the pain they caused him, but as scientists they were committed to ignoring it. Dr. S., working from a more flexible, inclusive conception of causality that allowed for many causes operating at once, was in a better position to assess the possible effects of his own actions, and to see them as part of an overall web of causes, which included K.'s prior experiences with his family.

Third, they failed to weigh the costs of their procedures (the stress to K.'s system brought on by testing) against the benefits. If five lumbar punctures had shown no positive findings, what did they expect to learn from the sixth? What was to be gained from subjecting K. to a small-bowel biopsy which, if it revealed anything, would likely reveal an incurable condition? Many of the tests performed were, in fact, designed to identify diseases for which there was no known treatment. If a primary immune deficiency had been shown to exist, it could not have been treated except by a bone marrow transplant, for which K., in his depleted state, was not a candidate. What, then, was the purpose of the testing? Was it to treat K. more effectively or to give the clinicians the reassurance of certain knowledge?

What was lacking in this clinical approach was any notion of probability. The questions that needed to be asked about each diagnostic or therapeutic procedure were "How likely is this to do good? How likely is it to do harm?" Similarly, there was no assessment of values. "What, in this situation, is good? Whose good are we working for? What is best for the patient? What does the patient want?" All of these questions were implicit in Dr. S.'s approach, where the assessment of probabilities and values formed the basis for estimating the probable costs and benefits of any action under consideration.

Without this framework for clinical decision-making, the diagnosis and treatment in the latter phase of K.'s hospital stay proceeded according to certain unexamined assumptions. The search for more information was seen not as a way of estimating probabilities, but of achieving certainty. All actions not directed toward that end were discouraged as "risky." When the psychiatrists faced the choice of keeping K. on their ward with a fever or sending him back to acute-care for further "observation," they didn't see it as a choice between two gambles. They saw it as a gamble versus a safe and sure alternative. So did the house officer who ordered a septic workup on K. during Dr. S.'s absence from the ward. The physicians who acted out the dominant clinical philosophy felt that it was "taking a chance" to treat K.'s infections empirically. They saw no serious risk, though, in relentless diagnostic testing, which they regarded as having either a good or a neutral outcome. If they discovered something, they were ahead of the game. If not, K. was no worse off than before. The problem was that with every exploratory procedure (though again, not necessarily because of it) he did get worse.

To Dr. S. it made more sense to consider *every* decision a gamble, and to choose what seemed the best gamble among the available options. Each time he ordered antibiotic treatment for K.'s infections (without having the slightest idea what caused the infections), he was playing the odds, since the treatment had worked whenever he had tried it previously. To him that was the scientific method. He reasoned that, as in playing cards, everything you do or don't do is a gamble. In blackjack do you take a hit and risk going over 21? In medicine do you accept the side effects of a diagnostic procedure in order to gain new information? If you believe, as did the other physicians, that diagnostic tests come just about free of charge to the patient's well-being, then you don't have to weigh the costs versus the benefits. If you believe, as did Dr. S., that you pay for each card you take, then you must weigh the price of the card against what you could win by taking it.

When the likely costs of playing out a hand exceed the likely benefits, you throw in your hand and pay for new cards. In medicine when do you give up on an unpromising line of treatment? Apparently never, judging by the physicians who performed six lumbar punctures (i.e., spinal taps) on K. without learning anything. You'd think they might have stopped after two or three. But although they knew how to work up a patient, they didn't know when to stop the workup. Even those who wanted to stop felt that somehow they couldn't. After all, they had to play the game by the rules, and the only rule they knew was to try to obtain a certain diagnosis, even if the diagnosis meant that nothing could be done. In their view, since K. was getting worse all the time, there was all the more reason to do the punctures. They had no criteria by which to stop testing, unless an incurable disease was discovered or the patient died. And so they went by the rule "Stop if nothing more can be done," rather than simply, "Stop if it's just not worth doing any more." With actions that were seen as "risky," however, their rule was to stop immediately when there seemed any possibility of losing the gamble. They accepted a degree of risk by letting K. be transferred to the psychiatric ward, but as soon as he developed a single complication there, they thought it necessary to bring him back to the (ostensibly risk-free) acute-care ward.

These physicians took every opportunity to exercise their considerable skills and were understandably reluctant to leave things to chance. They had to "Do something!"—a commonly felt imperative in medicine. It wasn't only the fear of malpractice claims. It can be frustrating for a highly trained person to have to just watch and wait. Dr. S. dealt with this almost universal anxiety by thinking of watching and waiting, and being with the patient, as "doing something," as skills in the same league as diagnosing and treating. Instead of struggling against the arbitrary power of chance, Dr. S. tried to develop skills for dealing with situations in which chance—probability—plays a major role. Thus in this instance he thought it best to let "tincture of time" make the diagnosis and begin the treatment. His successors on the ward decided otherwise.

This is not to say that if only the case had been handled differently, the patient would have lived. Dr. S. himself recognized that K. might well have had a genetically based immune deficiency or other organic disorder that would likely have killed him before long. Unlike some nurses who told Dr. S. that the cause of death for K. should read "institutional murder," Dr. S. did not claim that the hospital's treatment of K. "caused" his death. Believing as he did that our knowledge of causality is uncertain and that many causes may operate simultaneously, Dr. S. had to concede that if treated differently K. might well have died sooner, or not for another seventy or eighty years, for any number of reasons. But he understood what a philosopher friend of his had in mind when on hearing the story he commented, "In medicine, unlike elsewhere in life, you are considered much less culpable for killing than for failing to save a life."

2

UNCERTAINTY IN SCIENCE

The story of K. is not simply a case of one doctor being more humane and sensitive than other doctors. All those involved tried to be humane and sensitive. The two different ways of thinking, feeling, and acting that can be found in K.'s story have as their source two different conceptions of medical science. Dr. S. thought about the case differently from the other doctors. He also had a different way of coping with the emotions that anyone would feel when trying to treat a patient such as K. By thinking differently and feeling differently, he was able to act in a way that was as humane, sensitive, and effective as both he and the other doctors wanted to be.

Dr. S.'s way of thinking and that which was "standard practice" in the hospital differed so significantly that they can be said to represent two *paradigms* of thought: an old one, the mechanistic, and a new one, the probabilistic. The term *new paradigm* is today commonly used when what is meant is a new idea. A paradigm, however, is not just one new idea. It is a way of looking at the world, a way of perceiving reality and structuring knowledge. It marks the "burning questions" that people strive to answer in that area of knowledge called science as well as beyond. In particular

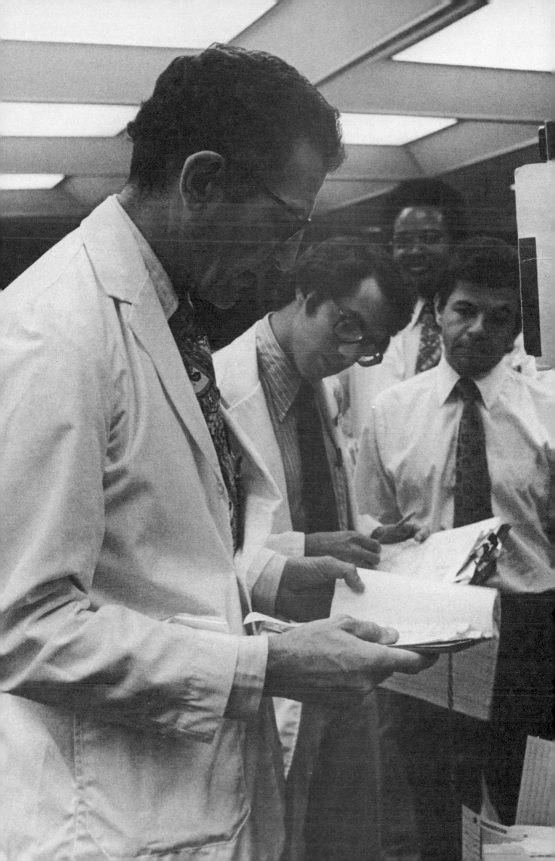

it focuses the energies of science by encouraging the asking of certain questions and discouraging others. It sanctions certain methods for answering these questions and rules out others. It even contains guidelines for what is an acceptable answer and what is not. In these ways a paradigm embodies the standards by which scientists decide what is legitimate and what is important.

We believe that the Probabilistic Paradigm represents not just a new way of doing physics, but a new approach to reality —that is, a new way of thinking, feeling, and acting. We shall explain what the new paradigm means—first in physics, then in medicine, and then as it extends to everyday life.

What we mean by paradigms, paradigm shifts, and the Mechanistic and Probabilistic paradigms in particular can be seen by analogy when we look at this drawing of two faces. Is it

FIGURE 2-1

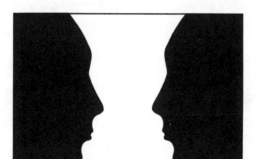

Vase or Faces?

two faces in profile or is it a vase? You may stare at the drawing for a long time and see only the faces. Once you discover (or someone points out) the outline of the vase, you will always be able to see it when you look at the drawing—but you will still be able to see the faces as well. The two images will come in and out of focus in a way that may be disconcerting until you get used to the idea of seeing two alternating images in a single drawing. Then you will have learned what to expect. You will have learned that the drawing will look sometimes like one thing, sometimes like another, and sometimes like both (but not like anything else). The instability of the image will have become stable.

Seeing the two images rather than either one alone opens up new possibilities for what images can be (i.e., stable or unstable). Similarly, a paradigm shift provides not only new knowledge, but new ways of thinking about what knowledge is. The Mechanistic Paradigm sought (and, in its day, found) answers that could be known with certainty, answers that were always the same—like a drawing that always conveys only one image. The discovery in modern physics that such certain, unchanging answers could not be found was at first disconcerting. Once physicists accepted the idea of uncertainty, however, they found that they could work with it and be comfortable with it when it was quantified in terms of probability. Even though they could not be certain, they could still have an idea of what to expect—as when the weather forecast predicts an eighty percent chance of rain for tomorrow. When you learn that a visual image can be unstable, your expectations of what an image is change, so that you are now able to understand an alternation between two images. Similarly, when the paradigm of physics shifted from the mechanistic to the probabilistic, physicists' expectations of what knowledge is changed to allow for probability, or *degrees* of uncertainty.

The Mechanistic Paradigm: Three Criteria

At least since the time of Sir Isaac Newton, physics has served as a model for other sciences, and science has been taken to be a model of rationality for society. Let us look at an everyday life situation and see how a "commonsense" approach to it reflects the assumptions of mechanistic (Newtonian) physics.

Imagine that an American newspaper sends a reporter to investigate the causes of unrest in a small foreign country. The reporter's mission is to get "the facts," or as they say in the trade, the "who, what, when, where, and why." The possibility that the reporter's presence in the country may affect what the people there say and do is not considered, since, after all, he is only one person in the midst of a population of several million. Besides, he's just an "outsider." As for the reporter's own opinions and reactions, he has been trained to suppress them as completely as he can, and in any case to leave them out of his reports. The editors are confident that they will be getting an "objective" descriptive account, as free from bias as is humanly possible, of what is going on "over there."

In 1686, in Book III of the *Principia Mathematica,* Newton (1953) explicitly set down what we can now understand as the three criteria of the Mechanistic Paradigm. That wasn't how Newton thought of them, of course. He regarded them simply as rules for good scientific practice. To him anything else was not science. But we can use Newton's rules to distinguish Newtonian science from what followed as well as preceded it.

Criterion #1:
Deterministic Causation

For every observed effect the scientist seeks to isolate a specific cause or set of causes, as if it alone can account for the effect. For example, Newton used gravity to account for the motion of the heavenly bodies. Suppose our reporter attributes the demonstrations and disorders he has observed to "economic deprivation." This is a *unicausal* (one-cause) explanation. If, on the other hand, he lists several causes and explains how together they have brought about political unrest, he is using a *multicausal* (many-cause) explanation.

The multicausal explanations (like the unicausal explanations) used in the Mechanistic Paradigm are *deterministic.* A scientist using such an explanation claims that it is complete

—i.e., that the list of causes is exhaustive and that the way they come together to produce the effect in question does not change. "Unfavorable economic conditions always cause unrest" is a unicausal deterministic explanation. An example of a multicausal deterministic explanation is this: "Unfavorable economic conditions, in conjunction with religious fervor, always cause unrest." In either case causal relationships in the Newtonian scheme are taken to be certain and universal. That is, "A causes B" means that we can completely specify the conditions under which A causes B. When we have such a complete list of conditions, then we can count on A causing B whenever those conditions occur. In the Mechanistic Paradigm both unicausal and multicausal explanations are acceptable as long as they are deterministic. Unicausal explanations are somewhat preferred, however, as they seem to give a more deterministic account.

Criterion #2:
The "Experimentum Crucis"

In our journalistic example the reporter is performing an *experimentum crucis,* or "crucial experiment," if he goes into the country with a specific hypothesis that he believes he can test by holding constant all other potential causal factors. For example, he might decide, "Either economic hardship or religious fervor is behind it all. I'll just wait and see what happens when economic conditions improve. If there is still unrest, then I'll know for sure that it's religious fervor."

The Newtonian "crucial experiment" is a test that establishes once and for all a deterministic causal relationship of the sort described by Criterion #1. Newton thought that his theory of light had been conclusively proved by a certain crucial experiment with a prism, since no matter who did the experiment, the result would always be the same. To "prove" that A causes B, the experimenter varies A, while holding everything else constant, and observes how B in turn varies. It is assumed that the experimenter can account for and control all possible causal factors. The experimenter is assumed to be a detached observer in the sense that, aside from his planned manipulations, he does not influence the observed effects. Since cause-and-effect relationships in the Mechanistic Paradigm occur with one hundred percent regularity, and since there is no distortion brought about by the act of observation, the results of an *experimentum crucis* can be reproduced by anyone who does the same experiment.

Criterion #3:
The Objective/Subjective Dichotomy

By any definition of science, scientific knowledge must be useful, and to be useful it must be reliable. If it is to be reliable it must be public, in the sense that scientists must be able to talk about it and agree on what it is they are talking about. In the Mechanistic Paradigm, where scientific knowledge must be *absolutely* reliable, the only knowledge that is thought of as being public (or capable of being made public) is "objective" knowledge—that is, knowledge of a world existing independently of the observer. Newton stated that all his evidence was objective and thus incontrovertible. Just as our foreign correspondent puts his feelings and reactions "out of his mind" when he addresses the reading public, so the Mechanistic Paradigm's experimenter dismisses from the realm of science his or her own beliefs, attitudes, and values. Since these are subjective (that is, not independent of the observer), they are assumed to be private (that is, not capable of being communicated and agreed upon). The strict separation of subjective and objective knowledge is consistent with the first criterion of the Mechanistic Paradigm, which requires that knowledge be certain and universal. The possibility of such a separation is consistent with the second criterion, which holds that what is observed is independent of any attributes of the observer. In this century, however, both of these assumptions have been called into question.

From the Mechanistic
to the Probabilistic

Since the 1960's the notion of objective, bias-free journalism has been looked at with growing skepticism. It has become only too evident that a reporter cannot be without bias, and that this bias cannot help but influence the way the reporter interprets and presents the news. The "New Journalists" of recent years have given a prominent place in their articles to themselves, their feelings, and their experiences, sometimes to the point of telling us more about themselves than what they are reporting on. Even so, the reaction against the mechanistic idea of journalistic objectivity has been useful.

Consider all the things that can happen when our American reporter tries to be objective about the politics of a small foreign country. True, one reporter wouldn't seem to have much impact on a whole country. But suppose he is arrested as a spy. Suppose the government seizes upon his intrusive presence as a pretext for rallying the country to unity. Even if nothing so dramatic happens, it is quite likely that the people he comes in contact with will speak and act differently when they are being observed by a foreigner. They may hide their feelings, or they may "show off," even staging demonstrations inspired by the presence of TV cameras. The reporter, meanwhile, in his effort to be objective may try to minimize the emotional effect on himself of what he sees and hears. He may affect a Hemingwayesque toughness that not only will be felt in the tone of his reports, but also will make the people of the country see him as "another one of those distant, impervious Americans." This stereotype will condition their behavior toward him, which in turn will help shape his view of them, and so forth. Finally, when the dispatches he sends home are published, the people he is writing about may be pleased or offended. These reactions, too, will become an ingredient in the complex relationship between the observer and the observed.

Such effects have been noted in science. In what was regarded as a classic experiment in learning theory, cats were trained to escape from a box by rubbing against a vertical rod in the center of the box, which opened a door at the front of the box. The front of the box was made of glass so that the experimenters could observe the cats. Not taken into account, however, was the fact that the cats could observe the experimenters as well. As later researchers pointed out, rubbing against vertical objects (animate or inanimate) is something that cats typically do when in the presence of people or other cats. Rather than learning how to get out of the box, the cats were simply "greeting" the experimenters in a way that came naturally to them (Moore and Stuttard, 1979).

It isn't just cats who respond to the presence and the interest of experimenters. The famous studies of worker productivity at the Hawthorne Plant of the Western Electric Company in the 1920's and 1930's showed that people do, too (Roethlisberger and Dixon, 1939). Initially the Hawthorne researchers found that small experimental groups of workers, some given better lighting and some not, all showed increased productivity. In fact, their productivity increased even when their work area was *less* well lit than before. Naturally the experimenters were puzzled by this "Hawthorne effect." They eventually found that the workers in all the experimental conditions appreciated the small-group atmosphere as well as the friendliness and leniency of the experimenters who acted as their supervisors. It was a lot better to work under the experimenters than to work under the regular foremen out on the factory floor. Again, what the experimenters unwittingly did just by organizing the scene for observation had more effect on the outcome than their deliberate experimental manipulations.

Characteristically, before one paradigm is replaced by another, scientists working within the old paradigm usually do everything they can to salvage it. First, they try to dismiss as illegitimate or irrelevant the problems that the paradigm can't solve. When the problems refuse to go away, scientists tinker with the paradigm to try to make it accommodate the new data or new issues. In the case of our hapless reporter the editors might try to reduce his bias in regard to the politics of his assigned country by briefing him extensively on the culture and values of its people. This, however, would still not eliminate his bias, which is what editors working within the Mechanistic Paradigm would want to do. So they might decide to send a second reporter to correct the bias of the first, a third to correct the bias of the second, a fourth to correct the third, and so on. By the time enough reporters had been sent, the reporters themselves would become a source of unrest. The country would no longer be what it was before they came.

Physicists went through similar sorts of contortions before they finally gave up on the Mechanistic Paradigm. Around the turn of the century physicists began to be troubled by a range of observations that did not fit into the paradigm. For example, according to mechanistic principles light had to consist of waves or particles, not both, just as the drawing at the beginning of this chapter would have to "be" either a vase or faces. Yet depending on how light was observed, it sometimes looked like waves and sometimes looked like particles. At first physicists discounted such observations as stemming from human and technological limitations. With bigger and better machines for observing, they thought, the problems would resolve themselves.

Einstein's theory of relativity was a last-ditch effort (on the part of a man who to the end of his days expressed the hope that "God does not play dice with the universe") to save the Mechanistic Paradigm by abandoning Newtonian conceptions of space and time. The decisive break with the paradigm came with quantum mechanics, for which Einstein (among others) laid the groundwork, although later he disavowed some of its implications. What Einstein resisted and what quantum physicists such as Niels Bohr and Werner Heisenberg accepted was that chance and cause were not mutually exclusive categories. Rather, to understand that "A causes B" was to see that there was some necessary degree of chance called probability in the relationship between A and B. Quantum mechanics placed probability right at the center of the universe (Bohr, 1969).

Not that probability in itself was a new idea. According to a half-confirmed legend the mathematical theory of probability came into being when two seventeenth-century mathematicians came to the assistance of a gambler. The gambler, Chevalier de Mare, asked his friend Blaise Pascal to advise him on some perplexing questions of strategy that arose in the course of what today would be called "shooting craps." Out of the ensuing correspondence between Pascal and Pierre de Fermat came the theory of probability.

Although Newton in the seventeenth century had little or no awareness of probability (Hacking, 1975), in the following two centuries the concept was easily incorporated into the Mechanistic Paradigm, but only as a "theory of errors," a way of accounting for imperfections of observation and measurement. People were fallible; instruments were inexact. Probability defined acceptable limits within which experimental findings could differ from what the theory predicted. Actual results, actual experiments, and actual scientists were, after all, only approximations of the ideal.

But the ideal was still Newtonian determinism. In theory one could know with certainty the state (position, velocity, direction of movement, etc.) of a given object at a given time. And if one didn't, it was only because the instruments of measurement were imprecise. Perfect the instruments, and certainty would emerge. If one knew the deterministic law governing the behavior of the object, one could then, simply by solving an equation, know with equal certainty the state of the object at any other time. It was a closed system.

As the twentieth-century physics of quantum mechanics emerged, however, the state of the object came to be understood to involve a degree of uncertainty. Even in areas such as planetary motion, where for most practical purposes classical mechanics sufficed, there were cases where the kernel of uncertainty predicted by quantum mechanics was precisely what was of interest to astrophysicists. Nor could there be any hope of eliminating that uncertainty with bigger and better machines that would locate and observe the object more clearly. For the uncertainty now was no longer a matter of perception, but of the very nature of reality. Previously it could be said that the world was certain, although human beings could only know so much about it. Now it was in the world itself that uncertainty resided.

Cause-and-effect relationships, being subject to change and chance, could now be understood only in terms of probabilities.

Probabilistic causality in turn made possible the discovery of the Heisenberg Uncertainty Principle, which holds that an object cannot be observed without having its position and movement affected by the act of observation. Subatomic particles behave in some ways like people whose feelings change on the spur of the moment when they are questioned by a reporter. When light is shone on them, subatomic particles change their position and momentum in such a way that both together cannot be predicted with certainty.

The Heisenberg Uncertainty Principle meant that the object or process being observed could no longer be treated as an isolated system. Now the observing subject (the experimenter) was as much a part of the system of causes and effects as the observed object. Thus Heisenberg's principle undermined the second and third criteria of the Mechanistic Paradigm—that is, the notion that there can be a decisive experimental test and the strict separation of the objective and subjective aspects of knowledge and of reality (Heisenberg, 1958).

The Probabilistic Paradigm: Three Criteria

When we sent our American reporter to investigate the causes of unrest in a foreign country, we learned that the search for causes continually creates as well as uncovers new causes. It is impossible to hold all these contributing factors constant by performing an *experimentum crucis;* they just won't stand still. And despite the best effort to use objective reporting techniques, the subjective bias of the reporter transforms what he observes. In other words, the Mechanistic Paradigm doesn't work.

How can we get around these problems so that we can find out what is going on in that small country? We can do so by accepting a degree of uncertainty in our findings. Instead of trying to eliminate the reporter's bias, we can acknowledge it and work with it. Having tried to understand how the reporter's values will affect his observations, we can see what, given those values, he says about the country. Or else we can choose two or three reporters for their divergent perspectives and interpret their accounts with their biases in mind. In either case a process of active interpretation rather than simply acceptance of revealed truth is required.

Ludwig Wittgenstein (1958), the modern philosopher who understood so well the delicate relationship between knowledge and uncertainty, compared the *experimentum crucis* to the sterile exercise of reading a second copy of the same newspaper in order to verify the content of the first. It is, of course, more informative to read two newspapers—say, a leftist and a rightist one—which is not to say that the reality will be found in between the two, but that, wherever it is found, it can be understood critically through contrast. Even a distortion, if understood critically, can shed light on the truth.

This approach to journalistic investigation is consistent with what we will call the Probabilistic Paradigm in science. Our analysis of the foundations of quantum physics yields three criteria (parallel to those of the Mechanistic Paradigm) which define this new paradigm of scientific investigation.

Criterion #1:
Probabilistic Causation

When we ask how something came about, we usually answer by saying either "This was what caused it" or "It happened by chance." In the commonsense reasoning that Newton made into a science, we don't think that something could have a cause or causes and *also* happen by chance. But this is just what happens in modern physics, where a world that is made up of causes and effects is still an uncertain world. It is not simply that we cannot know all the causes; it is that causes themselves operate to some degree by chance (Bunge, 1979).

In its more sophisticated applications the Mechanistic Paradigm allows that a particular effect may have many causes and that a particular cause may have many effects. Yet uncertainty is not allowed to come into the picture. The mechanistic scheme leaves out the possibility that causes other than the ones we are looking at may be contributing to the effects we observe. One of these causes, of course, is ourselves, since we change what we look at by the very act of observing it. The deterministic model (even in its multicausal form) also does not consider that causes may change with time, and may do so in a way that cannot be predicted. Things that were not causes may become causes, while things that were causes may cease to be causes. What was once a cause may become an effect and vice versa—the "chicken-or-the-egg" question. Causes may also have reciprocal effects on each other. As a result it is not possible to specify what will be or will not be a cause at any given moment.

Causal explanations that not only allow for more than one cause, but also acknowledge the degree of uncertainty inherent in causal relations, are referred to as *multicausal stochastic.* The word *stochastic* refers to influences changing probabilistically with time. Under the Probabilistic Paradigm, causes may act and interact differently at different times, the same effects may not always have the same causes, and the effects of a given cause (and vice versa) cannot be isolated with certainty.

Our reporter is employing a multicausal stochastic explanation if he understands that the political events he observes are subject to an ever-changing pattern of causation, with one cause being the way he interacts with the people he is writing about. The way they act toward him changes his attitude toward them, which in turn changes the way he acts toward them, which in turn changes their attitude toward him, and so forth. Often these changes may be very slight, but sometimes they are noticeable—as, for example, when the people become more intransigently anti-American because they read an article in which the reporter makes what they consider a slur on their religion. Even aside from the reporter's influence on events, the country's destiny is being shaped by a constellation of political and economic forces that is never fully revealed and never quite the same from one moment to the next. When one day's dispatch is filed, it is time to start working on the next.

Criterion #2:
Experimentation as Principled Gambling

In the Mechanistic Paradigm the idea of deterministic causation makes experimentation a simple matter: just manipulate the variables and record what happens. Working from the assumption that one or more causes can be specified with certainty, experimenters can hold some possible causes constant in order to measure the effect that others have (whether singly or as a group). The data dictate the result. In the Probabilistic Paradigm, on the other hand, multicausal stochastic causation negates the very idea of an *experimentum crucis.* If patterns of cause and effect are subject to chance and change, then no one experiment can be "crucial." As with our fast-breaking journalistic updates, no one experimental finding represents the "last word."

What method of experimentation is appropriate for a world in which (1) it follows from the first criterion of the Probabilistic Paradigm that causal relationships cannot be known with certainty and knowledge is subject to change, and (2) according to the Heisenberg Uncertainty Principle, one cannot observe without thereby affecting what is observed? Both of these conditions require that the experimenter interpret the significance of the data. Since the experiment itself does not provide absolute confirmation or refutation of any hypothesis, the experimenter must choose which hypotheses to accept and which to reject, just as we all must choose which newspaper accounts to believe. The experimenter makes this choice on the basis of the consequences of believing and acting upon one hypothesis rather than another.

By "consequences," however, we are not referring to external reward and punishment, as in the case of the scientists who found it useful to believe in the ideologically motivated scientific theories approved by Hitler or Stalin. Rather, what we mean is analogous to winning or losing a gamble. Gambling is, after all, making choices in the face of uncertainty. When we think in terms of the Probabilistic Paradigm, we can see anything we do as a gamble. We gamble on whether an experiment is worth doing, and we gamble (even after the experiment is done) on which hypothesis are worthy of belief. In the Probabilistic Paradigm we can choose a hypothesis to believe and act upon as we would choose a horse to bet on. Similarly, the decision to do an experiment is a gamble, and the results of the experiment present us with further gambles which we can choose to accept or reject. We then have a chain of gambles, any one of which can be called an experiment, or a chain of experiments, any one of which can be called a gamble.

On what basis do we make these choices? What consequences are we concerned with? We want to believe and act upon hypotheses that are true. We also want to achieve good outcomes (to win instead of losing). In the science of gambling that is practiced under the Probabilistic Paradigm, we do both; we seek both the true and the good. Since we cannot be certain of either, however, we must add a third stipulation—that of "justification." We can say that we are acting upon a true and good belief when we can justify our actions and beliefs to another reasonable person by explaining why they are true and why they are good. Thus we choose hypotheses that are "true, good, and justified."

This kind of gambling is both similar to and different from what we usually think of as gambling. Let's say you believe that a certain horse is going to win a race. The consequences of acting or not acting on this hypothesis (i.e., betting or not betting) depend on whether the hypothesis turns out to be true or false. If, for example, you act upon a hypothesis that turns out to be false (i.e., bet on a losing horse) or do not act upon a hypothesis that turns out to be true (i.e., fail to bet on a winning horse), you lose your bet. The same is true when a hypothesis is being tested in the laboratory or the doctor's office rather than at the racetrack.

As with any gamble, the consequences of choosing one hypothesis or another can be understood, up to a point, as a matter of costs and benefits. What do you stand to gain if your horse wins? What do you stand to lose if it doesn't win? How likely is it that the horse will win? Would you rather put your two dollars on an even-money horse (one that will return only two dollars if it wins because it is considered to have as much chance to win as to lose) or on a long shot? Would you still make the same choice if you were betting ten dollars or fifty dollars instead of two dollars? Similar questions are bound to occur to the scientist gambling that it will be useful to act on a given hypothesis.

We often try to understand the costs and benefits of a gamble by referring to probabilities and values. When we gamble we keep in mind the probability of something happening (e.g., our horse winning the race) and the value it would have for us if it did happen. But is that all we think of? Suppose, for example, you get inside information that a race has been "fixed" so that one horse is sure to win. Even though the probability (a "sure thing") and the value of winning are both high, you may decline to bet on principle. That is, you may believe that to win a bet by cheating is not a good outcome, in terms of its effects on others and on your own character.

Despite such examples of individual scruple, the gambling that people do for recreation and for profit can often be characterized as unprincipled. In science, on the other hand, our choice of gambles is guided by a number of principles. These principles grow out of some crucial differences between gambling under the Probabilistic Paradigm and what we usually think of as gambling. Normally gamblers bet against known odds for a definite reward. Most gambling games are structured so that some people win while others lose; there is a fixed pool of winnings that the players simply exchange (with the house, if there is one, taking its cut). In science it is not that simple. The probabilities, the rewards, the potential winnings, and the value of winning are discovered in the course of gambling. Indeed, finding out the odds can be the very purpose of the gamble, rather than merely a means toward gaining a material reward.

In science the idea of "winning" a gamble takes on a different meaning. Since what is to be won is knowledge, not money, there is no limit to what can be won over a period of time, and what is won by one person is not necessarily lost by another. As scientists make use of the knowledge they have won, they produce more knowledge. This knowledge is not only about the subject under study, but about how to gamble and what to gamble for. One experiments to get a better idea of the odds and of how the game works, so as to be able to gamble more consciously and more skillfully.

The principles of gambling under the Probabilistic Paradigm make it possible to gamble consciously and effectively in an uncertain world—the world described by the first criterion of the paradigm and by the Heisenberg Uncertainty Principle. They tell the scientist what to keep in mind while gambling, what rules to follow consistently (and when they may be broken) in order to have a good chance of a good outcome.

One such principle is that one must be aware of the context of uncertainty that surrounds experimentation and be ready to question one's observations, one's assessments of probability and value, and one's hypotheses. Even when the hypothesis under consideration has apparently been confirmed by experimental results, there remains the possibility that some other cause or causes, as yet unknown, have contributed to those results. A degree of doubt, of skepticism in interpretation, is called for.

As one doubts nature, so one must doubt oneself. According to Heisenberg's principle one cannot observe without affecting what one observes. In order to work within the Probabilistic Paradigm, therefore, one must keep in mind the possible consequences of one's actions as an experimenter. One must ask whether the apparent confirmation or disconfirmation of a hypothesis may have resulted from some unforeseen effect of the act of observation. In other words, one must be a self-aware experimenter. Whereas a gambler is primarily concerned with deception by others, a scientist is most concerned with his capacity for self-deception.

Actually, one may not have any problem learning to doubt the order of nature, or to doubt one's hypotheses, or to doubt one's own actions. The uncertainties that appear in one's very

observations and experimental results will give one ample reason to doubt. In a probabilistic world not every trial will work
out; not every piece of data will confirm a hypothesis; and even
when it does, it is not entirely clear what is being confirmed.
Under these conditions it is easy for doubt to become paralyz-
ing and for the experimenter to accept defeat at the hands of
what seems to be total uncertainty. Wherever there is doubt,
therefore, one must be prepared to give the benefit of the doubt
—to nature, to one's hypotheses, and to oneself as an experimenter.

In the first place, when dealing with probabilities one cannot
change one's hypotheses with every new piece of data. Just as
one cannot evaluate a new strategy for playing blackjack on
one trial, so in science one must be willing to pursue a line of
action that is not immediately rewarding in order to learn what
the probabilities are in the long run. Thinking in terms of
probabilities requires some faith that there is order in the
world. Under conditions of complete certainty such faith would
not be necessary; under conditions of complete uncertainty it

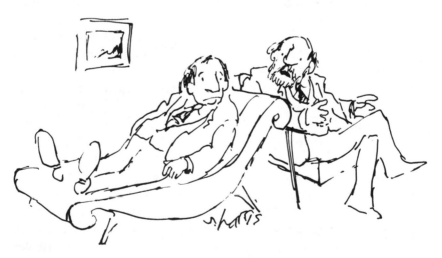

"But you can't go through life applying
Heisenberg's Uncertainty Principle to *everything*."

would not be possible. The idea of probability, on the other hand, implies that an uncertain world is not a chaotic one. Some things merit a higher degree of belief than others. If one trusts that there is an order, a probabilistic one, underlying phenomena, one will be able to stay with a course of action, even without knowing its consequences, long enough to learn its consequences in general and not just in one particular case.

Even when the probabilities have been established through a series of observations, there remains some uncertainty about what exactly has been proved. One must therefore give the hypotheses under consideration the benefit of the doubt before deciding which one to credit. Since there can always be some doubt left as to whether all possible hypotheses have been considered, one must be willing to act upon the one that seems most truthful and useful to act upon while at the same time being ready, if necessary, to reconsider previously discarded hypotheses. The Greek philosopher Heraclitus said, "You never step in the same river twice." For most practical purposes, however, the river remains the same. Just as the river flows downstream, so causes come and go, but very often not enough to make a difference. Where they do make a difference is a matter of judgment, experience, and interest.

Just as one trusts that one has not been out-and-out deceived by nature, so one must trust that one has not completely deceived oneself. While acknowledging that "observer effects" are intertwined with one's results, one must be able to suspend doubt at least long enough to act and then critically assess the results of one's actions. There is, for example, no question but that photographs are taken from the point of view of the photographer and reveal the interests of the photographer, but one can still look at a photograph and learn something about the world beyond the observer.

In summary, then, one must question reality, one's knowledge, and one's methods; and yet sooner or later one must trust sufficiently to choose. One can only interpret one's observations in a probabilistic world—in other words, comprehend the regularities as well as the irregularities of that world—if one extends to oneself as an observer and to what one observes a trust that is not blind, but critical. Being critical means being conscious of one's choices, getting some perspective on them, attempting to assess the consequences of various alternatives, and making choices by criteria that reasonable people can understand. This principle of critical choice, coupled with a degree of trust, sums up the principles we have considered.

Together, these principles give scientists a set of rules that they can agree upon as reasonable guidelines for their efforts and as a basis for communication between one scientist and another. At the same time, they enable the individual scientist to act in accordance with a long-range plan and agreed-upon goals and values amid inconsistent results and shifting fortunes. They help the scientist answer the crucial question, "When does one change one's mind?" For there are costs to giving up a hypothesis and starting over—costs that are referred to as "retooling costs." In a probabilistic world when does new information warrant one's incurring those costs? All one can do is to choose those experiments that seem most likely to yield the kind of information that will let one know whether or not it is worthwhile to change one's mind—and then to interpret the results in accordance with the principle of critical trust.

To understand the second criterion of the Probabilistic Paradigm in its broadest implications, we can start with Niels Bohr's interpretation of the Heisenberg Uncertainty Principle. According to Bohr (1969), Heisenberg's principle links the observer and the observed within a system of mutual influence in which the same laws apply to both. In other words there is not the absolute, unbridgeable difference between a scientist and an electron under the Probabilistic Paradigm that there is under the Mechanistic. The distinction drawn under the Mechanistic Paradigm between the straightforward behavior of physical objects and the complexities and uncertainties of dealing with people disappears under the Probabilistic Paradigm. No longer is the experimental situation set apart, in its precision and controllability, from the multitude of interactions among people as well as objects that occur throughout life. Under the new paradigm the same kinds of judgment apply. What it means to accept a belief about the motion of particles is much the same as what it means to accept a belief about a person. So we can look at the way we understand people as a model for the way we might learn to understand electrons.

When we meet a new person, we have to trust our observations about the person. When we see the person do something we don't understand, we give the person the benefit of the doubt —that is, assume that the person is acting rationally until we are shown otherwise. Similarly, we trust that the seemingly inexplicable behavior of subatomic particles can be explained —if not by a theory that we currently hold, then by another. When we see a person act in a way that isn't entirely consistent, we realize that nobody does the same thing all the time, and we trust that there is an underlying pattern of regularity in the person's actions. In physics, too, we look for relationships of probability, not certainty. We expect patterns to emerge, if not immediately, then in the long run. Finally, when we interact with another person we are self-aware. We realize that we affect and are affected by that person. Thus we ask, "Is part of what I observe in this person a response to my own behavior? Have I made this person act that way?" So it is in physics with the Heisenberg Uncertainty Principle.

It is not only the other person who is affected by the interaction, of course. When we decide whether or not to accept someone as a friend, for instance, we are certainly affected by our decision to look at that person in one way rather than another. To give a stark example, the Nazis, by seeing the Jews as subhuman and treating them as such, changed not only the Jews but themselves. Not only did some Jews act in subhuman ways when forced to live under subhuman conditions, but the characters of some Germans changed so that it became "all in the day's work" for them to treat other people as subhuman.

In science, too, our characters are changed by the decisions we make. Our methods of observing and understanding, the values we uphold, the principles we follow become habits that in part define what we are and how we see ourselves. Whenever we make a choice, we are strengthening or weakening our principles, or choosing new principles. In this respect as in others, the practice of science cannot be disassociated from what is normally thought of as ethics.

What scientific knowledge now requires is the ability to look at oneself as one looks at the objects of one's observation—that is, to see oneself as being made of the same matter and subject to the same laws as they are. What ethical knowledge requires is the ability to look at the objects of one's observation as one looks at oneself—that is, to begin by assuming that they are made of the same matter and subject to the same laws as oneself. Only for good reason should they be treated differently. Thus, although the second criterion of the Probabilistic Paradigm does not ensure that scientists will treat ethics as a part of science (for people can develop compartmentalized awareness), it guides the practice of scientists in such a manner as to encourage them to do so. This is further encouraged by the third criterion of the paradigm.

Criterion #3:
The Continuity of the Objective and the Subjective

In science, as elsewhere, whatever claims to be knowledge must be capable of being publicly discussed. Even if there is disagreement, there must be some basis of agreement so that public debate can take place. As we have seen, scientists working under the Mechanistic Paradigm take the view that such agreement and debate are not possible with subjective knowledge, since whatever is subjective is assumed to be inherently private and irrational. It is no wonder, then, that scientists under the old paradigm seek to experiment in a value-free manner. For such scientists the influence of subjective values upon their objective results is a contamination to be eliminated at all costs, since it threatens the claim that these results constitute knowledge.

We now know, however, as we saw under Criterion #2 of the Probabilistic Paradigm, that it is impossible to eliminate subjective knowledge from scientific inquiry. The effects of the experimenter's values (whether consciously or unconsciously expressed) on experimental methods and results have been noted in contexts ranging from Heisenberg's "observer effect" in physics to Robert Rosenthal's (1969) "experimenter bias" in psychology. As in our example of international news reporting, subjective knowledge is inseparably a part of what is considered objective knowledge. The question is whether or not scientists acknowledge its presence and try to account for its influence. Because scientists under the Mechanistic Paradigm have not dealt consciously with the influence of their values on their scientific practice, that influence has expressed itself through unconscious habit. But it has been there nonetheless.

If objective knowledge is not as fully objective as would appear from the Mechanistic Paradigm's strict dichotomy, what about subjective knowledge? Is it purely subjective? Are values private and irrational—and nothing more? The way values have been understood under the Mechanistic Paradigm is illustrated by the practice of public-opinion polling. Whereas poll-takers attempt to eliminate their own values and beliefs so that their "objective" interviewing techniques will not be qualified by subjectivity, they treat the values and beliefs of the people they interview as if these were unqualified by objectivity. The pollsters contact people individually, in isolation from the family members, fellow workers, and friends with whom they normally discuss public issues. The procedure, by implying that all values are equally private and equally irrational, encourages respondents to express the most selfish and individualistic of values. This is another "experimenter effect" understandable in terms of the second criterion of the Probabilistic Paradigm. What the pollsters look for—and what they get—is a collection of preformed opinions untempered by public discussion and shared experience. Private, irrational preferences become fixed as inert data ("hard figures") through the *experimentum crucis* of polling.

In real life, however, we do not hold our values and beliefs privately. We form and maintain them by living and working with other people. We share our values and beliefs with others and as a result may either change our minds or find our original beliefs confirmed and strengthened. In this way we try to establish what values rational people must agree on and what areas of disagreement and variation are reasonable. The town meeting embodies this kind of interchange. There people develop their values while seeing and hearing others (all of whom, unlike the "neutral" pollster, have an acknowledged stake in the outcome) defend their values and, by doing so, themselves. Through the give and take that occurs at such gatherings, the members of a community decide what rules they all must follow in practice and what differences will be respected. It is ironic that public-opinion polling, which reflects the assumptions of the Mechanistic Paradigm, is (with its trappings of science) a more recent development than the town meeting, which is closer in spirit to the Probabilistic Paradigm.

Just as there is a subjective aspect to objective knowledge (such as knowledge of electrons), as we saw under Criterion #2, so there is an objective aspect to subjective knowledge (such as knowledge of feelings). On the one hand, we find that we need to take values into account when we are being rational, as when we are practicing science. On the other, we find that we *can* be rational when we are dealing with values. Even in the realm of the subjective, reasonable people can find grounds to agree or disagree. It is not a case of "anything goes." For example, although a reasonable person may value his home over his car, or vice versa, it would be more difficult to understand his valuing his car over his life. Only when people reach some degree of agreement about what are reasonable values to hold can they practice science together according to an agreed-upon set of rules. Values that affect people collectively need to be created by people collectively.

Thus science under the Probabilistic Paradigm is more like a town meeting than a public-opinion poll. An experiment becomes an opportunity for the discussion and interpretation of values and beliefs, which are subject to the same kind of critical scrutiny and debate as experimental methods and data. Such values and beliefs, while subjective (in the sense that they are held by individuals and not "proven" by conclusive experiments), can and must be public, in the sense of being justifiable to other reasonable people engaged in the scientific enterprise. Through this process the subjective component of objective knowledge is revealed, and subjective values, by being articulated and explored rationally, become a form of knowledge. Thus the sharp dichotomy between the subjective and the objective under the Mechanistic Paradigm becomes, instead, a continuum, where knowledge may be more or less subjective and more or less objective, but not all one or the other.

It is an uncertain world that scientists study and that we live in. Therefore, as the philosopher Hilary Putnam (1978) reminds us, no one can afford to disregard such knowledge as is possible, be it of values or of electrons, just because there is some element of subjectivity in it.

What Is Probability?

Another area in which subjective judgment comes into play under the Probabilistic Paradigm is in the understanding of probabilities. Although mathematical probability theory has existed since the seventeenth century, we still don't know what probability really means. Everyone agrees on the rules for calculating probabilities. But what lies behind the numbers?

Imagine trying to decide between two interpretations of probability as the basis for science, one of which is identified with the experiment in the laboratory, the other with the gambler placing a bet with a bookmaker. Where one interpretation speaks with the authority of mathematics, while the other has its source in mere "belief," it is clear which one most scientists (or anyone, for that matter) would have more confidence in.

The two interpretations are the "objective," which flourished in the heyday of the Mechanistic Paradigm, and the "subjective," which originated in the eighteenth century but was neglected in the mechanistic era until its reemergence in the 1930's (Lee, 1971). (Since then it has been increasingly used.) The objective interpretation is based on "relative frequencies," the subjective on "degrees of belief." We can illustrate each by the way it arrives at the probability of a coin coming up heads.

Using the objective interpretation, you would flip a great many coins and see how often they come up heads. If you flip one coin, you cannot predict whether it will come up heads or tails. If you flip one hundred coins, you can predict that somewhere around half of them will turn up heads. The greater the number of trials, the closer the result is likely to be half heads and half tails. Thus the "objective" school defines probability as "a limiting value of a relative frequency as the number of cases increases to infinity." With a coin flip, of course, that value is fifty percent.

In the subjective interpretation the probability of a coin turning up heads is thought of in these terms: "How much do you believe that it will turn up heads? How much would you bet on it? At what odds?" The language of gambling expresses subjective judgment in numerical terms. We recall, of course, that the whole idea of probability had its origins in gambling.

It is understandable that the objective interpretation of probability was widely accepted under the Mechanistic Paradigm. It fit in with the mechanistic emphasis on objectivity, and its reliance on laboratory trials was consistent with the notion of an *experimentum crucis.* With its assumption that an infinite number of trials was needed to reproduce the ideal mathematical result, this version of probability gave scientists under the Mechanistic Paradigm a theory of errors which explained deviations from ideal experimental results.

The objective interpretation is not, however, consistent with the three criteria of the Probabilistic Paradigm. The inconsistency became apparent when paradoxes were found not only in quantum physics, but in the most mundane areas of science. These paradoxes can be expressed in everyday language by means of Gedanken ("thinking") experiments like the following (Putnam, 1979):

Gedanken Experiment #1:
"The Life or Death of Schrödinger's Cat"

In this paradox, named after the creator of the Schrödinger wave equation in physics, a cat with the regal name of

Mittendorf Plantagenet is placed in an opaque, soundproof box with a capsule of cyanide that will be released on the occurrence of a random "outside event" such as the detection of a cosmic ray. Mittendorf is left in the box for a time interval during which the probability of the outside event's occurring (by statistical laws) is fifty percent. If this grisly experiment is performed only once, what is the probability that "Mitt" will be found dead when the box is opened?

Part of the paradox here is that the cat's fate, while yoked to an event which has a known probability of occurrence, is itself decided only once. If probability is defined solely in terms of frequency of occurrence of a particular outcome over a series of trials, what probability can we assign to a unique event? According to the relative-frequency interpretation, the probability of a unique event such as Mittendorf's death is either one or zero. But this clashes with our theoretically derived probability of fifty percent for this unique event. We can thus see that the relative-frequency definition of probability is far too restrictive for physics today. This paradox disappears if we instead use a non–frequency-based interpretation of probability.

Many of the events to which physicists assign probabilities, such as some cosmic phenomena, are nonrecurring. Probabilities based on the notion of relative frequency are of little use here. Even in cases where relative frequencies *can* be calculated, some form of subjective judgment is required. In the case of the repeated coin flips the mathematical formulation of a probability that approaches fifty percent as the number of flips approaches infinity is useful, but it is based on the assumption that the coin is as likely to come up heads as tails on any one flip. It also presupposes that one coin flip is just like another. Both of these assumptions represent subjective judgments.

We can see this more clearly where the judgment of similarity is more difficult to make. When we say, "There is a ninety percent chance of rain tomorrow," are we just saying, "There is a ninety percent chance of rain on days like tomorrow"? How can we tell which days to put in that category? What days are just like tomorrow? Whenever we group things into categories for the purpose of calculating relative frequencies, we are making a subjective assessment of similarity based on our prior knowledge and experience.

In no case do the data alone dictate the probability. Always an element of human understanding is present. When we derive probability estimates from a theory, as in quantum physics, we are making a subjective judgment to the effect that the case in question is explained by the theory (and therefore by the probabilities generated from it) and that the theory itself is worthy of being held. When we apply probability estimates to a particular case, as in medicine, we make judgments based on our knowledge of that case. A patient who on the basis of available data is said to have a ten percent chance of having breast cancer is an individual. Our estimate of the probability must take into account our knowledge of the patient as an individual who may somehow differ from other patients in the ten percent category.

Here is a second Gedanken experiment, one that reveals another paradox in the use of "objective" probability estimates (Hempel, 1965):

Gedanken Experiment #2:
"How much would you bet on a raven being black?"

Imagine a law of the form: All ravens are black. You see a bird that you are certain is a raven but can't quite make out its color. But knowing the law you exclaim, "I'd stake my soul, by God, that that bird is black!" All of a sudden, a bolt of lightning strikes, the heavens darken, and a sinister yet familiar figure approaches you and sticks out his hand: "What would you like me to stake against this soul of yours?"

If we really knew with certainty that all ravens were black, it would be entirely rational to bet *anything* against *nothing* that this bird would fit the pattern. And yet no matter how many black ravens (and *only* black ravens) we saw, we would not be likely to make that bet. Moreover, we would not be considered irrational for refusing to do so, since people make an intuitive distinction between observational truths (such as "All ravens are black") and logical truths (such as "If all ravens are black, and if this is a raven, then this is black"). The former are considered risky to bet on; the latter are not. It seems that our subjective gambling decisions do not reflect a belief in a universe where everything is determined.

This is a case where our subjective probability estimate (say, the proverbial "99 and 44/100 percent") differs from the relative-frequency estimate, which, based on all ravens that have ever been seen, would be one hundred percent. Which is the more useful estimate? In the first place, to assign a probability of one hundred percent (certainty) to a statement based on observation rather than logic is legitimate under the Mechanistic, but not the Probabilistic Paradigm, whose first criterion (that the world is an uncertain place) it violates. So we would not make such estimates if we wish to work within the Probabilistic Paradigm. Beyond this, as has been shown by the philosopher Abner Shimony (1970), such estimates are inconsistent with the rules of probability. That is, a person who bets that statements based on observation are *always* or *never* true can be put in the position of having what gamblers call a semi-Dutch Book made against him. A *Dutch Book* is a series of bets set up so that the gambler must lose no matter what the outcome. With a semi-Dutch Book the gambler can only lose or break even, not win.

To illustrate how a Dutch Book works, we can use an example from boxing history. Let's say you and a friend agreed that Muhammad Ali should be a three-to-two favorite over Joe Frazier in a championship fight, and you bet six dollars on Ali against your friend's four dollars. Then another "friend" convinced you that Frazier was going to win, and you agreed to bet six dollars against four dollars on Frazier. If Ali won, you won four dollars on the first bet but lost six dollars on the second. If Frazier won, you won four dollars on the second bet but lost six dollars on the first. Either way, you lost two dollars. With your inconsistent probability estimates, you made a Dutch Book against yourself.

Our gambling phraseology gives us a way of answering the

question, "Does the subjective interpretation of probability mean that 'anything goes'? Is any probability estimate as good as any other?" Not quite. True, with subjective probability estimates there is no one correct answer, as there is when probabilities are calculated from relative frequencies. But when we think of our estimates as odds at which we would be willing to bet on something happening, we are giving ourselves a stake in the outcome and thus disciplining our choice of probabilities. If we stand to lose by making self-contradictory bets like the one on Ali and Frazier, we will avoid making such bets.

Consistency, then, becomes another principle that guides our choice of gambles. We limit ourselves to those gambles that do not allow a Dutch Book (or semi-Dutch Book) to be made against us. A variation of the consistency rule is the requirement of *transitivity,* which means that our choices should be consistent when more than one choice is involved. If we bet on horse A against horse B and also on horse B against horse C, in both cases accepting unfavorable odds, we'd better not be so foolish as to accept the same unfavorable odds on horse C against horse A (a sure loss no matter which horse wins). Finally, the same consistency rules that apply to our probability estimates should apply to our value assessments if we want to avoid a Dutch Book. As applied to values, transitivity, for example, means that if we prefer apples to oranges and oranges to pears, then at the same time we will prefer apples to pears.

Subjective probability assessment fits all three criteria of the Probabilistic Paradigm. It acknowledges that we cannot define categories so strictly as to exclude a degree of uncertainty even in those relationships where observation apparently reveals ironclad regularity (Criterion #1). It requires that people choose their probability estimates rather than have them revealed by an objective experiment (Criterion #2). It implies that probability cannot be clearly separated from other forms of knowledge, including values (Criterion #3). The Probabilistic Paradigm makes it possible to have a subjective understanding of probability and to make use of subjective probability assessments. The subjective interpretation of probability in turn provides an example of how we can use subjective knowledge. It thereby encourages us to look at feeling and value as additional sources of knowledge.

In practical terms the subjective interpretation assumes that people can and do arrive at reasonable probability estimates without necessarily having observed the outcomes of many similar trials. Moreover, it makes those estimates available to science. In medicine, for example, it allows probability estimates to be derived not only from tables of figures, but also from the subjective judgment of the doctor, patient, and family. It means that a doctor's knowledge of a particular patient's history may be more useful than statistical tables in assessing the likelihood that the patient has a particular disease or will respond to a particular treatment. And it means that there may be times when the patient or the patient's family are better judges of these probabilities than the doctor, especially a doctor who does not have prior knowledge of the patient.

Applying the Probabilistic Paradigm

Certainty is an age-old dream. It has taken different forms in different eras. Before the mechanistic age people sought comfort through ritual in the face of uncertainty. There were periods, for example, when people living at the mercy of uncontrollable natural forces gained a measure of psychological control by anthropomorphizing those forces and seeking to dominate them through the use of magic. Under the Mechanistic Paradigm people gained some real control over nature by acknowledging its separateness and learning how it worked. People watched—first with wonder, then with complacency—as diseases were wiped out one after another. It seemed as if the world were moving toward greater certainty.

In the twentieth century new areas of uncertainty have presented themselves: diseases that resist cure, irregularities in the movements of heavenly bodies and subatomic particles, the disruption of environmental balance, the threat of nuclear destruction. There is a renewed focus on things that human beings cannot control. To this we can respond in two ways. One is to recognize the usefulness—indeed, the necessity—of the Probabilistic Paradigm and to apply it as broadly as possible as a way of coming to terms with uncertainty. The other is to retreat into ritual—namely, the rituals of science and technology that so recently gave us the comfort of apparent certainty. Thus the continuing attraction and influence of the Mechanistic Paradigm in our time. There is always need for a little magic.

A paradigm that is dominant for generations puts down strong roots in the unconscious (of which it is a reflection). Despite the commonsensical ring of probabilistic thinking when we hear it in a weather forecast, much of what we call common sense is in fact mechanistic thinking. To overcome the inertial force that the old paradigm exerts unconsciously and implicitly, we need to apply the new paradigm consciously and explicitly. We also need to apply it systematically *as* a paradigm, using all three criteria in an interconnected way. When we try to apply one criterion at a time, the new way of thinking is easily undermined by the familiar habits of the old.

This is where applying the Probabilistic Paradigm differs from casually invoking the language of probability. To speak of using "part" of the new paradigm makes no more sense than to say that seeing only the faces in the drawing after seeing only the vase is a new form of perception. Yet the history of science offers many instances where some aspect of the Probabilistic Paradigm (such as probability) is used, but not the paradigm itself (Hacking, 1975).

However, once we see things in terms of a new paradigm, we can't go back to the old. When we have seen the vase and the faces together, we can't go back to seeing just the one or the other. When the new paradigm becomes familiar, it can exert a force equal to that of the old paradigm in its day. When this new way of thinking becomes so familiar as to be part of the consciousness of a culture, it will not only have revolutionized physics, but will also be a new world view. This vision will have particular impact in an area such as medicine where the concerns of science and the everyday meet.

3

UNCERTAINTY
IN MEDICINE

It is inconceivable, given what we understand a paradigm to be, that during a given era the effects of a paradigm shift would be confined to one discipline such as physics. There may be questions about how the new paradigm translates from one science to another, or beyond science altogether, but it is clear that such translations will occur. A world that understands Newton's laws as special cases of more complex relationships will sooner or later learn to apply the same perspective to the subtleties of social and emotional existence as to the physical.

Indeed, people who work in a wide range of fields have been announcing, predicting, or calling for the adoption of what amounts to the Probabilistic Paradigm in their disciplines. In *The Restructuring of Social and Political Theory* (1978), Richard J. Bernstein reports that the mechanistic "value-free" method of collecting facts and arranging them in the form of deterministic laws is being strongly challenged within the social sciences, which are becoming more hospitable to subjective interpretations and indeterminate causality. Economist Lester C. Thurow, speaking of "The End of Newtonian Economics," notes that "economics, along with much of modern science, is being drawn in a direction where events are perceived to be much more stochastic and much less deterministic

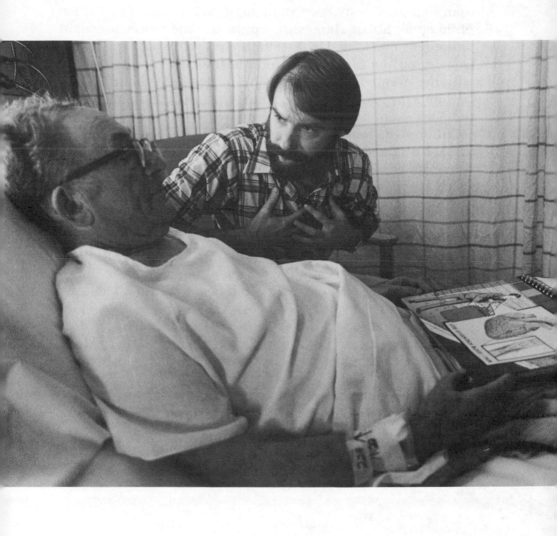

than had previously been thought" (1977, p. 86). The British philosopher Stuart Hampshire contrasts "the two centuries of philosophy dominated by Newton's physics," which "naturally transferred the idea of unalterable laws to human affairs," with the twentieth-century study of biological systems, which "exhibits the sovereignty of chance, luck, and contingency, and provides examples of sudden and substantial changes due to small unpredictable displacements, of little causes producing great effects, and of explanations by probabilities." Hampshire concludes that the human species "is no less exposed to risk than any other species of animal, except that human beings are better equipped to calculate some of the risks and to take out some insurance" (1979, p. 42d).

Where does all this leave medicine? Medicine as an applied science (both biological and social) has not kept up with these changes in scientific thinking. It is not helping people recognize uncertainty, calculate risks, and take out insurance—that is, gamble. In the words of G. Gayle Stephens, M.D., former president of the Society of Teachers of Family Medicine, "Medicine has not noticed that the tides of its intellectual fortune have gone out in the past seventy-five years. Now we are grounded on a shoal. . . . In comparison with physics we are in a pre-Einsteinian phase of existence. We still worship Newton. Physics was forced to deal with the dilemmas of determinism sixty years ago. In medicine it is not discussable even today" (1979, p. 18).

The Mechanistic Paradigm in Medicine and Its Breakdown

The mechanistic philosophy of medical practice which gained ascendancy in the nineteenth century (replacing what we now term the superstition and fancy of prior ages) and still underlies what we call "modern medical science" is expressed most clearly in Claude Bernard's *Principles of Experimental Medicine,* published in 1865. Bernard, one of the founders of modern medicine, made explicit and implicit references to Newton's work in expounding what we can now recognize to be the three criteria of the Mechanistic Paradigm:

Criterion #1:
Deterministic Causation.

I acknowledge my inability to understand why results taken from statistics are called *laws*; for in my opinion scientific law can be based only on certainty, on absolute determinism, not on probability (Bernard, 1957, p. 136).

Criterion #2:
The "Experimentum Crucis."

As a science, medicine necessarily has definite and precise laws which, like those of all the sciences, are derived from the criterion of experiment . . . the principles of experimental determinism must be applied to medicine if it is to become an exact science founded on experimental determinism instead of remaining a conjectural science based on statistics. A conjectural science may indeed rest on the indeterminate; but an experimental science accepts only determinate, or determinable phenomena (Bernard, 1957, pp. 139–140).

Criterion #3:
The Objective/Subjective Dichotomy.

Only determinism in an experiment yields absolute law; and he who knows the true law is no longer free to see a phenomenon otherwise (Bernard, 1957, p. 140).

These prescriptions—which express the nineteenth century's growing confidence that calculation and controlled experimental comparison would give man mastery over his environment, be it natural or social—have even today a satisfying ring of assurance and tidy rationality. In fact they guide much contemporary scientific research. Where they can lead, however, is intimated in the story of K., the twenty-one-month-old boy in Chapter 1. Without realizing it, the physicians who were responsible for K.'s care in the hospital practiced according to the three criteria of the Mechanistic Paradigm. They did so by thinking it inappropriate to treat K. until they could find *the* cause of his condition (deterministic causation), by believing that diagnostic testing would reveal this determining cause without itself affecting the state of K.'s health (*experimentum crucis*), and by disregarding K.'s obvious resentment of the testing and their own distress at having to cause him pain (objective/subjective dichotomy).

The case of K. is just one illustration of the medical problems that cannot be solved through the application of these three criteria. Doctors now confront a very different set of diseases from the ones they faced in 1900. Medical technology under the Mechanistic Paradigm has licked diphtheria, tuberculosis, smallpox, and polio, only to find that the people who aren't dying of these diseases are living to contract hypertension, heart disease, and cancer. Treating chronic degenerative conditions that take diverse forms and have no (or many) known causative agents can be as different from treating acute infectious conditions as measuring the velocity of an electron is from measuring that of a toy wagon. Here the diagnosis and treatment are much less clear-cut. The doctor, patient, and family may have serious differences about what is wrong and what to do about it.

Along with these different diseases have come other problems that frustrate the straightforward technological solutions of the Mechanistic Paradigm (which indeed may be helping to create them). There is the problem of cost—higher and higher medical bills, insurance bills, tax bills. Then there is the suspicion, the mistrust, that has come between patient and doctor. Many people, once they realize that a doctor is not the idealized mechanistic scientist who can be trusted blindly to come up with the right answer, seem not to be able to trust doctors at all. Patients sue for malpractice, while doctors gripe about patient "noncompliance" and devise manipulative strategies to make patients comply. Medical care suffers because patients and doctors don't get along with each other, and one reason they don't is that their expectations of each other are grounded in the Mechanistic Paradigm.

The Probabilistic Paradigm in Medicine: Three Criteria

Against Claude Bernard's three criteria of Newtonian medicine, we can set the three criteria of the Probabilistic Paradigm. Again we can take our illustrations from the case of K., but this time from the way Dr. S., the intern, handled the case.

Criterion #1:
Probabilistic Causation

It is recognized that a patient's condition may have more than one cause, that it may not be possible to separate the effects of each cause, and that the same observed condition may have different sets of causes at different times. In the case of K., Dr. S. put much less emphasis on diagnostic testing than did the other physicians because he thought it unlikely that the patient's condition had a single treatable cause that could be revealed by testing. Instead he looked for a number of possible causes (genetic, environmental, psychological) operating in combination with one another in a way that was affected by chance. Among those possible causes were his own diagnostic and therapeutic actions.

Whenever he observed K., Dr. S. realized that he might be contributing to some change in K.'s condition. So he observed, then acted on his observations, then observed the effects of his observations and actions as well as other known and unknown causes. He kept in mind that each effect that he observed could also be a cause, and vice versa. Finally, whenever he observed the operation of causes, he also was observing the operation of chance. Thus, although he was able to form some expectations about K. as he gained more experience with him, he was still open to being surprised.

Criterion #2:
Experimentation as Principled Gambling

Given that the relevant variables cannot be perfectly controlled through detached observation and manipulation, doctors and patients working within the Probabilistic Paradigm treat diagnostic procedures as gambles, to be evaluated according to how fruitful they may be for the patient. Dr. S. understood that extensive diagnostic testing (the *experimentum crucis*) had not revealed and was not about to reveal a determining cause or causes of K.'s illness. Even after all the tests were completed, the data still needed to be interpreted so that choices could be made as to which hypotheses to act upon.

The outcome of each diagnostic or therapeutic gamble did not dictate which gamble to choose next. S., the observer, had to make that choice on the basis of principles which included self-reflection. While trusting himself, he had to be critical of himself at the same time. This was what he did when he acted upon the observation that the testing he himself had ordered was having some deleterious effect on K.'s emotional well-being, eating habits, and ability to withstand infection. Instead of aiming for an illusory diagnostic precision, he undertook exploratory treatments designed to assess over a period of time the relative importance of possible contributing factors such as malnutrition, lack of parental nurturance, and the kinds of germs found in any hospital environment. Recognizing that his own actions would in any case affect the patient, he sought to make that effect a constructive one by whenever possible giving him love and food and protecting him from pain.

In this kind of empirical therapy, diagnosis becomes a form of treatment, and treatment becomes a form of diagnosis. Experimentation is extended outward through time and space as physicians and patients learn from their actions and consciously adjust their subsequent practice. The physician becomes part of the experiment and, along with the patient, changes in the course of the experiment. For example, S. saw the interns and residents around him become more "hard-boiled," losing the capacity to feel love for their patients, the more they did painful diagnostic procedures on children. But that is not the only way in which doctors are transformed. In a more hopeful vein, the experience of a medical practice—the shared experience of doctors and families—can create a growing understanding that is expressed in the form of subjective probability estimates. Medicine, instead of trying to live up to an outmoded model of laboratory science, can then become a science of action, a science of practice.

Criterion #3:
The Continuity of the Subjective and the Objective

Not only the doctor's knowledge, but the patient's knowledge, the patient's feelings, and the doctor's feelings are considered to be of crucial importance in diagnosis and treatment. The goals and methods of treatment, rather than being determined solely by the physician's conception of "scientific" (i.e., technological) efficacy, are evaluated in line with the patient's and the doctor's values. When the patient's values are different from the doctor's, they are still given the benefit of the doubt and considered to be reasonable unless shown to be otherwise. Not that "anything goes," of course. Both the doctor and patient need to apply critical scrutiny to their own and each other's values as these affect the issues at hand. For example, Dr. S. did not simply accept K.'s preference not to eat (even to the point of starving to death) as a reasonable value judgment, although he might have done so in the case of a patient dying of a degenerative disease. And many times S. questioned himself, saying, "Am I fooling myself? Could it be that all the other doctors are right and I am wrong?"

S. found it hard to draw a sharp line between the objective and subjective aspects of K.'s case, since feelings (both the patient's and his own) told him a great deal about the illness and its treatment. Instead of dismissing the feelings of pain that he shared with K. as an irrational concern, S. tried to make sense of them and to see what he could learn from them. The other doctors experienced such emotions too, but they neither paid attention to these feelings nor considered the effects that other feelings they had (e.g., their need for certainty) might have on their actions toward the patient. S., on the other hand, listened closely to his own reactions as well as to those that K. conveyed through his moods, behavior, and eating habits. He assumed that the feelings that the child was showing were basically the same kinds of feelings that he had. Even though it appeared that the way K. was acting wasn't doing him any good, S. conceded that maybe K. did know what was good for him. Maybe he was trying to tell the doctors something. It was clear, at least, that the way K. felt would have a lot to do with how well he responded to treatment.

Subjective Probability Assessment

The three criteria of the Probabilistic Paradigm encourage the use of subjective probability assessment, which K.'s case also exemplifies. Since relative-frequency statistics were not available for a condition like K.'s, the house officers had no way of making use of probability. Instead they did virtually every possible test in their search for certainty. Dr. S., on the other hand, made use of his subjective judgments (based on observation, experience, and empathy) about how much the testing was likely to reveal, what various treatments were likely to accomplish, and what would be good for K. and what would not.

Even where relative frequency statistics are available, they are only a starting point, not an end point, for clinical judgment. They must be translated into subjective probabilities for the individual patient. There is a saying in medicine that every patient is unique. But to what extent a patient is unique and to what extent similar to other patients is a matter of judgment. Anytime one uses relative-frequency statistics for a particular patient, one is making the subjective judgment that this patient falls into the category of patients to which the statistics apply. One is acting on the belief that there is nothing special about this patient, no extraordinary circumstances that one has overlooked that would put the patient in a different category. Such a judgment is another kind of gamble, another guess that is educated by experience and guided by principle.

Benefits of the New Paradigm

Taken together, the criteria of the Probabilistic Paradigm give us a new way to think about and practice medicine. If in some ways they seem to confound common sense, in other ways they reaffirm it, for they restore a respect for the many-sidedness of reality that was lost in the oversimplifications of nineteenth-century science. It is a wonder that medical practitioners ever could have thought that the causes of complicated conditions *could* be known with certainty; that the doctor-patient interaction would *not* influence the course of an illness; that knowledge about microbes and bacilli *could* be separated neatly from knowledge about attitudes, feelings, and values; that *people* could not also be pathogens (as in K.'s case). The prevalence of these myths in our time is a tribute to the staying power of the Mechanistic Paradigm. Its rigidities, which passed unnoticed through the era of triumphant microbe hunting and superspecialization, now prevent medicine from adapting to the needs of a more complex environment.

Suppose the Probabilistic Paradigm were widely adopted by people who provide medical care and take part in medical decisions. If doctors, patients, and families were to think in terms of probabilities rather than certainty (and observe the other criteria of the Probabilistic Paradigm), would the problems that beset medicine today, such as high cost and doctor-patient conflict, be closer to solution? There are good grounds for believing that they would.

1. Cost.   The passion for certainty keeps costs high. It leads physicians to use whatever technology is available to obtain an elusive diagnosis, and it leads patients (who have become "consumers" under the influence of the profession and the media) to demand such diagnostic overkill. Even when physicians themselves do not see a need to perform all the prescribed procedures, they may do so anyway to protect themselves against malpractice suits in which the courts apply medicine's own standards of certainty. By those standards a doctor must do everything necessary to be as certain as possible before acting.

The Probabilistic Paradigm, on the other hand, holds that certainty is unattainable not only in fact but in principle. Therefore we no longer need to use the ideal of certainty to judge how much uncertainty about a patient's condition is tolerable, how much greater certainty can reasonably be attained, and how much effort and resources should be spent in seeking more information.

Probabilistic thinking encourages people to adopt a broader definition of "cost," not only the monetary cost but other kinds of costs as well. Let's turn from the life-or-death situation of K. to the routine "lab work" that we perform or submit to during almost any office visit. If we think for a minute, we can identify several potential costs of laboratory testing:

— financial costs (whoever pays)
— costs to the patient in pain, feelings of violation, and risks of physical harm (such as radiation, allergic reaction, blood loss, and infection)
— costs of extra paperwork for busy personnel and overburdened facilities
— misdiagnosis and/or emotional stress resulting from laboratory errors
— the diversion of time, skill, and energy from other diagnostic modes (e.g., sensitive personal observation) to the reassuring rituals of impersonal diagnosis
— the risk of alienating both the physician and the patient from the diagnosis, which is no longer a product fashioned jointly by the physician and patient in the process of history-taking and physical examination, but a product stamped out by a machine which has access to a part of the patient hidden from both patient and physician

Of course, we can't think about all these things every time we take a throat culture; nor should we. We would never get anything done if we didn't form habits and routines. But while habits are necessary, it is also necessary that they be grounded in principle and on occasion critically reevaluated. Doctors and patients alike need to have an underlying consciousness of the costs and benefits as well as the principles at stake. They need to develop an instinct for asking, "What's it worth, and to whom? And am I fooling myself?" before reaching for the throat swabs. Looked at in this way, some of the lab work that is now routinely performed will turn out to be justified; some of it will not. And, in terms of this broader definition of "cost," the same will be true for other things that are done in the name of good health: office visits, hospitalization, medication, surgery, and so forth.

2. Doctor/Patient Conflict. The Mechanistic Paradigm has no notion of principled conflict. Indeed, it has no provisions for handling conflict at all. Diagnosis and treatment are regarded as a smooth, impersonal process—an *experimentum crucis* controlled by the physician and designed to yield objectively valid results. No allowance is made for any desire the patient may have to share control of the process. No allowance is made for values and feelings (either the doctor's or the patient's) and therefore for differences in values or feelings. Any conflict that occurs is outside the bounds established by the paradigm.

One way in which the Probabilistic Paradigm would help doctors and patients deal with conflict more constructively is simply by substituting more realistic, probability-based expectations for the mechanistic expectation of certainty. When people are led to expect a definite answer, a definite cure, they may quite understandably blame each other when things go wrong. The malpractice suit is the patient's way of blaming the doctor; the charge of "noncompliance" is the doctor's way of blaming the patient. Under the Probabilistic Paradigm the fact that things may go wrong, and that it may or may not be anybody's fault, is acknowledged from the start.

Conflict does not go away under the Probabilistic Paradigm. On the contrary, it is built into the paradigm. Since doctor and patient are both scientific observers whose observations are affected by the point of view from which they observe, their feelings and values are recognized as having a legitimate and necessary role in their decision-making. Where they differ, the conflict between them can be seen (though it may not always be) as a reasoned disagreement between people who, in order to be able to work together at all, have made a prior agreement about what actions are rational and ethical in an uncertain world.

There is then a basis for people in the midst of conflict to appeal to each other by rational means, and there is the hope that they will keep an open mind and be influenced by reason. When one learns to see oneself as one sees another and to see another as one sees oneself, one can have a sense of communality with another even amid disagreement. When doctor and patient work together under the Probabilistic Paradigm, each does not have to see the other as a different kind of person, a natural enemy in the jungle of mechanistic relationships. Each can trust (until shown otherwise) that the other is not out to "get" him or her, whether with a surgeon's knife or a legal judgment.

Six Medical Choices

Does the Probabilistic Paradigm's approach to medicine differ from that of the Mechanistic Paradigm in every case? Will the use of the Probabilistic Paradigm completely alter all the normal everyday procedures followed in physicians' offices and hospitals? Yes and no. Again we can look to physics for an analogy. In physics there is a range of problems for which the results obtained by using the probabilistic methods of quantum physics are the same as those obtained by using Newton's laws. In this category are all those high-school physics problems such as, "What is the speed at which a block sliding down a 3-inch plane inclined at 30 degrees, with a given coefficient of friction, will reach the bottom?" Here the effects of the observer, as well as other factors taken into account in quantum theory, are insignificant. They do not enter into the calculations. In these "limiting cases" of the Probabilistic Paradigm in physics, it is just as accurate—and much easier—to stick with the old methods. The physics of Newton is not valid for the problems that Einstein and Heisenberg addressed, but for practical pruposes it is still valid for the problems that Newton addressed.

A similar distinction can be drawn in medicine. Just as it would not pay to apply the principles of quantum mechanics to every homework problem in high-school (Newtonian) physics, so there are classes of medical problems for which the Probabilistic Paradigm itself would dictate, on grounds of principle and cost, what amounts to the mechanistic approach. In these instances people who have had some experience working within the Probabilistic Paradigm have concluded, after keeping an open mind to the possibility of applying probabilistic methods directly, that it isn't worth the trouble to do so, since they would end up doing essentially the same things as they would under the old paradigm.

"Essentially" is, however, an important word. Even when the same decisions are reached under the Probabilistic Paradigm as under the Mechanistic, they are made in a manner and spirit governed by the new paradigm, not the old. They are not dictated by the data, but chosen critically, with a consciousness of the context of uncertainty in which choices are made and a readiness to make different choices when necessary. A physicist today who makes use of Newton's formulas is not about to forget that such formulas have only limited application in the context of modern physics as a whole. Similarly, doctors and patients who have learned to think in terms of the Probabilistic Paradigm and to apply it fully—as a paradigm—cannot just put on blinders and go back to thinking mechanistically. Probabilistic considerations will be implicit in all their decisions, even those that could also have been reached by the mechanistic route.

Here are three pairs of cases that illustrate where the two paradigms lead to similar medical decisions and where they lead to different ones. For each of the three criteria on which the two paradigms differ, there is one case where the decisions reached under the Mechanistic Paradigm are adequate, and another where the Probabilistic Paradigm appears better able to handle the many ramifications of the situation. Of course, while each case primarily illustrates one of the three criteria, it also illustrates the other two, since the three criteria work together.

It will be noted that in the three "mechanistic" cases the doctor alone makes the decisions, while in the three "probabilistic" cases the patient and the patient's family are (or ought to be) involved. In the Probabilistic Paradigm, where values, feelings, and subjective judgment play an important role in decision-making, the doctor, patient, and family are all also "observers" whose points of view influence the outcome. With each patient being seen as an individual rather than a statistical unit, patient and family participation are necessary to give expression to the various causes, some of them unknown to the doctor, that may affect the patient's illness and its treatment. Even in our "mechanistic" cases, where standard medical procedures are clearly required, the Probabilistic Paradigm's focus on the patient's and family's feelings would still be useful in dealing with the special psychological circumstances that surround any "case."

Criterion #1:
Causality

Pneumonia is one of those infectious diseases to which the Mechanistic Paradigm's unicausal deterministic model is usually applicable. Hypertension is one of those noninfectious diseases to which it is usually not applicable.

Case #1.
Pneumonia.

A forty-three-year-old woman enters the hospital emergency room with a two-day history of fever and shaking chills, cough and rusty-colored sputum production, and, most recently, acute shortness of breath. Microscopic examination of a stained smear of the phlegm reveals numerous pus cells and pneumonia-causing germs. A chest X ray shows extensive lung involvement. When bacteria are grown in the laboratory, a diagnosis of pneumococcal pneumonia (pneumonia caused by a particular type of germ, the pneumococcus) is made. The patient is hospitalized and placed initially on intravenous penicillin therapy. With the results of the sputum culture in, this therapy is continued.

The assumptions of the Mechanistic Paradigm help the intern in a busy emergency room function well in the diagnosis and treatment of this case. In particular the intern can act as if pneumococci were the one and only cause determining this patient's illness. This simplifying assumption, though it may lead to ignoring other possible causes (e.g., environmental), is likely to do no harm here (Bursztajn and Hamm, 1979).

Simplifying assumptions of this sort are part of what is meant by *heuristics.* Heuristics are strategies with which people attempt, within the limits of their knowledge and time, to solve problems. Working from the assumption that this woman's illness has only one cause, the intern does not act upon the possibility that she may at the same time have a bronchial neoplasm (cancer of the large airways), which also can cause infection and accumulation of fluid in the lungs. (This possibility is considered only later as part of a differential diagnosis, a long list of possible diagnoses that is often produced in discussion with a senior physician the next day, but which does not affect one's initial choice of action.) Statistically this assumption is justified, but it still represents a judgment. It can be reconsidered if the illness does not respond to treatment in the time it would normally take for pneumonia to show improvement.

Case #2.
Hypertension.

A fifty-five-year-old man comes to his physician's office with a blood pressure of 160/100. History reveals that this is hypertension of over five years' standing. A hypertensive workup, consisting of diagnostic tests which involve taking X rays of the kidney after injection of dye, is undertaken. These tests include an intravenous pyelogram (IVP), in which dye is injected into a small vein in the forearm, and a renal arteriogram, in which dye is injected directly into the artery that supplies the kidneys. The results are negative. Treatment with medications is then initiated. The patient's blood pressure is reduced and becomes well controlled.

It sounds reasonable to test for the physical causes of hypertension, find none, and then begin treatment for "essential hypertension" (the name given to those cases of hypertension that are of undetermined origin)—until you realize that ninety to ninety-five percent of all cases of hypertension, having as yet no detectable cause, fall into the "essential" category. Thus the benefits of testing are questionable, whereas the costs of these tests may be considerable in terms of money, pain, and possible severe side effects. The IVP occasionally touches off an allergic reaction which in rare cases can be life threatening. As for the arteriogram, in one or two out of every thousand cases it causes the artery to thrombose (i.e., to clot at the site).

Why perform the tests, then, except in those special cases where they are clearly called for? To the physician trained in the Mechanistic Paradigm's model of causality, essential hypertension is not a very satisfactory diagnosis. Such a physician works from the heuristic principle: "Find the cause, then treat" (or the surgeon's "You can't cut what you don't see, and a chance to cut is a chance to cure"). Without a known cause there is no clear basis for treatment, and the physician is uneasy with whatever treatment he undertakes. For this physician it is worthwhile to find a definite answer for five or ten percent of the cases at the cost of unnecessary testing for all the others.

Some physicians, however, would not immediately perform an extensive diagnostic workup in this case, but rather would begin treatment with drugs and/or life-style changes (low-salt diet, exercise, stress reduction, etc.). If this regimen were to bring the patient's blood pressure under control, they would proceed no further with the diagnostic workup. Physicians using such a strategy would consider this a problem well solved, even though no "cause," in the Mechanistic Paradigm's deterministic sense, had been revealed. They would feel no particular anxiety in having to deal with a "mysterious" disease like essential hypertension.

By the standards of the Mechanistic Paradigm this strategy is "unscientific." A doctor who takes such an approach is considered—and may consider himself—an empiricist, or one who does "what works" rather than what science dictates. But according to the Probabilistic Paradigm this approach *is* scientific. Where illness is seen as having a range of possible but uncertain causes, it may be reasonable to deviate from the rigid two-step model of diagnosing a cause and then treating it. Therapeutic action may be scientifically based upon the estimated probabilities and values of possible outcomes. As a strategy of investigation it is reasonable to use the patient's response to clinical therapy as evidence for refining one's knowledge and thus one's actions. This was what Dr. S. did when he used K.'s response to being fed and nurtured as a kind of diagnostic test.

The difference between dealing with K. and a patient with hypertension is that the latter can work out the methods of diagnosis and treatment with the doctor before these are begun. Once the diagnostic imperative of the Mechanistic Paradigm is challenged, once it is recognized that there may be more than one right thing to do, once values and principles as well as probabilities are taken into account, then it is no longer only the doctor who can make the necessary choices. The patient's values and principles are every bit as important as the doctor's, especially when you consider who is on the receiving end of the tests and treatments.

Suppose, for example, that the patient thinks it worth the costs of testing to go for the five or ten percent chance of a more specific diagnosis. There are a number of reasonable grounds for such a preference. For one thing, some people value certainty more than others do. Besides, it isn't only the tests for hypertension that have costs, but the treatments as well. With drug treatment these may include money, inconvenience, a daily or even thrice-daily reminder that one is a medical patient (perhaps with a social stigma attached), and side effects. The most common side effect is drowsiness—a high cost indeed for an active person who may have experienced no symptoms and no apparent disability from the disease itself. To avoid these costs, the patient may accept the costs of the workup, which offers at least a slim hope of a surgical cure. Or the patient may choose to try life-style modification alone in an effort to control his blood pressure without drugs. If this is unsuccessful, he may decide that he would rather risk the long-term consequences of hypertension (which include an increased probability of heart or kidney failure, heart attack, and stroke, and therefore a shorter predicted life span) than put up with the medications.

Of course, the doctor will have something to say about these choices, and so will the patient's family. Since both the illness and its treatment are so closely tied in with the patient's daily life, the family needs to be fully informed about the choices and to participate by expressing preferences. For example, if the "diagnostic treatment" involves diet, family members will be buying, preparing, and perhaps eating somewhat different foods. If it involves experimenting with drug dosages, they may for a time have to put up with a "doped-up" breadwinner and assume some of the responsibilities that are normally his. If they are unprepared for these adjustments or unwilling to make them, they may exert pressure on the patient to give up the treatment and become what physicians under the Mechanistic Paradigm call "noncompliant." On the other hand, it is often the family that can persuade the hypertension patient to value his long-term responsibility to stay alive and healthy over the day-to-day inconvenience of taking medication.

Such treatment decisions and the manner in which they are made are part of the diagnosis and thus themselves become causes of the patient's condition. For example, by participating in the decision-making, the patient may become more relaxed and therefore may show a lower blood pressure reading. This, too, is part of the treatment to which the patient is observed to respond. Of course, in talking about diagnosis as a form of treatment and treatment as a form of diagnosis, we are moving from the question of causality to that of the nature of experimentation, which is the second of our three criteria of science.

Criterion #2:
Experimental Method

Here the issue is between the controlled, value-free *experimentum crucis* of the Mechanistic Paradigm and the more flexible, ongoing information-gathering techniques of the Probabilistic Paradigm, which presuppose that the information gained is observer-dependent.

Case #3.
Broken Leg.

A five-year-old boy is brought into the emergency room after a fall. The child's ankle is swollen, tender, and painful. Suspecting that it is broken, the doctor has it X-rayed. Discovering a fracture, he sets it and then puts on a cast.

In this case, the physician appropriately takes actions consistent with the Mechanistic Paradigm. He suspects a single determining cause of the patient's distress, one that can be located in the body: a broken bone. He verifies this with an X ray, which is the crucial experiment: the child is controlled by being immobilized; the doctor takes himself and his subjective hypotheses out of the room. The X ray reveals whether the bone is broken, and the appropriate action (which has been determined through previous experimentation) follows.

Here there seems to be no question of the patient's condition changing when the doctor looks at it. Of course, as the risks of radiation exposure have become better known, it has become clear that repeated X rays can themselves be a cause of future illness. In addition to such long-term effects there are immediate contextual factors that may deserve consideration. For example, a child who has been seen repeatedly for "falls" that result in broken bones, each broken bone having been treated properly but without regard to the context in which it occurred, may one day come in dead, a victim of child abuse. A doctor who suspects child abuse will have to make some sensitive subjective judgments about how far to pursue that hypothesis.

Case #4.
Juvenile Onset of Diabetes Mellitus.

A two-year-old son of a diabetic mother is admitted with coma, labored breathing, and dehydration, all signs of a system thrown out of balance by diabetes. Within a day careful management brings an end to the crisis. It is then decided to bring the patient's blood sugar level under tight control prior to discharge. To this end, morning, afternoon, and evening blood sugars are obtained daily by repeatedly drawing blood from the veins (when they can be found). Over the next two weeks tight control remains elusive in spite of increasing insulin dosages, with the patient continuing to show evidence of sugar and a small amount of ketones (a breakdown product of fat) in the urine. The patient's blood remains free of ketones and is not overly acidic throughout. The patient has become emotionally frazzled while in the hospital, with the three-a-day multiple venipunctures becoming regular battles between staff and patient. Finally the mother takes matters into her own hands and takes her son out of the hospital. His physicians then give up their original goal of tight control of his blood sugar levels. Instead they put him on an insulin regimen which keeps him from having either too low or too high a blood sugar. As the patient is carefully followed at home with minimal invasive testing, his insulin requirements decrease.

In this case the mechanistic approach was tried, only to be abandoned in favor of the probabilistic. Working from the hypothesis that the child's high blood sugar had one determining cause—not enough insulin—the physicians arranged an *experimentum crucis* to test this causal relationship by keeping the child in the controlled environment of the hospital. While every other factor that might affect the blood sugar (such as diet) was held constant, the insulin dose was systematically varied and its effect on the blood sugar level recorded. This is the ideal experimental method under the Mechanistic Paradigm.

Only it did not work. It did not take into account other causative factors—the hospital environment, separation from the mother, etc.—that also may have affected the child's blood sugar. By regarding these factors as constant, the doctors were unable to observe their effects either singly or in combination with one another. In the artificial experimental environment of the hospital the child felt uncomfortable. The factors which in his home made for his comfort and thus could have aided his recovery were controlled out of existence.

For this patient a satisfactory blood sugar level depended on both environment and insulin. As nearly as we can tell, it was lack of sufficient insulin that put him in the hospital, and lack of a proper environment that kept his blood sugar from stabilizing once he was there. In this case it was the patient's mother who decided to gamble. Her "experiment" consisted of taking the child out of the hospital and seeing how he did at home. This empirical treatment, which was not geared toward isolating any one variable, revealed more than did the attempt at an *experimentum crucis* in the hospital setting, which turned out to obscure important causal relationships.

Recognition that the hospital environment in this case was both a causal factor itself and a restriction on other causal factors calls into question another assumption of the *experimentum crucis*—that the act of observation has no effect on what is observed. Drawing blood from the child three times a day made him angry and anxious, which led to a release of adrenaline, which in turn increased the amount of sugar found in the blood that was drawn. The fact that the child fought desperately each time his blood was to be drawn finally led his mother and then the physicians to realize that the experimental conditions were making it impossible to find out what they were designed to find out. It took so long to reach this common-sense observation because the Mechanistic Paradigm, with its insistence on the separation of the observer from the observed, predisposes physicians to ignore the doctor-patient interaction as a possible source of scientifically valid diagnostic information.

The probabilistic approach eventually followed in this case took into account the various causal factors that might be present, including those growing out of the interaction of the observer with the observed. It also asked another sort of question. If this child felt and acted differently in the hospital than at home—i.e., was under increased stress, which in turn affected his blood sugar—what was the use of learning how his blood sugar responded to insulin in the stressful hospital when he was not going to continue to live there? Such knowledge might be of interest to researchers, but it would not do much good for this patient.

The question of what knowledge is worth obtaining cannot be answered without raising a question of value. Under the Mechanistic Paradigm questions of value in treatment are given consideration in the sense that in treating a patient the physician acts for the good. But it is assumed that scientific investigation (including medical diagnosis) is a value-free process of finding out "what is." Under the Probabilistic Paradigm the question of values forms a part of any inquiry. For one thing, the experimenter's values influence his or her choice of which of many possible causes are important enough to look for, and in what way. A doctor who pays attention to the patient's and family's points of view will see a different set of causes than a doctor who does not do so. Moreover it is not only the doctor but the patient and family as well who are observers, and so their values, too, will affect what is observed.

Under the Probabilistic Paradigm diagnosis is approached in the same way as treatment—with a consciousness of the values involved. The probable value of the information to be gained is weighed against the probable costs of obtaining it. In the case of the diabetic boy, practitioners working under the Probabilistic Paradigm could place a high value on such information as (1) the effect of the doctor-patient interaction on the hospital test results, and (2) whether the dose of insulin necessary in the stressful hospital environment might not result in a dangerously low blood sugar when the child is in his normal home environment. As things stand, although these considerations are often noted, children are still placed in the hospital to "determine" their insulin requirements. Under the Mechanistic Paradigm, which has no systematic way of dealing with values in scientific investigation (and in fact explicitly disregards them), the wrong questions are often asked.

Criterion #3:
The Subjective and the Objective

The question of values leads directly into our third scientific criterion—the legitimacy or illegitimacy of subjective knowledge in scientific investigation.

Case #5.
The Comatose Patient.

A thirty-year-old man is brought in, semicomatose, following a fall from a twenty-five-foot scaffolding. Although his blood pressure, pulse, and respiration are initially stable, his neurological status (as measured by level of consciousness, nerve function, reflexes, etc.) progressively deteriorates, with the pupil of the right eye becoming dilated. A neurosurgical procedure is initiated to relieve the pressure from the accumulation of blood between the surface of the brain and the skull.

The physician handled this case according to the diagnosis-treatment model of the Mechanistic Paradigm. Once one knows what *is,* one knows (or figures out) what one *ought to do.* The doctor determined what was wrong with the patient, using his observations of the patient's body as objective data. The diagnosis in some sense dictated the treatment.

Neither value judgments nor subjective information played a major part in this case. Objectivity was made possible by the complete separation of the observer from the observed. The patient alone was the object of scientific observation; the physician alone observed. Since the patient was not fully conscious and his family was not available, he did not participate as observer or decision-maker and did not express subjective knowledge, feelings, or values.

It should be noted that to find a case where subjective information did not play an essential role, we had to choose one where the patient was semiconscious and critically ill, and where the available choices were limited by the need to act quickly. In such a situation one must to some extent depend on habits dictated by custom. The doctor did have to make the subjective judgment that the patient fell into the category of "acute subdural hematoma" even though he did not have all the "classical" findings (which few patients ever show). Even when the doctor acted from habit in this seemingly mechanistic "limiting case" of the Probabilistic Paradigm in medicine, the doctor was making critical choices.

Case #6.
Cancer of the Large Intestine.

An eighty-five-year-old man with widespread cancer of the colon has previously indicated that he does not wish to have any heroic measures taken which would prolong his life. In the five-year course of his disease he has become progressively more confused. Now his bowel becomes obstructed, and he is rushed from the nursing home to the hospital. The surgeon who is called down to the emergency room exchanges greetings with the patient, performs a physical examination, and proceeds quickly to perform a colostomy. The operation involves having the intestine empty directly through a hole made in the skin, thus circumventing the obstructed area.

Clearly this case demanded careful attention from the physician. The patient may have had a number of good reasons not to want this operation. At worst the operation might have left him less comfortable and more dependent on medical aid (e.g., by having to empty his feces into a bag). Anesthesia disrupts an old person's life by leaving him confused, and some people believe that it also hastens the destruction of brain cells, pushing the person toward senility and—again—leaving him more helpless than before. Whatever the costs of the surgery, if it didn't stand a reasonable chance of making the patient *more* comfortable and better able to take care of himself, he may well have felt that at this point there would be little benefit in prolonging his life by such extreme measures. Given the patient's wishes and his condition, it is not at all clear that he should have been operated on.

Many people would find this decision worthy of serious ethical consideration.The lack of such consideration by the surgeon in this case may be considered an expression of the Mechanistic Paradigm. It is grounded in the assumption that, given a particular cause of distress, a particular procedure will cause its relief. The standard procedure for relieving a colon obstructed due to cancer is a colostomy. This surgeon did not think it necessary to consider other aspects of the particular case.

What he failed to consider were the patient's values, the patient's knowledge (in this case, the patient's prediction concerning whether he would survive the operation and what change it was likely to make in his condition), the doctor's feelings (which are important both as a barometer and a stimulus to the patient's feelings), and that part of the doctor's clinical judgment of probabilities that is not derived from objective fact and statistics. These are forms of subjective knowledge deemed irrelevant under the Mechanistic Paradigm. The surgeon deprived himself of all of these sources of potentially useful knowledge, which for him did not exist on the same plane as "objective" knowledge about the relief of colonic obstruction by surgery.

Within the Probabilistic Paradigm subjective and objective knowledge do exist on the same plane and are used in conjunction with each other. In keeping with the Probabilistic Paradigm, the surgeon could have used his own subjective knowledge and personal experience, along with the patient's, to estimate the probability that the patient would survive surgery and that the operation would effectively decompress the colon without debilitating side effects. The patient at some prior time could have been encouraged to estimate the value (for him) of continuing to live with cancer, as well as the costs of going through another operation. When the emergency arose, the doctor could then have gambled for the patient in keeping with a shared understanding of what his own and the patient's values were. Where these differed, he would tend to give the patient's values the benefit of the doubt, assuming them to be reasonable and consistent with general principles unless there was good reason to believe otherwise. Such deliberation might or might not have changed the surgeon's decision to operate. But whatever the decision, it would have been the patient's as well as the physician's, and would have taken into account a much wider range of considerations than did the decision that was in fact made.

Applying the New Paradigm to Medicine

Physicists look at such things as subatomic particles and heavenly bodies; physicians look at biochemical processes inside the human body and at the way human beings live. Is it reasonable to say that physicists and physicians can look at these very different things in much the same way? Although a physician does not do what a physicist does, a physician can appeal to the same standards of rationality that a physicist does. Physicist and physician both study relationships that when looked at superficially appear reassuringly certain, that when looked at somewhat more deeply become hopelessly uncertain, and that finally yield to understanding by means of probabilities. Neither can claim to find universal deterministic laws to explain the causation of a particular event. Both must recognize that they influence what they observe, whether the position and motion of a tiny particle or the well-being of a patient under examination. Indeed, the application of the Heisenberg Uncertainty Principle should be more intuitively obvious in the latter case than the former. (Obvious, that is, were it not for the pervasive influence of the Mechanistic Paradigm.) Of course people change when they interact with others. Of course the way people feel affects whether they are sick or well.

The recognition of these simple and yet complex truths would make medical science and medical practice very different from what they have been for the past hundred years. It would bring what are called the "art" and "ethics" of medicine into the realm of the science of medicine. There has always been a place in medicine for clinical judgment that is based on personal experience and intuition and that takes into account intangible factors such as the physician's knowledge of a particular patient or family. Traditionally this kind of skill has been thought of as "the art of medicine." Under the Probabilistic Paradigm, where it is known as subjective probability assessment, it is taken as seriously and utilized as fully as any other scientific tool. Similarly, although individual doctors may do their best to practice ethically, medical ethics will continue to have only a limited effect on practice as long as doctors are trained and rewarded for practicing a science that does not include ethics. It is as a science that medicine is respected and listened to, and it is within a scientific framework (that of the Probabilistic Paradigm) that the art and ethics of medicine can be practiced with impact.

If anything will bring about the participation of patients and families in medical decision-making, not as a charitable gesture or a response to political pressure but as an unquestioned part of scientific medical procedure, it will be the adoption of the Probabilistic Paradigm. Those who campaign for doctor-patient equality will note that in the Probabilistic Paradigm the patient and the patient's family have equal status with the doctor as scientific "observers" whose observations contribute to the outcome, even though they do not observe in the same way as the doctor. Three of the studies in this chapter show the disadvantages of leaving out patient and family participation, which would have fit naturally and inevitably into the probabilistic procedure.

Case studies later in this book show the advantages of practicing by the Probabilistic Paradigm for all concerned. Patients and their families gain the opportunity and the responsibility to participate in decision-making and influence decisions in accordance with their values. Doctors gain the benefit of the patient's and family's knowledge and the support that comes from sharing the diagnostic and therapeutic dilemmas which previously they have borne alone. More flexible decision-making strategies, together with the consideration of a wider range of possible causes, lead to better decisions and better health care, and the mutuality of the process increases trust between doctor and patient. Costs are reduced in some areas (e.g., by cutting down on unnecessary testing), increased in others (e.g., by having doctors spend more time working with patients and their families). However, even the costs of using the new paradigm—particularly the cost in time and effort—may not be as great as they now appear. Once the use of the paradigm becomes a matter of habit, doctors and patients can carry out the requirements of probabilistic thinking naturally and smoothly as they go about their work, just as they now do in the case of mechanistic thinking.

The problem is that the use of the Probabilistic Paradigm has not yet become a habit. It is the Mechanistic Paradigm that conditions our habits, in medicine and elsewhere. It is easy to feel superior to the physicians who took so long diagnosing K.'s illness that they had no time left to treat him. In retrospect our criticisms of them seem only commonsensical. But at the time it seemed only commonsensical to do what they did; anyone might have done the same. By almost unanimous consensus of the personnel involved, what they did was what a conscientious doctor "should" do; it was the essence of good sense in medicine. It is, in fact, how doctors are trained to do their work. And not only doctors. Almost all our experience in life directs us toward seeking certainty.

Some physicists believe that learning Newtonian physics is a handicap to learning relativistic and quantum physics. The same effect can be seen wherever the two paradigms are applied. To use the Mechanistic Paradigm even where it seems to work satisfactorily (as in the first of each of the three pairs of cases in this chapter) is to gain a short-term benefit at a long-term cost—the "retooling cost" spoken of in the previous chapter. Our minds get used to thinking in terms of whatever tools we use. When we use a crude tool such as the Mechanistic Paradigm, we become less able to take up a more subtle instrument such as the Probabilistic Paradigm when we really need it. Using an outmoded way of thinking even "for convenience" is not without its side effects. The overworked intern in the emergency room may find the Mechanistic Paradigm useful in many instances, but the doctor who is thus trained may find it hard not to treat the whole world as an emergency room.

What is true for doctors in the emergency room is true for all of us throughout our everyday lives. If the Probabilistic Paradigm is such an effective tool for medical decision-making, why don't we use it? As the next chapter will show, we don't use it because the way we live—at home and at work—reinforces the habits of mechanistic thinking, feeling, and acting.

4

UNCERTAINTY
IN EVERYDAY LIFE

Dr. S. understood the way his patients thought from the way he himself thought when he wasn't being a scientist. "Damn table!" he would blurt out when he stubbed his toe against a table leg. It was the table's fault. Then as he hopped around in pain, he would shake his head and think, "Boy, am I a klutz!" It was his fault. It was hard for him to think about more than one cause at a time when his foot throbbed with pain. As a doctor S. saw himself as a scientist who practiced consciously by the Probabilistic Paradigm. But when he wasn't giving special attention to the way in which he was thinking, he would fall back into thinking *un*consciously, as others did, in terms of the Mechanistic Paradigm.

In dealing with his patients and colleagues and in critically examining his own practice, S. realized that thinking takes place in contexts—contexts of feeling, contexts of prior experience and learning. People learn to make decisions long before they come to a doctor's office. They learn it at home and in school, at work and in the supermarket. There they learn to make decisions that "feel right" to them. Whether those decisions are right or are being made in a reasonable way is another matter.

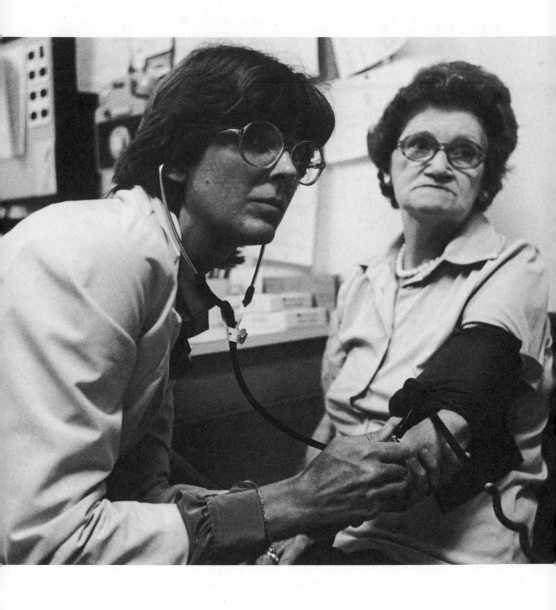

Science serves as a standard of rationality for society. When people seek to do what is right in their daily lives, they look to science for guidance. This has been true, at any rate, since science assumed a dominant place in Western society in the era of the Mechanistic Paradigm. The Social Darwinism of the late nineteenth century illustrates the ease with which science (in this case the illegitimate extension of the biological theory of evolution as "the survival of the fittest" to social and economic survival) replaced the fading "Protestant ethic" as a justification for competitive business practices. The era of Social Darwinism was also the era of Claude Bernard in medicine, the period when the influence of the Mechanistic Paradigm began to reach out beyond science to business and industry, the consumer marketplace, and the family. The notion of a scientific paradigm, in its narrowest construction, refers to the conditions under which scientists work. As we shall see in this chapter, the Mechanistic Paradigm has come to represent the conditions under which everyone works and the conditions under which everyone lives.

Why does the Mechanistic Paradigm rule everyday decision-making at a time when it has been fundamentally questioned in the sciences? It survives in part because it has helped to create social institutions that in turn help to perpetuate it—for instance, a profit-oriented economy and a weakened family. Clearly, changes in these institutions would have an impact on the way people think, in medicine and elsewhere. But the reverse is also true—that by learning a different way of thinking, people can begin to create new social institutions and new living conditions for themselves.

As realistic as he was about the odds against people learning to think probabilistically, Dr. S. didn't think that people's actions were determined by their socioeconomic or family backgrounds. If he had thought so, he would have been thinking unicausally. People have the capacity and the responsibility to make choices. Indeed, this book is about the way S. and his patients learned to make choices and how other doctors and patients can do the same. But to learn to make choices effectively, one needs to be aware of the conditions, favorable or unfavorable, under which choices are made. To understand how people think, one needs to consider the mind that thinks, the family that transmits one way of thinking or another, and the society that generates and sustains that way of thinking.

When people get sick and go to a doctor, they don't stop thinking the way they normally do. When people are in pain, they seek explanations for what caused the pain. The explanations that are right at hand are those that people learn throughout their lives—i.e., those supplied by the Mechanistic Paradigm. Moreover, even people who are capable of thinking rationally most of the time tend to fall back on rigid habits of thought when in the presence of the pain and fear that accompany illness or injury (like S. when he stubbed his toe). If S. was going to teach people to think probabilistically, he would have to keep in mind the reasons why people are sometimes afraid to be rational even when they have the capacity to be, as well as the reasons why people often are not capable of being rational even when they are not conscious of fear.

Labor Without Love:
The Workplace

At fifty-four Eleanor Perk had a chronic cough which was not responding to treatment. She had had asthma on and off for eight months. It surely wasn't doing her any good to sit in on those smoke-filled meetings every morning at the prestigious law firm where she worked as an executive secretary. Eleanor had developed a special role in her twenty years with the firm. Every morning she was called in to the meeting, where she took notes which she then organized, summarized, and gave out to the people who attended the meetings—several of whom smoked cigars. S. sought to relieve Eleanor's plight by giving her a note telling her employers that she should not be required to work in a smoke-filled room.

A month later, her cough having subsided, she was back with a new complaint. Her employers had responded to S.'s note by telling her, "You don't have to be in on the meetings. There's other work to do in this office." There was—but it was the work of a junior secretary. "Sure, Doc," Eleanor lamented, "I still get the same pay, but when I go home at night it feels as if something is missing. I mean, all I do is type letters. The way they speak to me now, it's as if they don't know me from one of the 'temporaries'; it's as if I haven't been doing this job for twenty years. They specify how to type everything down to the dotting of the *i*'s. And when I'm finished, someone is always looking over my shoulder. I won't get fired, mind you, but I am made to understand that if I don't do things just the way they want me to, consequences will follow."

"Consequences?" asked S. "Is this anything new?"

"Well, in some respects it's always been this way, I guess. The fellows I was working for before, if they didn't like something I did, they'd let me know about it."

"Then how is this different?"

"It's this way. Now that I'm just one of the girls again, I'm expected to produce just so much by the end of the day. If I don't type my share of this or that report, the girl who's waiting to work on it the next day is going to be stuck. That's part of it. There's also a different feeling now. Before it was as if the rules didn't apply to me. Now it's 'company policy this,' 'company policy that.' For instance, I've been told that it's against the firm's policy for me to change one word of what I type. It used to be that I had some responsibility. Oh, I put down what was said at those meetings, but I also put my two cents in when I wrote those reports. I felt as if I was making something of my own, not just recording what somebody else said.

"Maybe it's okay for a lot of the girls there. After all, they're being promised a career. Stick with the firm, and the firm will take care of you. But there's nothing for me in starting over at the bottom at this point in my life. It's no fun doing what I'm doing. Doc, I need something for my nerves, you know, some of that Valium stuff. Look, we tried it your way, and look where it got me. The firm didn't change. They just put me in a different place."

Eleanor Perk's words illustrate the way the management of a modern labor force discourages critical thinking by exerting control over workers. In his book *Contested Terrain* (1979), Richard Edwards lists three forms of control exerted by management: direction (specifying task requirements—or, in Eleanor's words, "They specify how to type everything down to the dotting of the *i*'s"); evaluation (assessing performance and correcting mistakes—". . . someone is always looking over my shoulder"; and discipline (rewarding and punishing to reinforce compliance—". . . I am made to understand that if I don't do things just the way they want me to, consequences will follow").

Edwards goes on to identify three styles of control (listed in order of their historical appearance). In *simple* control the boss or bosses exercise power personally, through direct contact with workers (". . . if they didn't like something I did, they'd let me know about it."). *Technical* control, epitomized by the assembly line, occurs when work is paced by a mechanical or technological process rather than by immediate human command ("If I don't type my share of this or that report, the girl who's waiting to work on it the next day is going to be stuck."). *Bureaucratic* control is exercised through an impersonal rule of law ("Now it's 'company policy this,' 'company policy that' ") and through the firm's power to bestow or withhold long-range rewards ("After all, they're being promised a career. Stick with the company, and the company will take care of you.").

By employing these three styles of control, management places itself at a progressively increasing distance from the labor force. As this distance increases, managerial authority can take the form of deterministic laws, as it did in Eleanor's case ("company policy"), or else can become so arbitrary in interpreting rules that uncertainty reigns ("who knows what they'll come up with next?"). Either way, workers are unable to challenge authority as they did when the boss was right there giving orders and hearing complaints. As in Eleanor Perk's case, they are taught that it is futile to try to think for themselves in order to influence the process of production. Thus one effect of Eleanor's old job on her health was a cough. Her new job had more serious, long-range effects, such as a dulled capacity for thinking (or at least a habit of not thinking) and a sense of losing control of her life. Here Eleanor learned a way of thinking, feeling, and acting—the mechanistic way—which would affect the way she made choices (or left them to chance) concerning her health as well as other aspects of her life.

Links between a way of thought and a type of economic system have been pointed out before, for instance, by Max Weber in his demonstration (1930) that Protestant religious beliefs were conducive to the development of what we call the free-enterprise system. Similarly, it was no mere coincidence that the Mechanistic Paradigm established itself in science in an era characterized by an expanding, increasingly industrialized market economy, for its three criteria admirably serve the needs of such an economy. This is not to say that the profit system can flourish only under the Mechanistic Paradigm, or that only a profit-oriented economy can tolerate a mechanistic science. Rather, it is to observe that mechanistic science had both tangible benefits in the applied science of industrial production and intangible benefits in the molding of industrial society. With its exaltation of the "objective" (the production and accumulation of material resources) over the "subjective" (feelings that were potentially disruptive to a smooth-running order) and its insistence on single causes, the Mechanistic Paradigm was well suited to a society single-mindedly pursuing the goal of rapid economic development.

How is the paradigm inculcated and critical thinking discouraged in the worker? The classic example of modern industrial production is Henry Ford's assembly line. In *Captains of Consciousness* (1976) Stuart Ewen (quoting a 1939 Federal Trade Commission report) characterizes Ford's "line production system" as using "expensive, single-purpose" machinery run by "quickly-trained, single-purpose" workmen to mass-produce a standardized car. In the juxtaposition of expensive machines with inexpensive workers, we see the worker being fitted to the machine rather than vice versa. When the relationship between worker and machine is modeled on that of machine and machine (or machine and product), the operation of the three criteria of the Mechanistic Paradigm is evident.

In the term *single-purpose* we can discern the deterministic causation of Criterion #1. Or in Henry Ford's own words (from *My Life and Work*):

> The net result of the application of these principles is the reduction of the necessity for thought on the part of the worker and the reduction of his movements to a minimum. He does as nearly as possibly only one thing with only one movement (Chandler, 1964, p. 39).

Each worker's contribution is reduced to a single repetitive act designed to produce a single invariable effect. The worker is not expected to influence the process, but simply to do what is asked, to comply. In this way the worker is not seen as a cause, but as one more variable (along with capital, raw materials, and machines) to be manipulated as if in a scientific experiment (Criterion #2).

This last analogy is not ours. While Ford was pioneering the assembly line, factory owners were introduced to "scientific management" by Frederick W. Taylor, who advocated "taking the control of the machine shop out of the hands of the many workmen, and placing it completely in the hands of management, thus superseding 'rule of thumb' by scientific control" (Hofstede, 1978, p. 453). Taylor divided the workers in a factory into isolated experimental groups. He observed them, timed them, and manipulated their working conditions to determine how they could be motivated to work most efficiently. Years later, ironically enough, the discovery of the "Hawthorne effect" (discussed in Chapter 2) demonstrated that Taylor's application of the *experimentum crucis* to the workplace had been fatally compromised by experimenter effects that could have been anticipated under the Probabilistic Paradigm.

Workers who ran the new machinery were trained and controlled in the same manner as the machinery itself—by the cookbook rules that then constituted "science." No mutual influence between worker and management was allowed for. Moreover, what the scientifically managed worker thought or felt was of no interest to management except insofar as it affected production. The worker was being paid to act in an "objective" manner, not to question the values and goals of production. If a worker was bored, alienated, tired, or ill, performance would be reduced. These subjective states, therefore, like the worker himself, became objects of concern to management, to be dealt with through the evolving science of industrial psychology.

In the myth of "disinterested" observers, devoid of feelings, scientifically manipulating workers "uninterested" in their jobs, brimming with distracting feelings, we have the objective-subjective dichotomy that is Criterion #3 of the Mechanistic Paradigm. By that criterion the objective and subjective aspects of knowledge can be neatly differentiated, "and never the twain shall meet." Scientists and their methods are considered to be objective. Furthermore objective data traditionally were thought to be the only suitable objects of scientific study. By the twentieth century, however, it became possible (or so it was thought) to study subjective, irrational feelings by objective, rational methods. Sociologist Richard Sennett, in *The Fall of Public Man* (1978), traces the historical development by which emotions became "facts" that could be detached from the contexts of living in which they occurred and placed under the microscope of mechanistic science. In such science objectivity is seen as a strength, a resource for gaining knowledge and control, while subjectivity is seen as a weakness by which people can be manipulated. This point of view was enthusiastically taken over by managers who saw themselves in the objective, scientific, controlling role vis-à-vis their workers.

Of course, Ford's assembly line and Taylor's "scientific management" represent the industrial practices of 1910 or 1920 rather than those of today. Taylor's crude manipulations in the name of science have given way to "human relations" management, which is thought to be *more* scientific in that it embodies a subtler understanding of psychology. Today's managers are prepared to take into account a range of subjective factors in job satisfaction (which they still consider irrational) and to allow for considerable interchange between workers and management in establishing company procedures. Still, there is reason to question how much things have really changed. The methods may be flexible, but the goals of production and profit remain fixed and are not open to question. Although workers are encouraged to ask, "How can this be done?" the question, "Is this worth doing?" is not considered a legitimate one. The control exerted over the work force may be subtler than in the past, but it is control nonetheless, and by its very subtlety less accessible to modification. The "enlightened" workplace can still be seen as being run on mechanistic lines, in that workers are denied the opportunity to think and make critical choices about what they produce, as well as the subjective satisfaction that comes from doing so.

It isn't only the factory or clerical worker who is subject to this system of control and its unquestioned goals. Another of S.'s patients, Jerry Matthias, found that being promoted from a stressful assembly-line job didn't do him any more good than being demoted did for Eleanor Perk. Jerry had begun to develop high blood pressure at a time when he was having trouble keeping up with the pace of the assembly line. He wasn't lazy or negligent; on the contrary, his insistence on taking proper care with each piece caused him to linger over it until the next piece was upon him. A competent and intelligent worker, Jerry thought he could put the stress of his job behind him when he moved up to a junior management position. As a manager Jerry was now responsible for making this area a "profit center" for the company. Instead of having to keep up with the pace of the line, he had to set the pace for others according to standards set by higher management.

The new job was no easier on his blood pressure. "I used to think it was the guys on the line who were under pressure," he told S., "but I feel like I'm still on a treadmill. You want to know who's under the most strain? Not the guy who's actually putting the machines together. It's the guy you see standing around with a cup of coffee. Take a good look at that guy. He may not have to be at a particular place at a particular time, and he may not have to produce x number of widgets per minute, but he does have to produce x number of dollars per month. Only he doesn't always know exactly how to do it, and nobody can tell him. That's what he's standing around trying to figure out, and that's where the stress comes in."

Food Without Nourishment:
The Marketplace

S. was looking out the window as his last patient of the day, Jerry Matthias, drove up for his blood pressure check. The car Jerry was driving was a model that had recently made the news as having been recalled to remedy a potentially life-threatening defect in the fuel storage system. S. wondered whether Jerry had taken his car in yet. So when Jerry came into the office S. remarked, "Bet you're not the only one who's been in for an exam lately."

Jerry looked at him.

"You've probably had your car in for a checkup too."

"Oh, that recall. Yeah, I got a notice in the mail about it a few weeks ago. Haven't gotten around to it yet. Don't know if I will."

S. looked—and was—astonished. "What do you mean? From what I read in the paper, that gas tank business is a pretty serious thing. Aren't you concerned? What about your family?"

Jerry was getting angry. "And suppose I miss half a day's work to get the car fixed? That's half a day's pay gone, down the drain. What about my family then? They have to eat, you know."

S. thought that the exchange he was having with Jerry was likely to affect the blood pressure reading he was about to take, but he persisted. "What about doing it when you get home?" S. inquired. As a doctor he was genuinely curious about why someone wouldn't do a "simple little thing" that might beneficially affect his health or safety.

"Yeah, I guess I could do it then," Jerry answered slowly. "But by then I'm too damn tired. When I'm tired, the odds don't feel the same. Look, Doc, you're the one who always talks about costs and benefits. When you weigh the probability that my gas tank is going to blow up against the sure loss of half a day's pay, which would *you* choose?"

"I guess it depends on how much money you have to begin with. If you have enough money, the value of half a day's pay goes down some."

"Besides," Jerry said, "I don't know how seriously to take this recall stuff anyway. Sometimes I think it's just a lot of government red tape. That's a good little car I've got out there. Like they say on TV: 'Build your own car to your every desire.'"

S. had seen the ad. He had seen lots of them. "You" as a consumer could "build your own car" by taking your pick from among the selection of options offered by the company to create the illusion of choice, the illusion that you were producing instead of consuming. Speaking of options, one option Jerry couldn't choose was the option of not driving. "Don't get me wrong," said S. "I know all about the hassles of owning a car when you're too busy working to maintain it properly. Sometimes I wonder if it's all worth it—were it not that I absolutely need it." S. suddenly wondered whether "absolutely" was quite accurate. "How about you, Jerry? Could you do without your car? Would you consider taking a bus to work?"

"A bus? You think I'm crazy? Listen, Doc, I'm so goddam dog-tired when I get out of work that I don't want to get on any bus. I want to get into *my* car and stretch out and hit the road. That car is the only thing I've got that's really mine."

"With all these recalls, though, you've got to admit they don't make them like they used to."

"I know that, but I need a car that looks new. People see me in the parking lot. I'm in management now, and everything about me has to look good, including my car. You know how it is these days, Doc. It's not what you are; it's what you wear."

Whatever this conversation did for (or to) Jerry's blood pressure, it set S. to thinking. Jerry's "noncompliant" response to the auto recall notice told S. something about all the patients who (much to his exasperation) didn't bother with their physical exams and other preventive health-care measures. They were probably just as tired as Jerry. They, too, must be concerned about the half-day's pay they would lose by coming to the doctor. And what better way to rationalize these real concerns than by an appeal to the odds? "It won't happen to me." "My car won't be the one to blow up." "I won't be the one to get breast cancer, so why bother with the monthly self-exam?" Why bother to take care of yourself, or your car, when you didn't have to? It was hard enough to take the time when you were really sick or when the car wouldn't run.

In medical school S. had been taught to expect two things from patients. They would come, and they would pay. But he was beginning to realize that, for many of his patients, coming and paying were not simple things. Paying was not simple because they had other things to spend their money on. Coming was not simple because they had other things to do with their time, such as earning a living. Most of his patients needed to earn a living, especially when "really living" meant having to buy the kinds of things they spent their working hours making.

Jerry's plight illustrated the production-consumption cycle in which so many people were trapped. Jerry had to have a new car so that he could keep up appearances on the job—and keep the job. Once he had the car, he needed the job all the more so that he could pay for the car. People have been willing to "buy" a lot more than cars in order to keep their jobs. On January 5, 1979, *The New York Times* reported that five women employees of a West Virginia chemical plant had had themselves sterilized after a company official told them that they might lose their jobs because of the danger of exposing unborn children to lead poisoning. "He even said he felt sure our health insurance would cover the operation," said one of the women. "We did it because we were afraid," said another. For the sake of their jobs these women "consumed" a medical procedure approved by their insurance companies. If Eleanor Perk had known what was in store for her when she gave up a job that put her health at risk, she might have gone on consuming cigar smoke against medical advice.

In order for goods to be produced at a profit they must be consumed. In an economy of scarcity people are valued for what they produce. In today's economy of artificial abundance, as described in Stuart Ewen's *Captains of Consciousness,* people are valued for what they consume. From the point of view of the corporate producers people should see themselves as having needs that can be met by commercial products. That is, they should see themselves as consumers. Richard Sennett's account of the rise of the department store in the latter half of the nineteenth century shows how people who previously expressed their social identity by haggling with merchants were induced to gain satisfaction from the passive, impersonal "act" of buying standardized, fixed-price merchandise. By various stimulating presentations mass-market retailers persuaded people to think of products for which they had no practical use as representations of their own personal experience and character. That was the beginning of the consumer society.

In motivating people to consume, the economic system organizes consumption, as it does production, according to the three criteria of the Mechanistic Paradigm. Criterion #1, deterministic causation, is reflected in all the advertising that promotes this or that product as a source of certainty. The Mechanistic Paradigm creates the need for (and expectation of) certainty; manufacturers and advertisers purport to answer that need by packaging certainty in brand names: "You can be sure if it's Westinghouse." How easy it was, in K.'s case, for hospital personnel to turn that habitual way of thinking into "You can be sure if you take a blood culture (or do a spinal tap, or whatever)." In the simplistic, mechanistic world of advertising a single cause has a single effect; one stimulus elicits one response. If you have a headache, take Anacin. If you have underarm odor, use Ban. If your life could use a "shot" of power and glamour, get a Mustang. It is hardly a model for learning to think probabilistically.

Advertising does not mention uncertainty or multiple causation. It is not in the interest of General Motors or Ford to encourage consumers to question whether one needs a powerful, flashy car rather than some alternative means of transportation. It is their business to make and sell cars, and the choices among cars that they offer a consumer like Jerry Matthias correspond to the limited choices among tasks and working conditions that the more enlightened factory managers offer their workers. Nor is it in the interest of the drug companies to portray headaches as a multicausal problem so that people might see themselves, their family lives, and their jobs as being among the causes of their headaches. Instead, a magic pill or other product is sold as a "technical fix" for medical, personal, or social problems.

Criterion #2, the *experimentum crucis,* is invoked throughout the system of consumption. First, there are the crisp "scientific" findings that advertisers cite in support of their claim of superiority for their product: "Studies show that Aspirin Plus is better than aspirin." "With Fluropaste you get twenty-seven percent fewer cavities than with Brand X." Second, it is with the detachment of the mechanistic scientist that advertisers manipulate the market by influencing people, creating "new markets," and then "responding" to the needs they have helped to create. To the advertiser the consumer is an object to be experimented upon, and thus the advertiser's relationship to the consumer is the same as the "scientific" manager's relationship to the worker. Finally, advertising instructs the consumer to do his or her own *experimentum crucis* by buying the product and observing its effects. "Try it; you'll like it" is the message, with its neat juxtaposition of experimental manipulation and determined outcome. "Try our product," the advertisement is saying, "and it will have a planned, predictable, demonstrable effect on your life." The message aims to limit the consumer, like the worker, to a series of repetitive, single-purpose acts (in this case buying and using products). It ignores the fact that the effect of using a product depends on how and when one uses it; it is context-dependent. While the product may make one feel good, it may also damage one's health, put one deeper into debt, or give one a false sense of security.

A person who understands both the headache and the headache pill in context (the context of a person's life in society) can see himself or herself as a cause and as acted upon by other causes. This complex awareness, however, will have to come from a source other than consumer advertising, which usually portrays causation in all-or-none terms as being "out there" in the objective world ("take this pill, and your headache will vanish") or within the person in the subjective world ("build your own car to your every desire"). Advertising plays on these extreme emotional reactions by giving people a fantasy of omnipotence in response to a world where what happens to them is too often beyond their control.

According to Sennett, "The celebration of objectivity and hardheaded commitment to fact so prominent a century ago, all in the name of Science, was in reality an unwitting preparation for the present era of radical subjectivity" (1978, p. 22). As psychoanalyst Joel Kovel (1978) points out, the two extremes complement each other in the interest of the economic system, which requires that people be "objective" enough to do what is required of them at work, but "subjective" enough to want the income they get from working and the consumer goods that their paychecks can buy them. The subjective desires of the consumer not only guarantee a market for industry's products, but also ensure a compliant work force, since people must keep their jobs to be able to gratify their desires.

In other words, people must be objective as producers, subjective as consumers. The Mechanistic Paradigm, with its clearcut separation of the objective and subjective realms (Criterion #3), is the ideal vehicle for maintaining a radical distinction between producer-consumer roles. This radical distinction allows people to be easily controlled in both roles. Indeed, the very word *consumer* puts people in a passive role, so that even when they assert themselves, it is only to seek "consumer power."

When Jerry Matthias decided some months later to approach his employers for a position of greater autonomy, he realized that he would first have to get off this treadmill of worker-consumer dependency. As he told S., "You better sit down. I sold my car last week, the day before I went in to talk to them. I knew that unless I had some money in the bank, I wouldn't have the guts to quit if they turned me down."

S. couldn't believe it. "You're kidding. So what happened?"

"They gave me what I wanted. I could have gambled and kept my car, as it turns out. But who's to know?"

The drastic step Jerry had taken was an attempt to get out of the economic corner in which he had found himself. By facing up to the power of the economic system, he had taken a step toward freeing himself from it. If he wanted to enjoy his work more (i.e., get more subjective gratification out of it), he might have to be a little more objective in restraining his desires as a consumer.

Industry pays close attention to the feelings of consumers, like those of workers, so as to manipulate them. Hunger must be converted into a craving for Cheerios, natural cereals, Mc-

Donald's hamburgers, cookbooks, or diet books. Among the needs that industry capitalizes on (without pausing to consider their origin) are those created by the conditions of life in our society, such as Jerry Matthias's need for a car that would impress his clients and Eleanor Perk's need for a tranquilizer to counteract the frustrations of her job. Advertising also *creates* needs which it then supplies products to satisfy: the need for junk foods, the need for elaborate cosmetics, the need for a slender physique, the need for flashy cars. Those who manufacture and market consumer goods sometimes claim that they are simply responding to needs that are rooted in human nature. People do need food, clothing, and shelter to survive; they need to sleep, eliminate waste, be with other people, and sometimes receive medical attention. It is when the survival not of people but of corporations is at stake that the list of human needs becomes much longer.

Given most people's lack of control and fulfillment in the productive sphere, it is understandable that for many people these consumer needs take the form of an addiction. When people are uncertain of their relationship to the physical and social environment—uncertain about how much (if any) control they have over their destinies—they seek compensatory sensations that *are* certain. If one can't really do anything, if one can't make meaningful choices, one can at least feel good. So Eleanor Perk pops a Valium pill, and Jerry Matthias tears about in his car ("the only thing I've got that's really mine"). But there is no nourishment in this kind of consumption; it is a fleeting satisfaction that does not remove one's basic uncertainties or equip one to make critical choices.

Eleanor Perk asked S. for Valium because she wanted a drug to suppress the critical thinking which she had learned to use in her previous job, but for which there was no place in her new job. The drug would also deaden the pain and anxiety that came with not being able to think critically and be a productive human being. "Look, Doc, can't you just give me the Valium?" she exclaimed. "I'm getting a lot of flak for speaking up to those guys. I can't just shut off. I can't shut off the way I've been working for the past twenty years. Maybe the Valium will calm me down so I can do things their way. Look, I try to shut off, I try to be just a cog in the machine, but then I get panicky. I get panicky when I don't feel alive. Maybe this pill will help me with that feeling, too, huh, Doc?"

What could S. tell her? "You could change jobs," he suggested. "At my age?"

For S., who would have preferred to change the world, there was sadness as he reluctantly gave Eleanor the prescription for Valium. With it he gave her the best explanation he could of why things were the way they were in her life. He suggested that she join Nine to Five, the organization seeking better working conditions for secretarial and clerical workers. With the group's support she just might be able to change things in her own office, and she would in any case gain a sense of purpose in working with people who had similar grievances and similar goals. S. also arranged for Eleanor to come in periodically and speak with him about her job and her habits of consumption, so that he could work with her in preventing her from developing an addiction to Valium. And he didn't doubt that she *would* keep coming back, if only for prescription refills.

Turning the pages of the latest medical journals, S. wondered whether things ever really changed. Nearly a decade before, S. and a group of like-minded physicians had protested the sensationalist advertisements for tranquilizing drugs, such as the one showing a frustrated driver stuck in traffic, that appeared throughout the most prestigious medical journals. These advertisements implied that the way to deal with problems in society was to make people less anxious rather than to seek solutions for the problems. Appealing to the professed standards by which the journals evaluated articles for publication, S. and his colleagues prevailed upon the editors to require more responsible content in the text and illustrations of advertisements. S. was proud of this success; he had helped change the system. But had he? There were still just as many tranquilizer ads, even if they were more subtle. They no longer had such imflammatory pictures, but the names of the drugs were still printed in big, bold letters designed to register in a harried physician's mind. The drug companies still expected doctors to comply with the ads by prescribing their latest products, and doctors still expected patients to comply with the prescriptions. In the marketplace, as in the factory, the message was still the same.

Exchange Without Trust: The Family

The message is the same at home too. A person's capacity to think critically is developed and exercised in the course of being with other people. The workplace and the marketplace are two of the social contexts in which people learn an implicit paradigm of thought, feeling, and action. The doctor-patient relationship is another. But the first and most important of those contexts is the family. The family is where a child learns strategies for dealing with uncertainty, with pain and fear. These strategies can be mechanistic or probabilistic; they can deny uncertainty or make use of probability.

In a world in which both science and industry follow the mechanistic paradigm, it would be surprising if the family did not transmit it as well. Furthermore the operation of the Mechanistic Paradigm has served to weaken the family by isolating its members from one another and reducing their capacity to take effective action together. Thus weakened, the family can still transmit ingrained habits of mechanistic thought, but it cannot (and indeed is not encouraged to) provide the experiences necessary to teach the critical thinking and the trust required under the Probabilistic Paradigm.

A number of social institutions have contributed to bringing the Mechanistic Paradigm into the home and weakening the family as a social unit. The economic system as a whole has colonized the family, made it fair game for profit-seekers, and reduced it to a cluster of individual producers and consumers playing specialized roles (including that of the professionalized homemaker practicing "home economics"). Such a family cannot be a productive community in which family members gain self-respect and strengthen their ties with one another by producing goods together. As Christopher Lasch has noted in *Haven in a Heartless World* (1977), the "helping professions" (medicine, psychology, education) have substituted their own ministrations for traditional family ties and thereby undermined family authority.

Finally, the mass media, particularly television, have taught the family to see itself in mechanistic terms. According to Sennett, over the past two hundred years a society of actors (people creating and playing public roles in relation to one another) has given way to a society of *voyeurs* (strangers passing one another on the street, trying to find out as much as possible about one another while revealing as little as possible about themselves). Television represents the culmination of this historical development. Its version of mechanistic authority (which goes along with the boss, teacher, doctor, and Lasch's emotionally absent parent) is the face on the screen that a child or adult can turn on or off, but not argue with, persuade, or engage in a process of mutual influence. This mechanistic, on-off choice is the only kind of choice possible in the world of passive consumption. Even when family members watch a TV program together and talk about it, they can't change the next episode.

The mechanistic thinking which the family absorbs from science and society centers around the notion of the single determining cause (Criterion #1). This scientific version of the primitive belief in single causes expresses itself in the illusion of total power and the dread of powerlessness. Unconsciously one tends to attribute causality entirely to oneself ("I did it") or to forces outside oneself ("It/they did it to me"). At their extremes these two habits of belief characterize the aspects of personality called *narcissism* and *paranoia* respectively. Although these terms are used in psychiatric diagnosis, where their focus is on abnormal instances, their existence in everyday life illustrates the mechanistic thinking that can manifest itself in anyone. We all have streaks of narcissism and paranoia. Like Dr. S., we all tend to blame ourselves or the table when we stub a toe or bang a knee.

These tendencies within a family are reinforced by the mechanistic vision of experimental manipulation (Criterion #2), where people are left thinking of themselves as either the controlling experimenter (narcissism) or the controlled experimental subject (paranoia). Whichever role is assumed, other family members are seen in the opposite role. Daily existence then becomes a struggle over who is going to be in control. There is no wonder that there is fear of losing, since the stakes are high.

Criterion #3, too (the subjective-objective dichotomy), finds its way into family life. People may identify with their subjective wants and needs and see themselves as alienated, helpless victims at the mercy of powerful objective forces beyond their control. Or they may identify with these objective forces (science, "hard facts," industry, money, disease germs, and technological cures) and thereby distance themselves from their feelings, including their feelings toward family members.

What are the effects of this mechanistic thinking on the family and its members? What follows is an extreme portrait, one that may not apply literally to any particular family, but that applies in greater or lesser degree to all families whose members face the considerable uncertainties of today's world without being able to do so consciously and thus be able to share the risks in a mutually supportive way.

Family relationships governed by the Mechanistic Paradigm resemble the relationships of the workplace and the marketplace. To apply a distinction made by psychologists Margaret Clark and Judson Mills (1979), they tend to be *exchange* rather than *communal* relationships. In an exchange relationship (as represented, for example, by a business contract) people gratify their needs individually in a spirit of pragmatic cooperation. They give one another benefits in order to get comparable benefits in return. Such benefits create reciprocal obligations. They must be paid for, if not in money, then in kind. "What's in it for me?" is the ever-present question. In a communal relationship (for example, the mutuality of a loving relationship) no such obligations are incurred. Benefits are given and received, but not on a quid pro quo basis. It is, in fact, considered inappropriate to "pay off" one benefit with another. Rather, the people involved are understood to care about one another's well-being and to respond to one another's needs as they arise. In a relationship of this sort to satisfy another's needs is also to satisfy one's own.

The love and mutual support that exist in a communal relationship transcend any mathematical distribution of goods. In an exchange relationship, however, people bargain for their share of a supply of goods, or benefits, that is viewed as constant. The concept of exchange fits nicely into the Mechanistic Paradigm, every criterion of which implies a dichotomy. Hypotheses are either true or false (Criterion #1). One is either an experimenter or an experimental object (Criterion #2). Knowledge is either objective or subjective (Criterion #3). Thus mechanistic thinking is "either-or" thinking. Something is either yours or mine, not ours. All that can be done is to divide up the spoils (whether in a civilized or a cutthroat way). Sheila M. Rothman, in an article entitled "Family Life as Zero-Sum Game," speaks of the current tendency of psychologists, feminist leaders, and various organizations to champion the cause of one family member against all the others:

> Since the family is a battleground, every member should have, and now does have, its own Clausewitz . . . Whatever the precise nature of the advice, one assumption is common to all of it: family life is a zero-sum game. Some interests must be sacrificed to others. What is good for wives is not necessarily good for husbands and what is good for mothers is not necessarily good for children. Where our predecessors saw harmony, we see discord. Where they saw mutuality of interest, we see conflict of interest (1978, p. 397).

The Mechanistic Paradigm predisposes people toward exchange rather than communal relationships because, unlike the Probabilistic Paradigm, it does not provide for trust. When nothing between complete certainty and complete uncertainty is acknowledged, there is no use for trust and no way for trust to occur. Without trust people cannot cope with the uncertainty that they do face. And they face a great deal of uncertainty—including uncertainty about the people around them.

In a world where the economic system and its subsidiary institutions tend to split up families into atomized individual units, and where the Mechanistic Paradigm provides a way of thinking by which families split *themselves* up in the same way, family members tend to see one another as competitors. In the mechanistic world view the family's nurturance (the food, love, and care symbolized by the mother's breast) becomes the single cause of one's well-being, an object to be fought over and consumed. The family members do not see themselves as participating in and helping to produce support for one another in health and illness. Instead they see that support as an object to be received, and they fear the loss of what they depend on as an infant fears the loss of the breast. Seeking to control the source of nurturance, one sees others in the family as objects to be dominated lest one be dominated by them.

An extreme example is what is called the "addictogenic" family. People who become drug addicts often have a childhood history of inconsistent treatment, of being kept in perpetual uncertainty by emotionally distant parents. Addiction can be seen as the perpetual search for certainty of experience through the pill, shot, or bottle that eases the pain. In the relationships through which the addict obtains the desired substance, he manipulates as he felt himself to be manipulated, exploits as he felt himself to be exploited, to get the nourishment that he never had (and never has) quite enough of. As with narcissism and paranoia, the pathological example has its everyday counterpart. In the addict's desperate clinging we can see the addictions of everyday life that social psychologist Stanton Peele and Archie Brodsky analyze in *Love and Addiction* (1976). The addict's fear—of his own weakness, of being close to other people, of uncertainty—is everyone's fear.

Alienation within the family and fear of uncertainty set up a vicious circle. The less people can be sure of, the more they fear the unknown. The more uncertainty (lack of trust) people

experience in their closest human relationships, the more emotional pressure they feel to deny uncertainty generally. Fear of
uncertainty in the outside world can lead people to compensate
by being more rigid and blindly trusting in their family relationships. Once this blind trust is shattered, as it must be in an
uncertain world, what comes to take its place is blind mistrust
and cynicism. With less trust to fall back on, people become less
able to face uncertainty. Thus they require even greater certainty in their interpretation of the world and in their conduct
of their relationships. They think, feel, and act more rigidly. In
the absence of critical thinking people have a difficult time
breaking out of this cycle, and it tends to perpetuate itself in
ever-worsening degrees.

Faced with fear, faced with pain, faced even with the degree
of uncertainty involved in everyday decision-making, people
revert to primitive means of warding off the demons. One of
these is to retreat into the fantasy of certainty. People tend to
be most rational when they are with other people, for it is then
that fantasy is continually corrected by reality. In the mechanistic family, with its isolation and emotional distancing, people are not really with one another very much, and fantasies of
both the narcissistic and paranoid types are left free to grow.

How do people keep these fantasies from becoming utterly
debilitating and destructive? How do they keep the fear within
bounds? By applying the simple strategies of the Mechanistic
Paradigm for warding off uncertainty. By doing "what's always
done," people can achieve a superficial certainty that carries
with it the hope of averting an uncertain future.

Forming exchange relationships in the family is one such
strategy. That way, at least, the potentially deadly family com-
petition will be civilized, and one will be sure of repayment if
not of love. Within these mechanistic relationships family
members play rigid roles, i.e., formulas for repetitive action that
reduce the individual to a single purpose or a set of disconnected
purposes. These roles may be permanent or semipermanent
(e.g., breadwinner, homemaker/hostess, child-development expert, specialized teen-age consumer), or they may rotate among
family members, as in the case of the stereotyped "sick role" and
nurse/doctor roles that people assume in times of illness. Either

way, there is no capacity or opportunity for flexible responses. One can only act out the script, follow the rules.

By understanding the impact of the Mechanistic Paradigm on family life, we see the origins of the modern family as described by Christopher Lasch: emotionally distant parents who, having power only in the family, have no power even there; children who, having nothing else around which to build an identity, cling to phantom parents. This is a family that lacks the authority to give children principles by which to orient themselves in an uncertain world. Without meaningful authority there cannot be the kind of meaningful rebellion that tests the limits of assurance and discovers the consequences of action.

When the family is a community of trust, when its members share the losses as well as the gains, the pain and fear as well as the pleasure and hope, it is safer for the individual to go out in the world and gamble. Even when out in the world alone, one still has one's family to fall back on. And if we assume that people can tolerate uncertainty only up to a point, then the less uncertainty one has about one's family—the less uncertainty that the family will be there when needed—the more uncertainty one can accept and cope with elsewhere. Thus the presence of love and trust in the family makes it more likely that children will learn to think critically and make rational decisions.

The gambling that is practiced under the Probabilistic Paradigm, the leap of faith by which one transcends one's immediate interest and commits oneself to a communal relationship—these require a flexibility of mind and spirit that few people achieve without close trusting relationships. A family that lacks strong mutual trust cannot transmit the habit of active, critical thinking, but only the passive consumption (whether of television programs, ideas, or decision-making strategies) that is its mode of existence. In sum the family that has been formed by the Mechanistic Paradigm can teach its offspring only the Mechanistic Paradigm.

According to social psychologist Herbert Kelman (1963), there are three ways in which children learn from their parents (and people influence each other generally). The first, most primitive way is through *compliance.* Compliance is based on the hope of reward and the fear of punishment. To obtain compliance from a child, the parent must be actively present, ready to impose sanctions. The second, *identification,* occurs when the child follows the parents' teachings not so as to obtain the parents' approval, but to have a satisfying relationship with the parent by being like the parent or being what the parent likes. The child is influenced not by the parent's actual physical presence, but by an inner presence, a favorable image of the parent that the child adopts as a model: "I want to do it the way Daddy (Mommy) does" or "I want to be what my parents think of as a good child." The final, most developed stage is that of *internalization,* in which the child (adult) acts so as to achieve his or her own ends and maintain his or her own values. The parent's teachings are kept in mind, but it is no longer the parent's power or the parent's image that maintains them. Having internalized the parent's description of what actions lead to what consequences, the child is doing not "what Daddy (Mommy) does," but "what I do."

Normally, a child learns by all three processes in turn. The child accepts parental dictates (compliance). The child follows the parents' example (identification). The child shares experiences with other family members and draws conclusions which sometimes confirm and sometimes challenge parental authority (internalization). But in the modern family as described by Lasch, children do not have the experiences that lead to internalization. Children listen to their parents not because the parents have something to teach them that will help them face uncertainty (internalization), but because not to listen calls forth the primitive fear of pain, loss of nourishment, and death (compliance). There is nothing to do but to comply —or not comply. Children who do not learn what it means to apply rules flexibly can only apathetically comply or cynically "get away with" not complying. At best they can identify and "do what Daddy (Mommy) does." Alternately, they can identify with cult heroes outside the family and in so doing devalue the family.

In the mechanistic family, then, learning proceeds by compliance and sometimes identification. But the Probabilistic Paradigm and the decision-making strategies it entails are sufficiently complex that they require internalization. They must be learned by taking action and interpreting the consequences, not by playing roles and following rules. They cannot, therefore, be taught by many families today.

Thinking in the Midst of Pain and Fear: The Doctor's Office

The case of K. points to the close connection between the mechanistic pattern of family life and the way people think, feel, and act when they or others are ill. K.'s family, overwhelmed by the conditions of their lives, denied their child the nourishment he needed to survive. Hospital personnel, seeing a child crying out for a mother, wanted to do right by him. But they could not openly act on their desire to give him loving support in an uncertain situation. Instead they had to act out the professional role of objective experimenters pursuing a diagnosis. Themselves afraid of uncertainty, they took so much care to avoid the loss they feared that they created a situation where little could be gained. And yet in so doing they only acted (as well as thought and felt) as almost anyone else would.

There are a number of parallels between family relationships and the doctor-patient relationship. Both are intimate relationships in which people must together confront uncertainty, pain, and fear. Both involve decisions that require a capacity for critical thinking. In the doctor's office as at home people learn to make these decisions through compliance (with instructions), identification (with the doctor as gambler), and internalization (of strategies of critical thinking). The relationship between patient and doctor, like that between family members, can be an exchange or communal relationship.

The two relationships also intersect in several places, such as the "sick role" and caretaker role that family members take turns playing. The doctor's office can be a place where family relationships are either reproduced or changed, since the doctor's authority as a representative of science and as one who can heal pain can provide a model, whether mechanistic or probabilistic, for authority in the family. Today the dominant pattern is the mechanistic one. The science practiced in the doctor's office is usually mechanistic science, and healing proceeds along the lines of "One shot and it will all be gone." Pain here is not seen as something complex, something that may have many causes, something that one may have to live with. Rather it is seen as an offending particle to be surgically removed. From such experiences with physical pain the child learns to deal with other pains, other losses. If a finger hurting from a splinter has a single cause and a simple remedy, perhaps a broken heart does as well. Or so we think.

Not surprisingly, mechanistic thinking is especially evident in people's explanations of how they come to be ill. Traditional medicine has until recently focused on germs "out there in the air" as the primary if not sole cause of disease, as if people were powerless against such external causation. In the most extreme form of this kind of thinking—a paranoid thought disorder—one may find a person accusing others of poisoning him by injecting or implanting him with germs. Some exponents of holistic health swing equally wide in the opposite direction, claiming that the way a person lives is what brings on or prevents illness. Here the all-powerful "I" of narcissism becomes the sole cause of all that one experiences. Both sides are abstracting half-truths from a context of multiple causation, a context that includes (in addition to germs and personal lifestyle) environmental factors and people's relationships with one another in the workplace, the neighborhood, and the family.

Even when people do think in terms of multicausal explanations and probability, they may still revert to mechanistic thinking in the context of medicine, where life and health are at stake and pain and fear (particularly the fear of death) are ever-present. Even the most intelligent, well-informed, self-possessed people get scared when they are in a doctor's office.

Probably the doctor is a bit scared too. It is difficult for people to think rationally when they are scared. Instead they become rigid in their thinking. They go back to the way they used to think when they were children, a way of thinking that is less than fully conscious.

In speaking of narcissism and paranoia, we have noted an affinity between mechanistic thinking and unconscious processes. The fixation on single causes, the stark "either/or" quality of all three criteria of the Mechanistic Paradigm—in these elegant formulations of Newton's we hear echoes of a primitive response to life. Is it the case that the Mechanistic Paradigm during the past few centuries has shaped unconscious as well as conscious thinking, or that the Mechanistic Paradigm simply formalizes unconscious tendencies that are fixed in the human psyche? For our purposes it does not matter whether the chicken or the egg came first; the effects we observe are reciprocal. What matters is that when the fear of death is touched off, the unconscious reaction that occurs takes the form of mechanistic thinking. This close connection between thought and feeling means that a doctor who is concerned with the way patients think must also be concerned with the way patients feel.

Although it is in medicine that we find mechanistic thinking at its most extreme, it is also in medicine that there may be a hope for change. If people learned from their families how to cope with pain and fear without resorting to mechanistic ways of thinking, they wouldn't need to learn it in the stressful moments of illness. But since most people do not learn this in the family, they need to learn it somewhere else. The doctor's office (or wherever doctors and patients meet) provides a setting where people can confront these issues consciously and gain practice in probabilistic thinking. Both the efforts of probabilistically minded physicians like Dr. S. and the energy coming out of the "active patient" movement suggest that the doctor-patient relationship may be just the place to break old patterns of thought, feeling, and action and try new ones that will then make themselves felt in the family, the workplace, and the marketplace. Medicine has been very effective in teaching the Mechanistic Paradigm; perhaps now it can teach the Probabilistic Paradigm.

PART II

CHANCE
AND CHOICE

5

DECISION ANALYSIS IN MEDICINE

When Dr. S. began his practice, he thought to himself, "No more K. cases!" In reviewing the case of K., he saw how mechanistic thinking could defeat the best of intentions. From hindsight the outcome had a tragic inevitability. What had been missing in that case was probabilistic thinking. S. would have to learn to think probabilistically and share his understanding with patients. He and they would have to learn to modify uncertain knowledge on the basis of new information (in the hope of making it less uncertain), while acting on the basis of information that would still be uncertain. Since one way of gaining new information was by acting, decision-making would become a matter of acting, understanding the results, and reevaluating; acting, understanding, and reevaluating—always with an awareness that a degree of uncertainty would remain, fluctuating but never disappearing.

This was easier said than done, especially for people who were not already comfortable dealing with uncertainty by means of probabilities. How could the Probabilistic Paradigm be translated into decision-making methods that people could use? What would those strategies look like when set down on paper? What would they sound like in discussions between husband and wife, parent and child, patient and doctor? What

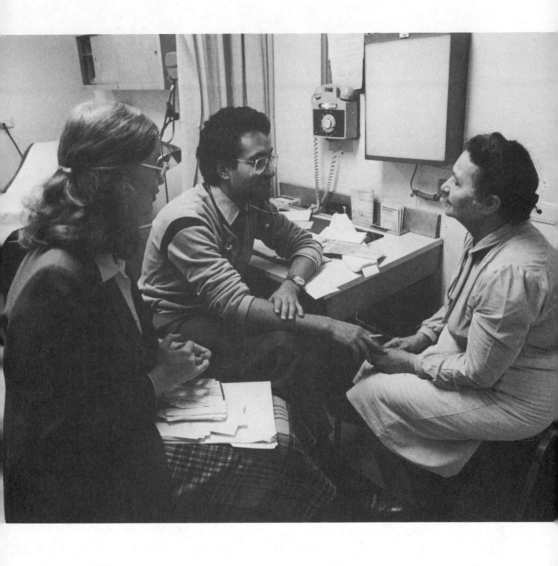

would they feel like to someone who was just learning them?

S. and his patients needed tools for turning the abstractions into concrete plans of action. When one such tool, decision analysis, first presented itself in medical publications (and in some medical-school curricula), S. naturally was receptive. Decision analysis had its origins in World War II when the Americans and British found that mathematicians could solve certain strategic and tactical problems better than the generals could. Out of this experience came a series of attempts, in which the mathematician John Von Neumann and the economist Oskar Morgenstern (1944) were pioneers, to apply systematic mathematical methods to decision-making. Decision analysis has been one outgrowth of these efforts. First used in economics, public-policy planning, and business investment and marketing, decision analysis is now being applied to other fields, including medicine. It is used in situations where one faces a sequence of choices, each having more or less uncertain consequences—a sequence so complex that people doubt their capacity to make the best decision intuitively (Raiffa, 1968).

In a medical situation, for example, one might test for one disease, get a negative result, try a treatment for another disease with no noticeable improvement, try another treatment, gain a partial alleviation of symptoms, and so forth. How can one keep all the relevant variables in mind simultaneously? How can one tell at the beginning of the sequence which choice is likely to lead to better outcomes several steps down the road? Decision analysis provides a way of laying out on paper the sequence of choices and their possible outcomes. By estimating the probability of each outcome at every step of the way and the desirability of the possible outcomes at the end of the sequence (e.g., death, complete recovery, partial disability, daily medications for life), one can mathematically calculate what, consistent with one's values, is the best action to take.

Some doctors look upon decision analysis as a promising tool because it seems to offer a way around all the factors that confuse people when they make decisions in medicine: economic pressures, family conflicts, and the pain and fear that accompany anyone to the doctor's office. With decision analysis it seems that, just by sitting down and working it all out on paper, a doctor and patient can coolly detach themselves from the hurly-burly of these pressures and just abstract the elements necessary for making a rational decision. Now that decision analysis (and its products, e.g., recommended approaches to particular diseases) is being made available to doctors and patients as the vanguard of probabilistic thinking, it is possible that each of us will meet up with it sooner or later in the doctor's office. Even if we don't use decision analysis ourselves, people around us will be using it, and their use of it will have consequences for our lives.

By learning about decision analysis, as S. did, we can decide intelligently whether, when, and how to use it. We can do so by seeing to what extent it is an aid and to what extent a barrier to thinking critically. In this and the following chapter we will be looking at S.'s experiences with decision analysis in order to see whether it can be of much day-to-day use to doctors and patients and whether (both in itself and as it is commonly applied) it is compatible with the three criteria of the Probabilistic Paradigm.

Whether or not we decide to make much use of decision analysis, it can still be a good learning tool (like the training wheels on a bicycle) for probabilistic thinking. Its formality can be helpful for the beginner (Dreyfus and Dreyfus, unpublished). Chance, choice, probability, value—all these are laid out in black and white. By going through the steps of decision analysis at least once we will know better what to keep in mind when we make decisions probabilistically in the more informal way that we refer to as gambling.

A Test Case

As the brief case example in Chapter 3 suggested, it doesn't make much sense to say, "Find the cause, then treat," when it comes to hypertension. As of now ninety to ninety-five percent of all cases of hypertension have no known cause, and in the remaining cases a cause may be discovered only with great difficulty. Nonetheless, in almost all cases elevated blood pressure can be reduced to acceptable levels, with a consequent reduction in complications and deaths. Still, treatment remains problematic. In a given case there may be reasons to consider drugs, life-style modifications, surgery, or no treatment at all. Moreover the effectiveness of treatment for a particular patient may vary greatly over time. For example, if an irregularity in the artery leading to one kidney *(renal artery stenosis, stenosis* means "narrowing") is corrected by surgery, the condition may recur a few years later in the artery leading to the other kidney. A drug regimen may keep a person's blood pressure controlled under some circumstances but not others. Indeed, it may take considerable experimentation before a combination of drugs is found that will stabilize the condition for a time. Even when an effective treatment is found, the patient, preferring the illness to the side effects of the drugs, often will stop taking the medication. Paradoxically, with hypertension it tends to be the treatment rather than the disease that initially brings unpleasant symptoms. Without treatment (except in severe cases) the patient may feel fine for many years. With treatment the patient may suffer side effects, such as drowsiness.

Hypertension is a very common chronic condition that people can live with for years without knowing they have it. A severe case may be brought to a doctor's attention when a person complains of headache, chest pain, dizziness, or shortness of breath, but the illness is most often discovered when a person's blood pressure is taken during a routine physical examination. It can have dramatic, sometimes fatal consequences, such as heart attack or stroke, but these typically do not occur until middle age or later. The doctor may be primarily concerned with preventing these harmful consequences of the illness in the future, whereas the patient may be primarily concerned with minimizing the inconvenience of the medication in the present. The very complexities involved in the diagnosis and treatment of hypertension together with its prevalence and potential consequences make it an important testing ground for decision analysis.

In his early years as a family doctor, at the time when he was investigating decision analysis, S. came up against an unusually challenging case of hypertension, that of Mrs. Pinelli, a thirty-five-year-old bookkeeper and divorced mother of three school-age children. When Mrs. Pinelli began to have severe headaches and chest pains, she went to S.'s nearby office, where a nurse took her blood pressure. "Just wait here a minute," said the nurse as she back-pedaled out of the examination room. "You can tell me!" Mrs. Pinelli called after her. "I know all about it! I've had it before!" Indeed, her blood pressure was 240/120, a dangerously high reading. (Although "normal" blood pressure depends on such factors as a person's sex, weight, and history, readings below 140/90 can roughly be considered normal.) She told Dr. S. that a few years earlier she had had another outbreak of severe hypertension, which had been "cured," according to the surgeon who operated on her, by a renal artery bypass operation. In taking her history it became apparent to S. that Mrs. Pinelli had been working at a furious pace. To make sure that she would rest, he hospitalized her. He was mainly concerned that she might have a heart attack or stroke at any time, and in the back of his mind he was also aware that he did not want to be held responsible for what might happen to her at home.

This was not the typical sort of hypertension (the kind that cannot be treated surgically) that S. was accustomed to dealing with. There was, therefore, some uncertainty, but there was also the fear that, should anything dreadful happen to this woman, he would be blamed. S. felt vulnerable, which was no surprise in the current climate of unreason, where controversy brings fears of malpractice claims.

In the hospital Mrs. Pinelli's blood pressure was quickly brought down with medications taken by mouth. Once back home with her children, Mrs. Pinelli began seeing Dr. S. at his office to work out a plan for controlling her blood pressure. He wanted to stabilize her condition with medications and then consult a specialist to see if this unusual case warranted further investigation.

After some delay he was able to obtain the records of Mrs. Pinelli's previous hospitalization. As is so often the case, he had to make decisions before the patient's records even arrived. The records told him much (though not all) of what he wanted to know about her medical history. Three years earlier Mrs. Pinelli had been found to have hypertension and had been placed on medications. But, as she put it, she "didn't have such a hot time with the pills," which made her drowsy. Because of her young age and severe hypertension, an X-ray study (arteriogram) of the arteries supplying her kidneys was performed. It revealed that a surgically correctable condition was present in both arteries, but was more severe in one than the other.

At that time surgery was looked upon as the preferred method of treatment for renal artery stenosis. "The way it was told to me," Mrs. Pinelli reported, "it could be cured by surgery. So why stay on pills the rest of my life?" She was referred to a surgeon at a leading teaching hospital, who successfully performed the renal artery bypass, and her blood pressure came down to normal. A few months later she had a falling-out with her doctor and stopped going back for follow-up visits. It was thus impossible to tell just when in the three intervening years she had relapsed.

S. had mixed feelings about being Mrs. Pinelli's doctor. He wanted to support her every step of the way, as long as she needed him, but he realized that to do so would require a good deal of work on his part. He knew that Mrs. Pinelli couldn't afford to pay for a fraction of the time he would spend making referrals, obtaining information, and so forth. Still, he wanted to give her complete care. If he gave her anything less, he would feel as if he were abandoning his patient.

His forebodings increased when Mrs. Pinelli began to express the same discontent with the medical regimen that had led her to have surgery the first time. The pills were making her dopey, she said. She couldn't do a good day's work, and she couldn't take proper care of her children. Besides, she insisted, it made no sense to try to treat her condition without looking at her kidneys, where the cause of her hypertension had previously been found.

Dr. S. agreed that she had a point, but did not want to rush into expensive and painful tests that might well not show anything. Instead he suggested that Mrs. Pinelli use decision analysis as an aid in making an informed decision. He delegated the task of conducting the lengthy briefing in this method to Jeanne Aaron, medical student then in training at his practice, who did some preliminary research to clarify the choices and the probabilities. She would then sit down with Mrs. Pinelli and lay out the options, so that Mrs. Pinelli could reach a decision on the basis of her own values and principles.

When Mrs. Pinelli returned for her next visit, Jeanne was ready. She explained to the patient the principles of decision analysis and the main courses of action open to her. "We all agree, don't we," Jeanne said, "that it doesn't pay just to do nothing about this." She looked up at Mrs. Pinelli for confirmation. Mrs. Pinelli gave the expected nod, but did she agree? From her earlier episode to the present she had shown a clear preference for doing nothing except when she developed symptoms that she couldn't ignore. Then, when she had to do something, she looked for a quick and total solution through surgery. S. and Jeanne, notwithstanding their own belief that drug therapy probably was the best choice for Mrs. Pinelli, would need to be aware of her tendency to oscillate between avoidance and the search for a magical cure.

Jeanne, however, tried to deal with Mrs. Pinelli on a rational level without first working with her to establish a shared sense of what it meant to be rational. She reviewed with her the problems connected with surgery. The fact that one renal artery had been bypassed was no guarantee that the artery to the other kidney (which was also, but less severely affected) would not become narrower in the future. Progression of such lesions (pathological distortions) commonly occurred only up to about the age of forty. Until then the picture could always change, and not for the better. If Mrs. Pinelli stayed on drugs for another five years before having surgery, she stood a much better chance of avoiding having to go through the operation yet again. Furthermore there was now a clear preference to turn to surgery at any age only as a last resort. The issue of recurrence after surgery did indeed concern Mrs. Pinelli. "I was never even told that there was any chance of its recurring," she said bitterly. But she had something else on her mind as well. "Someone" *had* told her that "no one knows anything unless the arteriogram is done."

A tension developed between the two women as they staked out their positions:

J.A.: Tell me how you feel about taking medications.

MRS. P.: I don't like it.

J.A.: How much don't you like it?

MRS. P.: A lot. It just seems like every time I turn around I'm popping pills.

J.A.: Would you feel better with just one pill?

MRS. P.: Better than with what I'm taking now.

J.A.: So it's the number of pills that's bothering you.

MRS. P.: Yes, and the idea that I have to depend on them for the rest of my life. But I'll take them for the rest of my life if the arteriogram says I have to.

J.A.: What if you only have to depend on them for five years, and then have surgery when it's more likely to cure your hypertension for a longer time? How much would it bother you to have surgery now and then have your blood pressure go up again, the way it did this time?

MRS. P.: Couldn't it be that this thing just flared up again? I mean, do I have to keep taking all these pills, or can we cut down on them once my blood pressure is down?

Throughout the session Mrs. Pinelli's hopes for a quick and simple answer were heard (and who could blame her?). She and Jeanne discussed the possibility that she was not having a relapse of renal artery stenosis at all, but rather a completely unrelated episode of essential hypertension (i.e., hypertension with no known anatomical cause or surgical cure). Both of them jumped at this explanation—Jeanne because it would mean that an arteriogram would be useless, Mrs. Pinelli because she mistakenly thought that a form of hypertension that didn't require surgery might be cured, not just controlled, by medication. She clung to the hope of someday being able to stop the medications.

When Dr. S. returned, Jeanne summed up the discussion for

him. "Mrs. Pinelli's main concern about the pills is the number she has to take," said Jeanne. "It really bothers her to take all these different pills every time she sits down to eat." Indeed it did, for as Mrs. Pinelli put it, "Sometimes you don't eat at all when you're taking all those pills." But her *main* concern, as she had made clear, was with having to be dependent on pills for the rest of her life. Jeanne also told S. that "Mrs. Pinelli is frustrated by the way her first operation turned out. She went into it thinking it was a permanent cure. So she's not sure she wants to go through surgery a second time until there's a better chance that this won't happen again." This was all very logical to Jeanne, but it was not Mrs. Pinelli's logic.

Mrs. Pinelli was indeed frustrated and bitter. Although her surgeon years earlier might have told her that her hypertension could recur, all she had heard was that she was "cured." That was all she had wanted to know while she was enjoying the luxury of not having to worry about doctors and pills. Now she felt betrayed. She paid no attention to the fact that her chances for a surgical cure would get better in years to come. Rather, she demanded all the more insistently the surgical cure that she still believed in, but felt she had been cheated out of. She had in fact raised several objections to Jeanne's idea of waiting until she was forty to have surgery, but it was as if Jeanne had not heard her. People have their own ways of talking and their own ways of listening.

With Dr. S. in the room an uneasy truce took hold as both the student (who had been doing most of the talking) and the patient deferred to the doctor. Mrs. Pinelli, who was not as anxious to confront S. as she had been with Jeanne, appeared more open to considering all the options. Taking his cue from Jeanne, S. indicated that newly developed medications might make it possible in the coming years for Mrs. Pinelli to get by on one or two pills a day. Mrs. Pinelli tried to bargain with him, saying, "If we can just get it down *close* to normal, can't we stop the pills for a while and see what happens?" S. told her, "With the kind of hypertension that you have it would be very unlikely that that would work." But he assured her that she had a right to have surgery if she so decided, and that whatever decision she made need not be considered permanent. "It's not as if it's signed, sealed, and delivered once and for all," he told her. "There are new drugs, new operations, and there is new information coming out all the time. The idea is to make a good decision now and then review it from time to time. And there's never any one right thing to do. For the time being you're safe, because your blood pressure is controlled. As long as that's the case, you can take your time and be sure you know what you want to do before you do it. You don't have to rush your decision."

Jeanne added, "Just wait till we do the decision analysis! That'll clear everything up." The three of them closed ranks around that sentiment and went through the decision analysis that Jeanne had prepared.

The Procedure

When Jeanne Aaron did the decision analysis with Mrs. Pinelli, she went through a standard procedure, parts of which involved the patient's participation. We will not draw full detailed diagrams or work out all the calculations here. Rather, we will outline the procedure and suggest what each step entailed for Mrs. Pinelli, Dr. S., and Jeanne.

Drawing the Tree

Jeanne's first step in preparing the decision analysis was to construct a *decision tree*. A decision tree is a diagram that shows a set of possible actions to take, the possible results of each, another set of choices stemming from these results, their possible results, and so forth. The tree consists of a series of "choice points," where the decision-maker decides what to do, alternating with "chance points," where the world (or reality, or fate, or nature) responds to the decision-maker's action in one of a number of ways. In the treatment of hypertension at least four initial courses of action might be considered: (1) drug therapy; (2) life-style modifications such as diet (e.g., low salt), exercise, or stress-reduction techniques such as meditation; (3) testing for surgically correctable causes; (4) doing nothing now and living with the subsequent consequences of the illness.

Jeanne wanted to present Mrs. Pinelli with a decision tree that would be easy to understand, yet would do the job. She and S. went over the four main options and decided, without consulting Mrs. Pinelli, that doing nothing would be unacceptable and life-style changes alone would be insufficient. Jeanne accordingly began her tree with two basic choices, as shown in Figure 5–1. She then filled out the branches with possible results and subsequent choices. "It will be simpler for her this way," she told S. "We'll make it easy for her."

This diagram is simplified for demonstration purposes, since the actual tree might involve taking more than one action at a time. For example, S. undoubtedly would give Mrs. Pinelli drugs to control her blood pressure while she was undergoing tests. Moreover, "drug treatment" represents many possible choices, not just one. However, S. and Jeanne began the "drug" branch of the tree with what seemed from their experience to be the best choice of drugs; they drew later branches on the tree to represent other combinations of drugs in case the first did not keep Mrs. Pinelli's blood pressure controlled. Most doctors, for example, begin the treatment of hypertension with diuretics—drugs which, among their several effects, promote salt loss from the body. Once S. and Jeanne had mapped out the possible diagnosis and treatment on the decision tree, they had to ask themselves and Mrs. Pinelli some questions about probability and value and perform a few calculations to come up with a strategy for action.

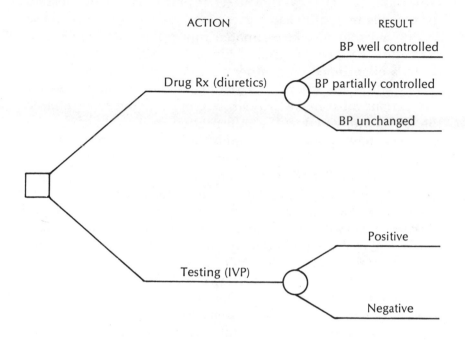

Partial Decision Tree
for Hypertension—Mrs. Pinelli

ACTION

RESULT

BP well controlled

Drug Rx (diuretics)

BP partially controlled

BP unchanged

Testing (IVP)

Positive

Negative

FIGURE 5-1

Prior Probability Estimate

S. and Jeanne first asked: "What is the prior probability that the patient has the disease in question?" In order to figure out which tests have the best chance of revealing useful information and which treatments have the best chance of success, it is necessary to estimate how likely it is that the patient has one disease or another. In some cases the doctor and patient must estimate probabilities for several possible underlying conditions so that they can direct their diagnostic and therapeutic efforts toward those that are most likely to be present.

Probabilities may be estimated with the help of statistical

tables on the frequency of occurrence of the disease in question for patients in certain categories of age, sex, symptoms, and so forth. They may also be estimated subjectively, on the basis of the patient's understanding of his or her past history and the doctor's experience with other patients and intuitions about this patient. Even when tables of data *are* consulted, the doctor and patient must make critical judgments about how reliable the tables are, whether the information in the tables is up to date, and how the statistics apply to the unique case of this particular patient. Even when one looks up numbers, one is still at best making educated guesses.

Mrs. Pinelli knew that she had hypertension. What she wanted to know was whether she had one of several rare types of hypertension that could sometimes be corrected by surgery. In particular she wanted to know if she still had the condition that was diagnosed at the time of her previous episode: *renal artery stenosis* (RAS). When one or both of the renal arteries is partially pinched off, high blood pressure can occur.

Given that at least ninety to ninety-five percent of all cases of hypertension are of the "essential" variety, it follows that renal artery stenosis is not very common. Its statistical frequency among both men and women with hypertension is only four percent. Since Mrs. Pinelli had a prior history of this condition, S. and Jeanne judged the probability of its being the cause of her hypertension now as seventy-five percent.

Revised Probability Estimate

The second type of assessment that S. and Jeanne had to make was: "Given additional information, what is the revised probability that the patient has the disease in question?" In an uncertain world we are always adjusting our probability estimates on the basis of new information. Today's newly revised probability estimate becomes a prior probability estimate for tomorrow's information-gathering. For example, before Mrs. Pinelli had her blood pressure taken or showed any symptoms of hypertension, the probability of her having RAS was practically nil. Once she was found to have high blood pressure, the probability jumped to four percent. That figure could in turn be revised by looking at her history as well as by undertaking further tests and treatments. The "risk factor" charts that appear on doctors' waiting-room walls testify to the fact that many different kinds of "signs"—age, sex, weight, family medical history, personal medical history, occupational stress, exposure to disease carriers or disease-causing agents, diet, exercise, alcohol and tobacco use, appearance of symptoms—can raise or lower by a few percentage points the probability of a person's having a particular disease.

By the time a medical decision analysis is begun, many of these factors (vital statistics, life-style, symptoms, prior history, family history, preliminary tests) are already known. These are incorporated into the estimate of the probability that the person has the disease. Further refinements tend to come from test results and from the observation of how the disease responds to treatment (or what "natural course" it takes without treatment). S. knew how Mrs. Pinelli felt, how old she was, how much she weighed, how she spent her work and leisure time, whether she had previously had RAS, and what her blood pressure reading was. What remained was to prescribe medication or administer more sensitive tests and then see what happened. S. still wouldn't be *certain* whether or not she had RAS, but (at the cost of time, money, and possible side effects of testing or treatment) he would have more to go on.

The ways in which choice and chance combine to bring about good or bad outcomes are shown in general terms by this simplified decision tree (Fig. 5–2). This tree presupposes, just as doctors and patients usually do, that test results are always accurate. It shows that the decision to treat or not to treat (without testing) may be right or wrong, but it makes it appear that the decision to test is never wrong. Indeed, if test results were always accurate, testing would always be the best choice (provided that there existed some real doubt to be resolved by testing, that the condition the test might reveal had some known means of treatment, and that the costs of testing—time, money, pain, risk of complications—were not excessively high). Under the Probabilistic Paradigm, however, it is recognized that no

Outcomes of Testing and Treatment Options
(when accuracy of test is assumed)

ACTION   RESULT   ACTION   OUTCOME

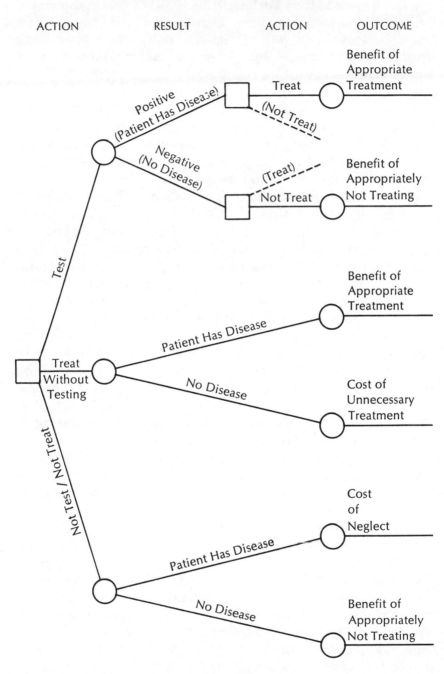

FIGURE 5-2

one test constitutes an *experimentum crucis* that resolves the diagnosis once and for all. A lab result is just another piece of information, and does not guarantee certainty. Most diagnostic tests are marketed with reminders of how often a test result will be in error. However, in practice many physicians do not pay sufficient attention to this information.

This state of affairs can be represented on the decision tree by substituting the branch shown in Figure 5–3 for the "test" branch in Figure 5–2. Along with the costs of unnecessary or inappropriately withheld treatment, the tree now shows the costs of inaccurate or misleading test results—those which identify a disease that isn't there (false positive) or fail to identify one that is there (false negative).

Even a small percentage of false positive results can make a test almost meaningless in cases where the prior probability of the patient's having the disease is low. Here is a case that S. remembered from his decision analysis course. Suppose that a certain type of cancer occurs in five out of every thousand people. Now assume that ninety-five percent of the people *with* this cancer will have a positive test result for the disease, while ninety-five percent of those *without* cancer will have a negative test result. On a National Cancer Day testing program at work you get a positive result. What do you estimate is the probability that you have the disease?

Most people's estimates are way off. Out of a large group of practicing physicians, more than half thought the probability was greater than fifty percent. Actually it is just under nine percent. Among all the people taking the test, most of those who get positive results do not have cancer. Common sense doesn't seem to work very well in interpreting test results of this sort. We can, however, make use of a mathematical formula that the Reverend Thomas Bayes proposed for just such purposes in 1763. We will not spell out Bayes's Theorem here; it can be found in any textbook of probability theory. What is important for understanding Mrs. Pinelli's case, and decision analysis in general, is the fact that test results must be interpreted in conjunction with other probabilistic information. When we make use of a diagnostic test, we are going from one probability esti-

Outcomes of Testing
(when accuracy of test is uncertain)

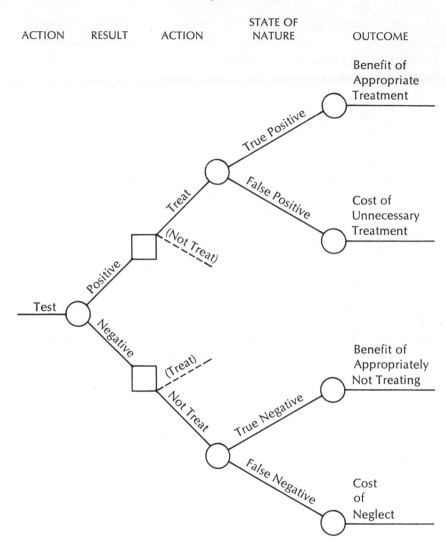

Definitions:

State of Nature: underlying reality
True Positive: disease is present; test result is positive
False Positive: disease is not present; test result is positive
True Negative: disease is not present; test result is negative
False Negative: disease is present; test result is negative

FIGURE 5-3

mate (the prior probability) to another (the revised probability) via a third (the information yielded by the test).

For renovascular hypertension the tests in question are the *intravenous pyelogram* (IVP) and *arteriogram,* two X-ray procedures (using injected dye) described in Chapter 3. Usually a doctor who suspects RAS or a related disorder will first do an IVP, which can reveal kidney malfunctioning. If the IVP suggests that there may be an insufficient blood supply to the kidney from the renal artery, the doctor may proceed to do an arteriogram, an uncomfortable and slightly risky procedure that gives an X-ray picture of the artery itself. The two tests are part of what is called a "hypertensive workup." In some cases they can provide grounds for going ahead with renal artery bypass surgery.

On the other hand, the accuracy rate for these procedures must be taken into account. With the IVP, for example, we can estimate from past experience that only seventy-eight percent of hypertensive patients *with* RAS will have a positive IVP (which means that there will be twenty-two percent false negatives), while ninety percent of those *without* RAS will have a negative IVP (which means that there will be ten percent false positives). Using Bayes's Theorem, we can calculate that a positive IVP would increase the probability of Mrs. Pinelli's having RAS from seventy-five to ninety-six percent, while a negative IVP would reduce the probability to forty-two percent. For Mrs. Pinelli a positive IVP would suggest that an arteriogram might be useful diagnostically. It would not, however, dictate the decision to do an arteriogram—especially since the arteriogram has its own error rate and since even a positive arteriogram is no guarantee of a successful surgical cure. Most doctors, in fact, now would advise against surgery for people whose hypertension can be controlled with medication. Because the primary purpose of the IVP and the arteriogram is to identify a surgically correctable condition, and because at Mrs. Pinelli's age the probabilities do not favor surgery, she and S. would choose the workup only if her values strongly favored either having the diagnosis for its own sake or seeking a surgical solution (which, as before, might only be temporary) (Pauker, 1976).

Probabilities of Outcomes

Having made the best estimates they could (using all the available information) of the probability that their patient had each of the diseases in question (in this case, renovascular versus essential hypertension), S. and Jeanne then made a third kind of assessment: "Assuming that the patient has a given disease (or no disease), what is the probability of each of the outcomes that may occur if a given test or treatment (or none at all) is administered?" In other words, on the decision tree each "state of nature" (e.g., the presence or absence of a disease) leads to a "choice point" (e.g., taking or not taking a particular action). That choice will have further "chance" outcomes—i.e., outcomes for which probabilities can be estimated. The estimating is done in the same way as with diagnostic probabilities, that is, by subjective, critical judgment, sometimes with the assistance of statistical data obtained from experimental studies or compilations of clinical experience. Subjective judgment, based on the doctor's own clinical experience and the patient's personal experience, is needed to decide which statistical categories are relevant to the case at hand.

These probability assessments, together with the patient's eventual value assessments, constitute a way of measuring the costs and benefits of each action under consideration. Costs and benefits include not only the true or false information gained from a test and the success or failure of a treatment, but also such factors as lost time, physical strain, and the risk of infection. Some of these side effects (e.g., whether a patient will have an allergic reaction to a medication) must be assessed probabilistically. Others, such as the monetary cost of the test or treatment, occur so dependably that they can be entered on the decision tree as "tolls" along with whatever other outcomes the test or treatment may have. A bottle of pills, for example, might or might not bring down Mrs. Pinelli's blood pressure, but she would have to pay the pharmacist to find out.

On Mrs. Pinelli's decision tree the two initial branches split off into many smaller branches as choices led to outcomes that necessitated further choices that led to new outcomes, etc. If one drug or combination of drugs didn't work, another would be tried. If the IVP or the arteriogram did not reveal an operable condition, then a nonsurgical option would have to be pursued. At those points the "test" branch of the tree, which had one branch leading all the way to surgery, split off into other branches that looked like the initial "drug treatment" branch. On all the branches "choice points" alternated with "chance points" until a set of final outcomes was reached, these being the estimated levels at which Mrs. Pinelli's blood pressure would eventually be stabilized given various combinations of actions and consequences.

Finally, since S. and Jeanne could not reasonably expect Mrs. Pinelli to assign values to blood pressure readings like 180/120 or 130/90, they had to translate these figures into descriptions of probable consequences for her life. Included in the overall picture were such factors as life expectancy, degree of disability, discomfort, and cost. Mrs. Pinelli could attach a value to a scenario such as "normal life span without stroke or heart disease" or "$——— a year in medical expenses, ——— side effects of drugs, and ——— probability of stroke or heart disease."

Value Assessment

The fourth kind of assessment required by decision analysis, one that Mrs. Pinelli had to make for herself, was "What value does the patient place on each possible outcome?" (In some cases the values of the patient's family or the doctor may also be relevant.) Mrs. Pinelli had to give numerical value assessments. One way to obtain them would have been to ask her to rate each possible outcome, for example, on a 0 to 100 scale. A score of 0 could be given to the worst possible outcome (immediate death, which is a four percent probability with renal artery bypass surgery and a one-tenth percent probability with the arteriogram), while a score of 100 could be given to the best possible outcome (living out her life without serious complications from hypertension). She then would assign numbers between 0 and 100 to descriptions of the other possible life scenarios.

It was not so easy, however, for Mrs. Pinelli to evaluate on a one-dimensional scale such diverse scenarios as "one month of urinary frequency, then stably controlled hypertension," "$180 per year, drowsiness, plus controlled hypertension," "develop nonfatal coronary artery disease in two years," and "develop fatal coronary artery disease in twelve years." How could she compare all these things on one scale? And how could S. and Jeanne be sure that she really thought that an outcome she called a "60" was as much better than a "40" as an "80" was better than a "60"?

A procedure called the "lottery method" (Raiffa, 1968) has been devised to help people assign numbers to outcomes in a meaningful way, as well as to take account of people's attitudes toward risk. The procedure involves setting up a hypothetical lottery between the best and worst possible outcomes and asking the patient to choose between playing the lottery and having the outcome that is being evaluated. The probabilities of the two extreme outcomes in the lottery are adjusted until the patient is indifferent to the choice between taking the outcome under consideration and taking his or her chance on the lottery.

The lottery method can be presented as a game, "The Devil and Mrs. Pinelli." A mysterious stranger with an uncanny resemblance to Dr. S. appears before Mrs. Pinelli and says, "Would you like to play a game?" He then produces a big jar full of black and white marbles. From the jar he takes out various combinations of them, always totaling one hundred marbles, but in different proportions of black to white. He then mentions one of the possible outcomes that Mrs. Pinelli faces. "If I give you a choice," he tells her, "between developing nonfatal coronary artery disease in two years and playing a lottery in which you have as many chances of the best possible outcome (living the rest of your natural life without serious complications) as the number of white marbles I hold out, and as many chances of the worst possible outcome (immediate death) as the number of black marbles I hold out, which do you choose?"

Clearly if the Devil holds out a hundred black marbles and no white ones, Mrs. Pinelli will choose the certainty of developing nonfatal coronary artery disease in two years. If he holds out a hundred white marbles and no black ones, she will choose the lottery. But as he tries various proportions of white to black between these two extremes, she becomes less sure of her preference. Finally he hits upon a combination—say, sixty white marbles and forty black—where she just doesn't care whether she gets to play the lottery or the certainty of the intermediate outcome. The two are of equal value to her. Getting coronary artery disease in two years is worth as much to her as a sixty percent chance of living out her life without complications due to hypertension and a forty percent chance of immediate death. In doing this procedure she will have assigned a value of 60 to the outcome, "developing nonfatal coronary artery disease in two years." Continuing in this way, she estimates the values of all the listed outcomes.

Calculating Expected Values

Once the four kinds of probability and value assessments have been made, probabilities can be entered on the decision tree for all possible outcomes along the various branches, along with values for those that represent "final," real-life consequences for the patient. The next step is to calculate the *expected value* (or expected utility) of each possible outcome. In commonsense terms, the question, "How much is this outcome worth to me?" boils down to "How much would I like or dislike this if it happened?" *and* "How likely is it to happen?" The expected value, then, is the value of a possible outcome multiplied by the probability that it will happen. If, under a given set of conditions, "developing nonfatal coronary artery disease in two years," to which Mrs. Pinelli has given a value of 60, has a ten percent probability of occurrence, then its expected value is 6. If it has a probability of twenty percent, then its expected value is 12. If we could repeat the same choice many times, the average result in the long run would be close to the expected value.

Making the Decision

At each of the final "chance points" on the decision tree the expected values of all the branches coming out of that chance point are added up to get an overall expected value for the choice that leads to that chance point. (For example, if at one of the final chance points of Mrs. Pinelli's decision tree there are three branches with expected values of 72, 18, and 3, the expected value of the choice leading to that chance point is 93.) There will be more than one such choice at that point on the decision tree. The choice with the highest expected value is kept, and its expected value is passed on to the branch that leads to that "choice point" from the previous chance point. Thus at any chance point we choose the action with the highest expected value. Occasionally there may be reasons for doing other than maximizing the expected value, as when we want to go for the best possible outcome or avoid at all costs the worst. Normally, though, we would choose to maximize the expected value, especially since to do otherwise would leave us open to having a Dutch Book (a sure losing bet) made against us, as explained in Chapter 2.

Working back along the branches of the tree in this manner, we chart a strategy for action that tells us the best choice to make at each choice point in response to whatever has happened at the previous chance point. With this strategy we are anticipating all eventualities that have been incorporated into the decision tree. The strategy indicates which of the initial options leads to the highest expected value. In Mrs. Pinelli's case, not surprisingly, it favored taking medications for blood pressure control, as opposed to testing for renal artery stenosis.

Algorithms

When S. had met Mrs. Pinelli, his first thought had been "If only there were an algorithm!" When decision analysis has been done for a number of similar cases, it is sometimes possible to "package" the resulting strategies in the form of an *algorithm,* a sequence of instructions for solving a problem. Algorithms are based on prior explorations of the probabilities and values involved in a given set of situations. An algorithm may take the form of a general decision tree (like the one for hypertension) which can be adapted to the needs of particular patients, thus saving doctor and patient the prohibitive effort of structuring a new tree for each case. Or it may simply be a table of therapeutic recommendations for patients classified according to age, sex, symptoms, diagnosis, and so forth.

Successful examples of the use of decision analysis in medicine have led some doctors to hope that medical practice in the future will be conducted increasingly with the aid of algorithms. Ideally, they speculate, a patient like Mrs. Pinelli should be able to "plug in" her values to a preexisting algorithm for hypertension and, whether by consulting tables or by feeding the data into a computer, come up with recommendations for action at each choice point. As yet, though, there was no algorithm for Mrs. Pinelli, and there might not ever be one. So Jeanne Aaron had to work out the decision tree from scratch and go through it with Mrs. Pinelli from beginning to end.

Decision Analysis Spurned

Mrs. Pinelli wasn't too happy with the "answer" (predictable though it was) that came out of the decision analysis. She agreed, however, to think things over for a week, during which Jeanne would find out whatever additional facts might help answer her questions. "This is quite a disease," said Mrs. Pinelli.

The next week, however, when Mrs. Pinelli came in, she immediately said, "Look, I want to see a specialist." S. sent her to Dr. Alan Berg, a prominent internist who specialized in hypertension and related conditions. He and S. were old friends and fellow students who had remained on the best of terms.

Dr. Berg chatted amiably with his new patient and then got down to business. He agreed to do some preliminary tests, including an IVP, but said that in all likelihood he would be treating her high blood pressure with medications. The interview proceeded smoothly until Dr. Berg concluded, "Unless I am satisfied that I have exhausted every possible avenue of medical treatment, I will not be comfortable sending you back to surgery. I think we can treat this thing well enough medically to prevent you from needing surgery again." Mrs. Pinelli shot back, "How are you going to prevent me from feeling like a zombie all the time?"

This was the first indication Dr. Berg had of Mrs. Pinelli's anger at doctors and medicine. Questioning her further, he soon realized that what she wanted was to exhaust every possible avenue of *surgical* treatment before going back to medications. Acting as the "good" doctor who was responsive to his patient's wishes, he went against his own judgment and put Mrs. Pinelli in the hospital for ten days. There he put her through a complete workup (including an arteriogram after a negative IVP) which he could have predicted would be inconclusive and wasteful—to the tune of thousands of dollars taken from the pockets of insurance subscribers. He did it to satisfy Mrs. Pinelli's desire to "know for sure" so that she might then become more amenable to taking medications.

S., meanwhile, wondered what was happening. When he found out that Mrs. Pinelli was in the hospital being tested, he was irked. His instructions, it seemed, had been ignored. The investment he had made in engaging Mrs. Pinelli in critical thinking was going down the drain. So he telephoned Dr. Berg and said, "Hey, Alan, I want my patient back! I only referred her to you for consultation."

It turned out that S., instead of writing Dr. Berg a note, had simply checked off on the referral form a box marked, "Please see and follow with us." Dr. Berg, who later said that he was too busy to read check marks on forms, had assumed that S. was giving him full discretion to handle the case. Although he often had patients referred to him by family doctors from upstate, he did not think of patients in the city as having family doctors. When local patients came to him, he usually ended up becoming "their doctor."

Dr. Berg apologized for the misunderstanding, sent S. the test results, and told Mrs. Pinelli that from now on she would be going back to her family doctor. This development was as big a surprise to her as it had been to Dr. Berg. She, too, had thought that Dr. Berg was now her doctor, her case being of the sort that required a specialist's attention. But she went where she was told to go.

The arteriogram showed that (as would have been expected after a normal IVP) Mrs. Pinelli's previous arterial bypass was still working properly and that there was no clear indication of any progression of stenosis in the other renal artery. There would be no surgery. Back in S.'s office, Mrs. Pinelli reported that, with the catheters and the hot dye going through her body, the arteriogram had been like "a torture rack." She didn't ever want to have one again. But at least it had reconciled her to taking pills for the rest of her life. Still, she made wistful allusions to new pills and new diagnostic tests that would be coming out in the next few years. (There was hope for surgery yet!) In the meantime, on Dr. Berg's suggestion S. was trying out some pills that didn't make her feel so sleepy as before. His strategy was to increase the dosage gradually so as to bring down her blood pressure without knocking her out. Her pressure was still only partially controlled (about 155/100), but he thought it better to achieve a partial success than to bring on disagreeable side effects that would lead the patient to stop taking the medication.

Mrs. Pinelli felt the same way. She was more comfortable with S. and Dr. Berg than with her previous doctor, who had threatened her with heart attacks and strokes if she missed taking one pill. "Dr. S. knows that I skip a pill once in a while," she confided to a nurse in his office. "He knows that it's my choice and that I know what I'm doing. Can you imagine what it feels like to have to walk around the room to keep from falling asleep—and then to hold a pill in your hand that you know will make you feel even *more* that way?"

Mrs. Pinelli indicated what her deepest concerns were when she said, "I'll be satisfied to keep my blood pressure not too far above normal. I'll chance what happens later. If I die when I'm fifty because of this, by then my kids will be able to take care of themselves. My youngest is six years old. Now is when I have to take care of her. If the pills make me so groggy that I can't work, or if my blood pressure goes so high that it kills me, what will she do?"

Mrs. Pinelli could have expressed these values through the decision analysis procedure. Her concern for her children would have had as much weight in her decisions as she chose to give it. Yet she didn't care to find this out. She was willing to lie still for the arteriogram, but she wouldn't sit still for the decision analysis. She viewed the procedure as biased (as Jeanne presented it), abstract, and irrelevant. When Jeanne had told her the four basic options, she had said, "Oh, I know all that stuff already." Somehow the procedure didn't give her the room she needed to express her own concerns in her own language.

Decision analysis assumes that a series of decisions extending into the future, although admittedly influenced by intervening events, can be anticipated and structured in advance. It is not easy to adjust a decision tree when people come to conceive of later decisions differently after having experienced the consequences of prior decisions. For example, in Mrs. Pinelli's case each decision introduced new psychological factors which predisposed the patient and doctors to make subsequent choices that were not anticipated by the decision analysis. In retrospect it is hard to see how they could have been anticipated.

Take, for example, Dr. S.'s decision to hospitalize Mrs. Pinelli immediately. Her blood pressure had to be brought down quickly, and S. wanted her to be in a place where she could be monitored. Nothing, however, was actually done in the hospital that couldn't have been done in her home or in his office. Even if she had confirmed his worst fears by having a stroke, it is not clear that she would have been much better off having it in the hospital. Yet S.'s reflex reaction was (as almost any doctor's would have been) to hospitalize her, not only because she somehow felt that she would be safer in the hospital, but also so as to protect himself against possible professional criticism. Since his decision *was* a reflex reaction, it is unlikely that he could have made his motivations accessible to decision analysis ahead of time.

That initial decision set in motion a chain of unintended events that led to the unnecessary arteriogram. When S. put Mrs. Pinelli in the hospital, he reduced his own contact with and influence over her and exposed her to the influence of house officers, nurses, and technicians who expressed their own version of an aggressive surgeon's mentality: "When you test, you can see, and to see is to know. Once you know, you can cut, and to cut is to cure." This visual, tangible imagery made a powerful impression on Mrs. Pinelli. Ironically, this woman who was so angry at doctors and hospitals accepted (as a result of her present and previous hospitalizations as well as her whole life experience in this society) much of their picture of reality.

By the time Mrs. Pinelli saw Dr. Berg, she had been given so much contradictory information (as when she heard Dr. S. arguing with another doctor in the hospital) that she felt all the more justified in her impatience and in her demand for a precise diagnosis, which Dr. Berg felt powerless to resist. When he implicitly reinforced her "visual" image of diagnosis by authorizing an IVP, he may have unwittingly made the next diagnostic operation, the arteriogram, almost a *fait accompli.* Although both he and Dr. S. had told Mrs. Pinelli that an arteriogram was not likely to be a useful procedure for her, the message she kept in mind was one that she got from a house officer: "You can see some things on the IVP, but you can see everything on the arteriogram. If you have gone this far, you might as well go all the way."

Going to the hospital, insisting on seeing a specialist, having an IVP and then an arteriogram—each decision almost automatically touched off the next rather than being viewed in isolation and made on its own merits, as in decision analysis. All concerned made decisions by and large unconsciously and sometimes irrationally. Their reasons for making the choices they did (e.g., S.'s concern that his actions be profes-

sionally and legally defensible, Dr. Berg's respect for "patient's rights," Mrs. Pinelli's sense of responsibility toward her
family) generally made sense at some level. Decision analysis
ideally would have reflected such concerns. It would have
been difficult if not impossible, however, for these three people to include in the decision analysis all the various and sun-
dry considerations that ultimately guided their actions, some
of which they were not conscious of, some of which they
would not have been comfortable dealing with explicitly and
publicly, and some of which they never could have predicted
would come up.

Throughout the case, decisions were influenced by unexpected events and situational factors. The patient and her two
doctors were operating in the context of disagreement, inadequate communication, and territorial conflicts among doctors;
a clash of assumptions and perceptions between patient and
doctor; a changing understanding of the treatment of the disease in question; and a health-insurance system that provides
no incentive for patients and doctors to consider the cost of
unnecessary procedures and no reimbursement for the time a
doctor spends speaking with a patient. These contextual issues
were not extraneous to the decisions at hand: they were essential elements in those decisions.

Mrs. Pinelli's "decision analysis bypass operation" left
Jeanne Aaron disappointed and frustrated. Jeanne was still
"high" on decision analysis. "It would have worked if she had
only listened!" she exclaimed to S. "After all, it gave her what
turned out to be the right answer!"

S. wasn't so sure. He realized that he and Jeanne, inex-
perienced as they were at the new technique, might not have
presented it as clearly as possible. Maybe they hadn't given it
a fair trial. On the other hand, what experience he had was
beginning to teach him that one cannot say much about any
tool or instrument without considering the contexts in which
people use it. It had required an expensive, futile technical
procedure (the diagnostic workup) to satisfy Mrs. Pinelli that
she didn't need surgery. S. had tried to satisfy her instead with
another technical procedure—decision analysis. It would have
been better, he realized, if he could have gotten through to her

in her own language. "People often say that a picture is worth a thousand words," he might have told her, "and you may think that a picture of your renal artery is worth a thousand dollars. But you know, sometimes you can see something and still not be sure what it is. There may be many ways of interpreting it. Even looking at a picture involves a gamble."

In the future S. would not take for granted, as he had with Mrs. Pinelli, that his patients' understanding of the decision-making process was—or should be—the same as his. Even in cases where he did use decision analysis, he would ask questions like, "What does this mean to you? What do you want to do with it?" Involving a patient like Mrs. Pinelli in decision-making might mean challenging her, as by saying, "So you think an IVP is worth doing? Well, what would you bet me, and what odds would you give, that it will reveal anything useful?" It would mean showing her and all his patients that they could work with him to create their own gambles.

6

DECISION ANALYSIS: USE WITH CAUTION

As time went on, S. found himself thinking of decision analysis more and more in the past tense. His patients' reactions led the way. Some, like Mrs. Pinelli, turned away from decision analysis altogether (and sometimes turned away from S. along with it). Others thought they had to follow it slavishly. Whenever S. would ask them, "What do you say about this?" they would throw the question right back at him: "What does the decision analysis say?" Although patients tended to be all too receptive to the "answers" that came out of decision analysis, it was often hard to engage them in the process of arriving at an answer.

For S., working with decision analysis had been a way of learning how to make decisions probabilistically over time. Somewhere at the back of his mind the formal decision-making framework still structured his thoughts (cf. Raiffa, 1968). Occasionally, when he wanted to clarify his thinking about an unfamiliar problem, he would "rough out" a decision tree, usually one that involved just one or two decisions rather than a long string of them. The procedure as a whole, however, turned out not to be flexible or efficient enough to handle the diverse situations he faced in his practice, where it sometimes seemed as if little remained the same from one day to the next, and

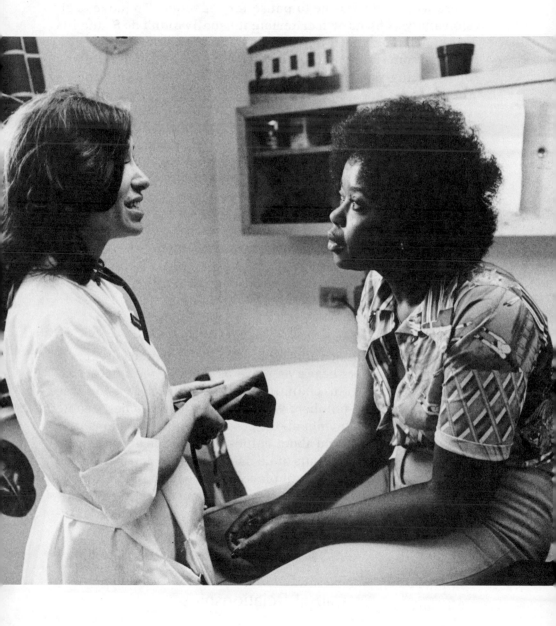

there wasn't much time to pause for reflection. To judge decision analysis by its own criterion: it usually didn't do S. and his patients enough good to justify all the effort it required.

S. had come to see that there are two major difficulties in using decision analysis. One is that the procedure is only as reliable as the various kinds of data that go into it, and those data all contain some degree of uncertainty. The other is that decision analysis involves some presuppositions that have their origins in the Mechanistic Paradigm. Not only do people tend to use decision analysis (like everything else) mechanistically, but it doesn't easily lend itself to being used any other way.

Garbage In, Garbage Out

Decision analysis ends with a set of exact-sounding numbers. By the time the calculations are finished, one can easily forget that those numbers began as more or less imprecise observations in an uncertain, changing world. Before a decision tree can be drawn and numbers written along its branches, people have to make judgments about possible causal relationships, about probabilities, and about values. The degree of confidence one can place in the results of decision analysis depends on the degree of confidence one can place in these human judgments, which are not made any more certain or permanently valid by being expressed in numbers and operated upon mathematically.

Causal Relationships

The very structure of a decision tree is based upon some assumptions about the world. Before one can estimate how probable it is that a given set of symptoms or test results has been caused by one disease or another, one must draw branches on the tree for whatever diseases have a *possible* causal connection with those visible signs. Similarly, one draws branches for those tests or treatments that have some relevance to the diseases in question, and for those outcomes (improvement, no improvement, side effects, etc.) that can reasonably be expected to follow from the actions taken. These choices, although they may be well supported by experience and knowledge, are still choices and need not be irrevocable, for one's knowledge of what causes can have what effects may change. If one examines standard decision trees (e.g., for hypertension), one can see where they might be redrawn on the basis of recently acquired knowledge. One must continually ask whether there is enough new information to warrant redrawing the tree.

Probability Estimates

"Four percent, seventy-five percent—what do those numbers have to do with me?" asked Mrs. Pinelli during a subsequent conversation with S. "Oh, I know that you changed them 'just for me' because I had had kidney artery trouble before. But how could you tell that the numbers you finally came up with out of your head were any more tailor-made for me than the numbers out of the tables?"

S. saw what she was getting at. It wasn't that there was anything illegitimate about either statistics or subjective judgment as a basis for probability estimates; after all, these were all that one had to go on. Rather, Mrs. Pinelli was pointing out the incompatibility between the exact numerical expression of probability estimates and their inexact origins. She saw through the precision of the form to the imprecision of the substance. What she said held for both objective probability estimates (those based on frequency data) and subjective ones (those based on individual or collective judgment). And indeed, S. realized that there were problems (not disabling, but sobering) with both kinds of probability estimation.

In the case of objective, frequency-based estimates, not only the numbers themselves but the methods used to obtain them have a reassuring aura of precision. For example, the data on which probability estimates are based may come from experimental studies comparing the efficacy of different treatments. In one type of study subjects are randomly assigned to experimental groups receiving one or another treatment (or a *placebo,* a physiologically inactive substance administered as if it were an active medication). Such *randomized* studies represent what we commonly think of as "exact science." Yet according to Criterion #2 of the Probabilistic Paradigm, the results of randomized clinical studies (like any other experiments) are affected by the process of experimentation. What the experimenters do and how the experimental subjects react are influenced by their knowledge that they are administering or receiving one treatment rather than another.

Such effects may be minimized through the use of the double-blind technique, in which neither the patients receiving an experimental treatment nor the doctors administering it are told which treatment it is. The double-blind procedure works well with drugs, which are easily disguised. It does not work in more complex situations that require conscious participation by patients and doctors (e.g., home versus hospital birth). Especially when the double-blind precaution is taken, randomized studies tend to be elaborate and costly. There is also the problem of how the results for both groups are affected by the knowledge that this is, after all, an experiment. Randomized studies also entail a potential ethical dilemma, in that half of the experimental patients do not get what may turn out to be the better of the two treatments being tested.

Given these shortcomings of the randomized method, even with double-blind controls, many investigators have searched for a better approach. There is, in fact, an experimental technique that is more probabilistic in spirit, more sensitive to the changing nature of the world, and fairer to subjects. This method assigns subjects to experimental groups on a *sequential* rather than randomized basis (Weinstein, 1974). In this "two-armed bandit" approach to clinical research the experimenters try out the treatments under consideration in the way a gambler might find out which of two slot machines pays off more often. Here patients are treated one at a time instead of all at once as in randomized comparison studies. The first patient is given Drug A. If this patient recovers within the number of days established as the criterion for "cure," then the second patient is also given Drug A. If the second patient does not show the requisite improvement, then the third patient is given Drug B. This drug likewise is used as long as it "works." If it doesn't work for one patient, the experimenters switch back to Drug A for the next.

The sequential method has the ethical advantage that the number of patients given each treatment is roughly proportional to the effectiveness of the treatment. The better a treatment turns out to be, relative to the other treatment(s) tested, the more patients will have received that treatment during the experiment. Moreover, this type of experiment embodies the principle of stochastic causality within the experiment itself. In contrast with the static time frame of a randomized study, sequential trials stretch over a period of time during which changes in probabilities can be picked up if they occur. Although changes in probabilities may not often occur in the length of time it takes to do a study, they can occur, say, if bacteria mutate so as to become resistant to a previously effective drug. In psychiatry, for example, new treatments (both drug and otherwise) tend to be very effective at first and then to become less so, whether because the doctors and patients using the treatments become less enthusiastic or less careful, or simply because the treatments are given to other patients besides the selected group of initially responsive patients (Tourney, 1967). An ongoing sequential study would be a good way to measure this psychiatric Hawthorne effect.

Notwithstanding the advantages of sequential trials, no experimental method can do away with the uncertainties of experimentation or the complexities of the world. Tables of data, whether obtained from research studies or recorded clinical experience, contain built-in layers of uncertainty. As psychologist Ward Edwards has observed:

. . . My friends who are expert about medical records tell me that to attempt to dig out from even the most sophisticated hospital's records the frequency of association between any particular symptom and any particular diagnosis is next to impossible—and when I raise the question of complexes of symptoms, they stop speaking to me. For another thing, doctors keep telling me that diseases change, that this year's flu is different from last year's flu, so that symptom-disease records extending far back in time are of very limited usefulness. Moreover, the observation of symptoms is well-supplied with error, and the diagnosis of diseases is even more so; both kinds of errors will ordinarily be frozen permanently into symptom-disease statistics. Finally, even if diseases didn't change, doctors would. The usefulness of disease categories is so much a function of available treatments that these categories themselves change as treatments change—a fact hard to incorporate into symptom-disease statistics (Edwards, 1972, pp. 139–140).

When it comes to applying the data to the individual case in practice, yet another layer of uncertainty is added. With both diagnostic and treatment probabilities, subjective judgment is required. For example, S. had a diagnostic probability table which gave the likelihood that a middle-aged male smoker who coughed had lung cancer. A patient of S.'s fit into this category, but he also had worked in a coal mine and had a family history of tuberculosis. There was no information in the table pertaining to such a patient; indeed the table could not possibly account for every variation and refinement of its basic categories that an individual patient might present. Yet S. had to account for these additional facts in estimating the probability that his patient had lung cancer rather than tuberculosis or black-lung disease.

He had to do the same when it came to treatment. Although hypertension, for example, is often associated with stress and anxiety, most of S.'s colleagues believed that elevated blood pressure could not be lowered by minor tranquilizers. In an algorithm for hypertension the probability that the condition could be successfully treated through the use of such medications would be listed as 0. S. disagreed. He regarded some of his patients with mild hypertension as anxious people whose blood pressure varied with their state of mind. Departing from the data, he explained to patients the costs and benefits of various treatment options, including minor tranquilizer use. Where this unorthodox treatment was chosen by the patient, it was successful about fifty percent of the time. In this way S., like any doctor, was able to build up a set of informal, mostly unwritten probability tables of his own which sometimes departed from the statistical norms so as to be consistent with his experience.

Whether or not objective probability data exist (all the more so when they do not), subjective judgment must play a part in estimating probabilities. Subjective judgment is no less fallible than tables of figures. An advantage, perhaps, is that it is less likely to appear infallible and to be thought of as such, especially in a world where people are not comfortable dealing with probabilities.

Mrs. Pinelli was not alone in finding the concept of probability not entirely compelling, and indeed a bit foreign. Most people, having been brought up under the Mechanistic Paradigm, have some difficulty even thinking in terms of probabilities, let alone training their senses to make good subjective probability estimates. And the estimates they do make can't help but be affected by the mechanistic assumptions that in varying degrees underlie everyone's thinking today. For example, by not taking into account the first criterion of the Probabilistic Paradigm (which holds that causes can come and go over time), people tend to estimate the probability of a future event based on their best guess as to the probability of its happening in the present. Moreover, people tend to be as confident in predicting events in the distant future as they are about events in the near future. This can lead to overconfidence. As patients and doctors gain practice in estimating probabilities, they will do better at it. But the numbers they come up with will still be no more than estimates.

Values

Values, too, can be estimated by objective and subjective methods. So-called objective techniques involve finding a numerical scale that exists independent of the observer and can be applied to any medical situation. The scale most commonly used is that of dollars and cents. On this scale the consequences of illness and treatment are measured in terms of how much future income the patient will lose. Such a monetary measure of values is rather obviously incomplete, for it does not include consequences other than lost work time, such as pain. It also values human lives in an unequal and unfair manner. On this scale a secretary's life might be worth only one fifth as much as that of her boss.

Since values have an inherently subjective quality (although by Criterion #3 of the Probabilistic Paradigm they are not *wholly* subjective), various measures have been proposed to take subjectivity into account. The "lottery method" described in the previous chapter is one such technique that takes into account subjective attitudes toward risk. Mrs. Pinelli, however, had some choice words to say about this "game."

"How can you talk about money and years of life in the same breath? Lottery, indeed! I don't play games where my life is involved. That was a big reason why I said enough to the whole decision analysis business. What I wanted instead was some solid information to sink my teeth into, like the information the arteriogram can give you: a picture that shows you what's wrong and how to fix it."

As S. understood, Mrs. Pinelli had her reasons for placing value on things, but Jeanne in her enthusiasm found it difficult to listen. Also, a measuring procedure that aligns all values along one dimension obscures the fact that many decisions call forth values that cannot be easily compared. These may involve principles that constrain choice, "thresholds" below which some values cannot be compromised. To use an example given by legal scholar Laurence Tribe (1972) in his critique of formal decision-making methods, social planners cannot bargain away one person's arms and legs because another person would gain more "satisfaction" in numerical terms by having them cut off than the first person would lose. The citizen's right to breathe clean air can be measured against the industrialist's right to pollute the air for a productive purpose—but not to the point where the citizen cannot breathe at all without suffering a severe health hazard. The value of the preservation of human life cannot be reduced to numbers.

Such discontinuities in values tend to occur where individual satisfaction clashes with the common good. They also can occur, however, within the value scheme of a single individual. How can numbers, arrayed on a one-dimensional scale, adequately convey a paradoxical attitude such as this: "It is unacceptable to me to lose my eyesight—I can't see how I could go on living; but then I guess I wouldn't just kill myself if I were blinded—not right away, at least"? This seeming contradiction is a common human sentiment, one to which we cannot do justice by saying that the person values death at "0" and blindness at "5" or "10." Mrs. Pinelli exhibited a similar complexity of response as she oscillated between trying to do something about the symptoms of severe hypertension and resisting the side effects of the medication. Yet she had an underlying concern that made sense of the apparent contradiction—namely, her fear of being disabled as a parent, whether by the illness or by the treatment. She had her reasons for valuing the things she did, but these became less clear when her values were reduced to numbers.

The lottery method is designed to enable people to express their attitudes toward risk. These attitudes, however, may not be consistent over the range of situations people face. Someone may be much more averse to risk in Russian roulette than with a roulette wheel. Someone may like to gamble at the racetrack, but not in the doctor's office. Another context that influences evaluation is that of the progression of items as they occur in thought or speech. In reflection or conversation there is a natural order in which various possibilities come up for evaluation. Presented in a different order, the possibilities might be evaluated differently. The lottery method, by setting up its own necessarily arbitrary order of presentation, may thereby affect the expression of basic personal values about life and death, health and illness (Bursztajn and Hamm, unpublished).

The lottery method is grounded in the belief that people can make better assessments of their values by making "choices" than when they try to state their values directly. While this may well be true, the kinds of choices people make in an imaginary lottery may not have much to do with the choices they would make in the context of their lives. "I don't care what the numbers say," Mrs. Pinelli said. "There are just some things I can't tolerate. Like walking around being drowsy all the time. I've got to work to support my family. I'm not going to take the slightest chance of leaving them without a home." Mrs. Pinelli's image of her children blocked out all other considerations. A decision analyst would be quick to point out that she could have used the procedure to express the overriding value she placed on her family's well-being. She could have, yet she didn't, because she didn't see the lottery method as a compelling representation of the choices she faced in "real life." It is when choices occur naturally, in the context of living, that people are best able to think about and act on their values.

Refining the Use of Decision Analysis

There are a few technical precautions that can serve to remind doctors and patients of the uncertainties of the data in decision analysis and help those who use decision analysis keep their minds open to new information. One is the practice (as yet not generally followed) of dating all decision trees and algorithms that are disseminated for general use. People who make use of such tools should have the opportunity to judge how likely it is that the information on which a decision tree or algorithm is based has been superseded by more recent findings. Ideally dates should be given both for the structuring of the options and their outcomes and for the data used in estimating probabilities, since both kinds of information can change. Although value assessments will not often appear on a general decision tree, some trees may contain hypothetical value assessments for "typical" patients in certain categories. These, too, should be dated, since the values assigned to outcomes can change on the basis of, for instance, the development of new pain relievers.

Irrespective of how recently the expected value was calculated, one need not and perhaps should not invariably choose the course of action leading to the higher expected value. In a world where perfect information is not available, it makes sense once in a while to check where the "road not taken" would have led one. As opposed to a *deterministic* decision rule, which keeps one on the "best" road, a *stochastic* decision rule recognizes that there is some value to exploring alternate routes occasionally to see whether in some cases one of them might be better than the "best" road. With a stochastic decision rule the greater the difference in expected value between the "best" road and an alternate route, the less often one would chance the latter.

A doctor might, for example, use a stochastic decision rule in treating patients with some kinds of coronary artery disease. For some such patients medical treatment has a higher expected value. For others the expected value of coronary artery bypass surgery is higher. Since these expected values represent "best guesses," it may be worthwhile to explore whether the one treatment really is better than the other for groups of patients for whom the expected value difference is small. How, though, would one allot patients to the treatment that is believed to have the lower expected value? The only ethical way to do so, it would seem, would be by sharing the decision with the patient, so that the patient could knowingly choose whether or not to accept the treatment with the lower expected value.

Tables giving the treatments with the highest expected value for various categories of patients with coronary artery disease have been developed by cardiologist Stephen Pauker (1976), who has pioneered in the use of decision-analytic methods in medicine. The tables indicate probability "thresholds" at which the expected value for one treatment becomes higher than that for the other. A stochastic decision principle can be applied to these tables in the following manner. Suppose, for example, that a particular man with an extremely devastating form of coronary artery disease has an eighty-eight percent chance of having his chest pain relieved by coronary bypass surgery. If this patient is in such great pain that he places a very high value on relief of pain, then Pauker's table of thresholds would recommend surgery as better for this patient than medical treatment. But the table also provides a threshold for changing that decision. It stipulates that surgery is better as long as the probability of a successful operation is above four percent. That is, this person finds his pain so unbearable that he would be willing to have surgery even if the chances of success were only four percent. Given this information, a deterministic decision-maker would choose surgery on the basis of its higher expected value. A stochastic decision-maker would probably choose surgery, on the grounds that the difference between eighty-eight percent and four percent is a decisive one, but might think twice about doing surgery in every such case if its probability of success fell closer to the threshold—say, below ten percent—because of the possibility of error in the probability estimates, as well as of patient-by-patient variation in expected values.

Whether or not one ever uses stochastic decision rules in a mathematical form, one needs to keep in mind the principle that underlies them. If decision analysis is to be used within the Probabilistic Paradigm, it cannot be used as an *experimentum crucis* that purports to make choice unnecessary. Decision analysis does not tell doctors and patients how to act; rather it contributes evidence to be considered in making choices critically. This is true whether one is using standard decision trees and algorithms or a decision tree constructed especially for a particular patient. Even after the structure of the tree and the data have been adapted to the circumstances, needs, and values of the patient, one cannot suspend critical thought. One must still say to oneself, "Okay, I've come up with a nice numerical 'answer,' but does it make sense? How does it match my understanding of the world? Does it jibe with my intuitions?"

Mechanistic Presuppositions
of the Method—and Its Users

Although to use decision analysis as an *experimentum crucis* is to defeat its purpose, that's just what people tend to do. Since people are trained to think in terms of the Mechanistic Paradigm, they are not likely to use decision analysis in a manner consistent with the Probabilistic Paradigm. Furthermore decision analysis itself is based on some mechanistic assumptions.

The Assumption of Fixed Structure

Decision analysis seeks to anticipate all questions. In reality, though, some questions arise only after other questions are answered. In Mrs. Pinelli's case it seemed that everything was turned upside down once the process got under way. The issue was decided by questions that never were anticipated when the decision tree was structured (such as whether it was Dr. Berg's job to take over Mrs. Pinelli's care or simply consult with Dr. S.) and questions whose meaning changed in the course of events (such as what having an arteriogram meant to Mrs. Pinelli). The strength of decision analysis as usually used is its commitment to answering a predefined question; its weakness is that it does not encourage one to redefine the question. Jeanne Aaron, for example, did not concern herself sufficiently with finding out what questions were important to Mrs. Pinelli.

Throughout his work with families S. saw how important time and experience were in changing both the questions and answers of decision-making. He observed that, in the process of making choices and acting on them, people explored what they were and defined what they wanted to be. As they chose one way of acting rather than another, they learned about and indeed changed their values. When a man and woman decided to have a child, they were choosing to become a father and a mother. They were changing themselves as individuals and creating themselves as a family. As the family changed in the course of the pregnancy, not only the decisions they faced but the way they thought about those decisions changed. Not only the values and probabilities but the mind-set within which these were perceived was being subtly altered by new experience. Decision analysis, with the mind-set neatly laid out in a tree, could not automatically accommodate these changes, nor those that subsequently took place when the man and woman decided, by making choices over time, what kind of father and mother they were going to be. When Mrs. Pinelli voiced her concern for her children's welfare as a crucial factor in her own decisions, she was defining the kind of person she aspired to become—and was becoming. This process occurred in the context of everyday life and everyday choices.

When S. began attending births, he tried to structure his own and the family's assessment of alternatives (hospital versus home, anesthetized versus nonanesthetized, etc.) as an ongoing decision analysis. He would draw flow diagrams with decision points throughout the pregnancy, labor, delivery, and postpartum period. But how could he talk about the "expected values" of "outcomes" when a large part of the value of the birth experience for the family came out of a nine-month process of making choices, facing uncertainty together, and accepting personal responsibility for these choices in a manner that would set the tone for their future decision-making? How could he measure the survival and health of the baby "against" the satisfaction the family derived from the experience when the meaning of the "outcome" was so greatly influenced, even created by the manner in which the family felt themselves to have brought about the outcome?

With Mrs. Pinelli, too, decision analysis assumed a stable set of values. Yet her way of dealing with her hypertension did not support this assumption. When she felt the symptoms to be unpleasant and disabling, she did something about the illness. When she felt the side effects of the medication to be unpleasant and disabling, she stopped doing anything about the illness. If her actual decision tree (as opposed to the one Jeanne laid out for her) could be visualized as having two main branches labeled "do something" and "do nothing," then each branch could be seen as leading her back to the beginning, whereupon she would take the other branch. Instead of a series of branches going in the same direction, her tree would look like a pair of linked loops. In this respect Mrs. Pinelli was not so unusual. Decision trees do not adequately represent the circuitous paths along which people may be led by their unstable values.

Ironically one of the experiences that contributed to changing Mrs. Pinelli's values and her actions was the experience of using decision analysis. "It's funny," she said in retrospect, "they told me that decision analysis would be a way to think about what to do. But by the time I was finished, the last thing I wanted to do was to think at all. All those boring questions, and those numbers—what did they have to do with anything? You might say I couldn't see the forest for the 'tree.' So when Dr. Berg talked about doing things that you could *see,* I jumped right up and told him that that was what I *wanted.* I was so tired of thinking, I just wanted to have something I could see, like when you've been working so hard that all you can stand to do is look at a movie for two hours." In other words, just as decision analysis is changed by the person who uses it, so in this case Mrs. Pinelli was changed by decision analysis.

As S. learned to observe and experience decision-making more consciously, he realized how well the process illustrates the first and second criteria of the Probabilistic Paradigm. In a world where information is shaped by the act of eliciting it, where the tool changes the user and the user changes the tool, where answers prompt new questions and decisions create further choices, people need decision-making procedures that are sensitive to change as it occurs. Decision analysis locks people into preexisting categories for decision-making. Of course, one can always redraw the tree, but that takes work. It is easier to deny the new perceptions, the thoughts and feelings that don't fit. With all its good intentions decision analysis can sometimes lead to what psychologists Buzzy Chanowitz and Ellen Langer (unpublished) call "premature cognitive commitment," or what S. would call a closed mind.

The Fact-Value Dichotomy

According to the third criterion of the Probabilistic Paradigm facts are perceived in terms of people's values, and values are facts about people that can be rationally understood and discussed as other facts can. Decision analysis, however, by its very structure separates facts—which are dealt with rationally through probabilities—from values—which are not considered to be rationally discussible. Mrs. Pinelli's outburst against "that silly game" (the lottery method) was a reaction to her feeling that S. and Jeanne were patronizing her by treating her values as completely irrational and therefore somehow childish. In her view her values were rationally justifiable, since they were grounded in her sense of the responsibilities of an adult.

S. could hardly fault Mrs. Pinelli, or any of his patients, for having trouble making the separate judgments of probability and value that went into calculating the expected value. In Mrs. Pinelli's words, "Jeanne multiplied the value by the probability to get the answer. But I think I was doing a little of that just to get the 'value' in the first place. So weren't we doing the same thing twice?" Of course, Mrs. Pinelli wasn't supposed to figure the probability into the value. The procedure called for her to evaluate first how good or bad something would be if it happened to her, and then how likely it was to happen. These two estimates together would make up the expected value. It is unrealistic, however, to expect people to be able to draw such a sharp line between probability and value. People evaluate a possible event in terms of its meaning for their lives. If she were asked, "What if the sky fell in?" Mrs. Pinelli would find it hard to focus on the seriousness of the consequences. Such a question would strike her as an abstract exercise, a "game." If, on the other hand, she were asked, "What if you lost your job?" she would feel the hypothetical consequences more intensely—not because they would actually be more dire than those of the sky falling in, but because they would be more likely to happen.

Bias Toward Quantifiable Data

There is a fable about a drunk who was seen groping around on the ground in the light cast through a doorway. A passerby asked him what he was doing. "I'm looking for my key," the drunk replied. "Where did you lose it?" "In the alley over there." "So why are you looking here?" the passerby asked with surprise. "Because it's light here." Similarly, decision analysts may tend, without even realizing it, to look where their method sheds light rather than where light needs to be shed. Where decision analysis sheds light is on "hard facts"—those that can be expressed in its own language of numbers and mathematical calculation.

As Laurence Tribe puts it, "Even the most sophisticated user is subject to an overwhelming temptation to feed his pet the food it can most comfortably digest" (1971, pp. 1361–1362). Taking an example from criminal law, he tells of two analysts ("one a legal scholar and the other a teacher of statistical theory") who, in estimating the probability that a palm print resembling the defendant's would be found on a knife used as a murder weapon if the defendant was or was not the murderer, simply equated the probability that the print was actually the defendant's with the probability that the defendant committed the murder. They disregarded the obvious possibility that the defendant committed the murder without leaving a print, or that someone else incriminated the defendant by using a knife which already bore the defendant's print. These possibilities did not easily fit into the analysts' formula, and therefore (apparently) were not considered.

If two highly trained observers could make such an error under the seductive appeal of "mathematical machinery," what about juries—and the rest of us? S. and Jeanne Aaron, two trained medical observers, may well have committed a similar oversight when they did not include a "life-style modification" branch on Mrs. Pinelli's decision tree. The effects of life-style modification on high blood pressure are no less real than those of medications and surgery. They are, however, less well documented statistically.

In a decision-making economy whose currency is numbers, measurable entities (e.g., "facts" with known probabilities, "values" based on financial costs and benefits) drive out unmeasurable entities (e.g., "facts" with unknown probabilities, "values" based on moral principles and sensibilities). Tribe suggests that if questions of guilt and innocence are rephrased as questions of mathematical probabilities, the scope of legal reasoning will be severely narrowed, and jurors may lose the capacity to draw upon a broad context of moral and social values in reaching their verdicts. The issue he poses is equally relevant to medicine, where patients, families, and physicians must make decisions as sensitive and as urgent as those made by juries. The child K.'s need for love could not be quantified as easily as could his diagnostic test results. Mrs. Pinelli's desire to remain alert and lucid while her children were growing up could not be quantified as easily as could her blood pressure readings. Were these concerns therefore not worthy of consideration? A society that implicitly answers in the negative by practicing a narrowly mathematical approach to decision-making or by holding up that approach as a norm is choosing to see itself in a technological light. The people who live in such a society will have difficulty seeing those parts of themselves on which the light does not shine.

Assumption That Reality Can Be Broken Down into Analytical Units

Things take on meaning from their contexts (Dreyfus and Dreyfus, unpublished). If you unscrew a ball-point pen and say, "This part is worth two dollars, and that part is worth one dollar, so I'll sell either part individually or sell the whole pen for three dollars," you are assuming that the whole is the same as the sum of its parts. But if you were on an island where there were no other pens with interchangeable parts, what would either part of the pen be worth individually? If you had nothing to write on, what would the whole pen be worth? What good is a brain without a heart? What would Mrs. Pinelli's life mean to her outside the context of her family?

When Mrs. Pinelli complained that it was not so easy for her to separate value from probability, she was pointing out that the context in which an object exists is part of what the object is, just as the object is part of the context. When decision analysis separates facts from values, one cause from others operating along with it, an individual's welfare from that of the family or community, an illness from a person's life history, one decision from the context of other decisions that define its significance, it turns decision-making into something rather artificial and academic. Of course, some such simplifying assumptions do have to be made if decision-making is to proceed at all, whether or not decision analysis is used. But those who do use decision analysis need to be aware of the special kinds of simplifying assumptions that it entails and the questions these raise when decision analysis is translated into actual decisions. For example, decision analysis will have a better chance to be used critically if the people to be affected by the decisions can create the categories of the analysis rather than simply assuming preformed categories.

Assumption That the Structure of the Tree Is "Given" Rather Than Chosen

Mrs. Pinelli was dissatisfied with some judgments that S. and Jeanne made both at the beginning and the end of the decision analysis. "Why didn't the tree have a branch for doing nothing and then seeing what would happen?" she asked. "Decision analysis is supposed to show *all* the options, but Jeanne only showed me the options that *she* thought were good." For their part S. and Jeanne had given Mrs. Pinelli the "standard" tree for her blood pressure level in order to make the work of decision analysis manageable for her. Since "all" the options would represent too long a list, some judgments had to be made. Still, S. and Jeanne didn't take into account the possibility that what was "standard" to them might not be acceptable to the patient.

When it came to interpreting the probable consequences of each of the "final" outcomes for Mrs. Pinelli's health, she again had questions. "I can't see the point of just saying, 'probability of a stroke in sixteen years.' What's a stroke? Why, they say my mother had three strokes before she finally died of a heart attack at the age of eighty. None of them slowed her down one bit. On the other hand, Uncle Joe had one stroke, and 'puff'—a vegetable. What I want to know is how likely I am to get the kind of stroke that Uncle Joe had. I don't care about any old stroke." Again, the categories that S. and Jeanne set up didn't meet the patient's needs.

Mrs. Pinelli's two complaints show that judgment is required in knowing how much to include in a decision tree. In the first place the decision to draw more or fewer branches is a matter of judgment (Raiffa, 1968). One must evaluate what is to be gained from further subdividing reality as well as from pruning options that may be irrelevant (such as, in Mrs. Pinelli's case, "doing nothing" and "life-style modification"). Second, there is nothing in decision analysis itself that dictates where to stop the chain of actions and results and declare a set of outcomes to be "final." It is not the causal structure of the world, but one's own sense of what causal relations are important, that brings about that choice. To S. and Jeanne "probability of stroke" was a reasonable stopping point. To Mrs. Pinelli it was not.

Again, the need for judgment does not invalidate decision analysis, since anything one does in a probabilistic world requires judgment. Nonetheless, the fact that Mrs. Pinelli threw up her hands at all the details in a procedure that she called a crude oversimplification suggests that the procedure may be at once too complex and too simple. It generates more distinctions than most people can comfortably work with, and yet it doesn't necessarily get to the distinctions that matter to people.

Mathematical Reasoning on Trial

In an article on the use of mathematical decision-making methods in legal proceedings, entitled "Trial by Mathematics," Tribe shows, on the basis of some of the theoretical considerations presented here, that these methods are not the unbiased, "value-neutral" tools that decision scientists would like them to be. Rather, they are full of unacknowledged biases. Mathematical evidence and mathematical arguments can be and have been manipulated so as to distort the legal process and subvert justice. Most people are familiar with the story of the French Captain Alfred Dreyfus, who in 1899 was accused of betraying state secrets to the Germans. The prosecution established its case by using "expert" witnesses who testified to the extremely low probability that certain resemblances between Dreyfus's handwriting and the writing on the incriminating letter could have occurred by chance. Subsequent review showed that the mathematical "proofs" contained in this testimony were worthless. Yet according to a historian quoted by Tribe, the defense counsel and the government commissioner, who admitted they had understood nothing of these arguments, "allowed themselves to be impressed by the scientific phraseology of the system" (Tribe, 1971, pp. 1333–1334).

In another case Tribe cites, this one dating from 1968, witnesses to a California robbery described the perpetrators as a woman with a blond ponytail and a black man with a mustache and a beard who drove a yellow car. A couple who matched this description were convicted after the prosecutor argued that there was only a one in twelve million chance that a randomly chosen couple would have all the characteristics listed. The California Supreme Court reversed the conviction on four separate grounds. First, the prosecutor's estimates of the frequency of occurrence of each characteristic individually were not supported by any evidence. Second, the prosecutor multiplied the probabilities for the separate occurrence of each characteristic to get the probability of the joint

occurrence of the combination of characteristics. This would
be valid only if the various characteristics occurred entirely
independently of one another rather than in relation to one
another, which in this case they clearly did not. For example,
men with beards often also have mustaches. Therefore, if one
out of every ten men has a beard and one out of four has a
mustache, the probability that a man has both a beard and a
mustache cannot be said to be one in forty, but is actually
closer to one in ten. Third, the quantification of these
probabilities diverted the jury from considering the more
difficult to quantify but equally crucial question of whether
the prosecution's witnesses were mistaken or lying. Fourth,
the probability that a randomly chosen couple would have the
same salient characteristics as the defendants did not (as the
prosecutor claimed it did) reflect the probability of the defendant's innocence. For in a sufficiently large universe of
suspect couples—say, twenty-four million, or thirty-six million—there might likely be several couples with these same
characteristics, each of whom would have an equal probability of guilt. In this case the prosecutor made opportunistic use
of mathematical probabilities, the defense attorney (at least
until the appellate hearing) was too bewildered to make effective rebuttal, and the jury was swayed from its better judgment by the spell of the numbers.

Tribe's concern is that the explicit use of mathematical
probability in legal trials, as well as in establishing standards
of legal proof, may undermine legal reasoning. Mathematical
proofs are subject to exploitive misuse because their valid use
involves complexities not easily grasped by lawyers and jurors. They also are likely to distract judges and juries from
deciding the simple questions of fact and the complex questions of moral intention that traditionally have been the prov-
ince of law. We may assume that jurors make implicit
probability estimates in arriving at their verdicts, just as all
of us do in daily life. To quantify such estimates explicitly
using Bayesian computations would, however, fundamentally
change the character of legal decision-making. It would put
into jeopardy, Tribe believes, two fundamental principles of
law: the presumption of innocence and the "reasonable

doubt" criterion for conviction. Thus if we choose to "try by mathematics," we as a society will be changing what we value and what we are.

From Decision Analysis to Gambling

In his discussion of the symbolic, expressive function of the rules of trial procedure Tribe makes an important distinction between dead ritual and what we might call rules to live by:

> Some of those rules, to be sure, reflect only "an arid ritual of meaningless form," but others express profoundly significant moral relationships and principles—principles too subtle to be translated into anything less complex than the intricate symbolism of the trial process (Tribe, 1971, p. 1391).

Rituals that are arid involve activities done mindlessly, repetitively, uncritically; i.e., mechanistically. Rules to live by, on the other hand, can ultimately enhance the possibility of critical choice rather than suppress it. They are similar to rituals insofar as they take some things for granted, but they do so in such a way as to allow one to keep an open mind. Even in the Probabilistic Paradigm, one begins with assumptions. One cannot keep an open mind if everything is open to question, for then chaos ensues. Where everything is taken for granted, or where nothing is taken for granted, the result is the same—the negation of critical choice.

Rules to live by embody principles used consciously and explicitly, so that they can serve as standards to be held up, lived up to, argued with, dissented from, and occasionally broken. The principles of the law are richer and more useful for having been derived from ethics rather than from the mechanistic science of the nineteenth century. They acknowledge the moral consequences and practical implications of uncertainty without lapsing into utter relativism, since in law something must finally be decided. "Reasonable doubt" is such a principle. For there to be reasonable doubt, there must first be doubt; then there must be reason.

It is thus apparent that similar principles can be arrived at from several different directions: from ethics, from the rules of law, or from the Probabilistic Paradigm of twentieth-century science. It is not surprising that there is often a convergence among the principles drawn from such different areas. For all of them represent human wisdom as derived from experience, wisdom that encompasses the good as well as the true.

Medicine has both rituals and rules to live by. There are, on the one hand, the savage rituals of contemporary medicine, like the unnecessary tests that K. was subjected to and that Mrs. Pinelli was taught to request. Doing things over and over again makes us less fearful, because then we know what to expect. It is a way to assert control in the face of uncertainty. But the assertion is strained, the control illusory, because the reality and the terror remain, though they may be inaccessible. And so, again and again, doctors and patients act out the ritual of "looking at the picture," so as to be sure not beyond *reasonable* doubt, but beyond all doubt.

There are, on the other hand, principles and rules to live by in medicine—the manners and mutual respect between doctor and patient along with consideration for their different areas of authority. It is these principles and rules—ancient in their ethics, modern in their acknowledgment of the unknown—and not the "arid rituals" of the present that need to be revived and strengthened.

Decision analysis, designed to help people free themselves from the dead rituals of medicine, came in S.'s eyes to look like a dead ritual itself. It was at once unconvincingly abstract and forbiddingly detailed. It aspired to a formal precision that broke down when one looked closely at its component parts. Decision analysis, it seemed, would be of little day-to-day use to doctors and less to patients. There might even be times when it would come between doctors and patients, if Mrs. Pinelli's reaction was any indication. "I just didn't trust myself after that whole business," she recalled. "The more Jeanne talked, the less I knew what to do. That's why I just nodded 'yes' to whatever she said and then asked to see a specialist. I just didn't know what to think, so I wanted to talk to someone who did."

For doctors and patients to face uncertainty together, S. realized, there had to be trust between them. If people became too uncertain about themselves and each other, they would flee from the additional uncertainties that medical decision-making presented. They would flee, presumably, back to the comforting rituals of mechanistic practice, the "seeing" and the "doing."

Rejecting the "elusive ideal of wholly objective, impersonal, and detached instrumental analysis" as "not only unattainable but destructive," Tribe has called for "a subtler . . . and more complex style of problem solving" (1972, pp. 107–108). Principles for decision-making are needed that can be used in the contexts in which people actually make decisions. What is needed is a way of thinking that doctors and patients can use together, one that seems natural to people because they already use it in their daily lives, one that encourages people to reason instead of diverting them with calculations, one that engages people in examining their own lives in order to create their own probabilities, values, and categories for making choices.

S. developed such a method through trying to explain to patients in their own language what it meant to make decisions probabilistically. He would say, for example, "It's like betting on the horses, or on a poker game. You're given the odds, but then you have to decide what you think the odds of winning really are. If you can get betting odds that you think are favorable, and if you can afford to bet, then you bet. How much you bet depends on how much you can stand to lose, how much you want to win, and what it's all worth to you. When you come here from now on, just imagine that you're going to the racetrack or the casinos in Las Vegas; but, of course, science will be there to guide you, and so will I."

Already in his mind's eye S. saw the big neon sign flashing in front of his office: YOU PAYS YOUR MONEY AND YOU TAKES YOUR CHANCES.

7

UNCONSCIOUS AND CONSCIOUS GAMBLING

To most people the word *gambling* suggests abdicating control of one's fate in the face of total uncertainty. The idea of "taking chances" with one's own or a loved one's life and health sounds foolhardy and irresponsible; the idea of a doctor's gambling with the lives of patients seems repugnant. Yet we recall that under the Probabilistic Paradigm everything a scientist does in order to gain knowledge is a kind of gamble. Acknowledging a degree of uncertainty in the world, the scientist gambles not as an abdication of control, but as a way of exerting a degree of control. The gambling that Dr. S. and some of his patients adopted as a model for medical decision-making wasn't the Las Vegas-style recreational or profit-seeking gambling, but rather this scientific gambling under the Probabilistic Paradigm. Although (as we shall see) the card game and the casino are models that are sometimes followed in medicine as it is currently practiced, our intuitions are correct when they tell us that these are not good models for gambling in medicine.

Making decisions under conditions of uncertainty is a form of gambling. Like the gambler the decision-maker (whether or not with the help of formal decision analysis) seeks informa-

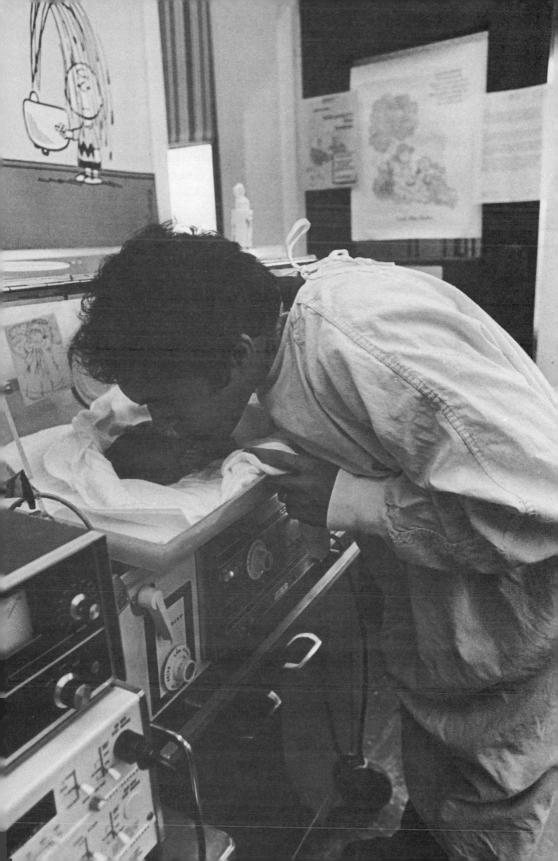

tion about possible gains and losses and then weighs the gains against the losses in terms of their probability and value. Nonetheless, there are some important differences between what we usually think of as gambling and the kind of gambling that is done in science, including the science of medical practice.

Clinic or Casino?

In casino gambling or in betting among friends, we can choose whether to play and how much to bet. We can set limits on the stakes, and we can quit while we're ahead or throw in our cards when the game gets rough. In medicine, on the other hand, the decision to gamble is not a voluntary one. In most cases we don't decide when to get sick. We can walk out of the doctor's office or hospital, but that choice is itself a gamble. Even if we stop going to the doctor, there is still uncertainty.

All choices in life are gambles. That is, we act with hope, but there are no guarantees. All choices that are worth thinking about (including many that we make without thinking) are worth thinking about as gambles—whether they are choices to act, to seek more information, or to believe something, or choices *not* to act, seek information, or believe. It is a gamble to go to the doctor or not to go to the doctor, to diagnose or not to diagnose, to treat or not to treat.

Moreover, in such real-life gambles the stakes may be higher than in recreational gambles—sometimes as high as life and death. Gambling in life is more than just a game. The consequences of our choices are not limited to an artificial sphere of activity, but are felt throughout our lives. We never know quite how much we are risking on each throw. We have all the more reason, therefore, to make those choices consciously, with some critical understanding of how we are gambling and what may be at stake.

Paradoxically, though, it is more difficult to gamble consciously in life than in a game that is set apart from life. In a game we at least know that we are gambling. In real life, where we are not deliberately doing something that is called "gambling," we may tend to gamble unawares. It is easier to gamble with eyes open when the stakes are limited and well defined than in the kind of real-life gamble where we don't know whether we've won or lost (or how long it will take before we will know), and where we rarely win or lose irrevocably. No wonder we don't always know, or want to know, that we're gambling. Gambling consciously would mean looking uncertainty in the face and acknowledging that we don't have as much control over our lives as we like to think.

Then, too, at the back of our minds lurk the distasteful images of the compulsive gambler, who is driven to seek the sensations of gambling regardless of the results, and the professional gambler, who lives by winning at others' expense. These are not images of how we want to live. No wonder Mrs. Pinelli didn't go along with the "lottery game" when she was facing life-and-death issues.

There is no simple antidote to our emotional discomfort with gambling, but we can describe what it means to gamble in science under the Probabilistic Paradigm and note how different this gambling is from both the compulsive and exploitive styles of gambling. In medicine, for example, one wins a diagnostic gamble by believing and acting on a correct diagnosis or by rejecting an incorrect diagnosis. One loses by believing and acting on an incorrect diagnosis or by rejecting a correct diagnosis. One wins a treatment gamble by trying a treatment that works or by not trying a treatment that would not have worked. One loses by trying a treatment that does not work or by not trying a treatment that would have worked. A correct diagnosis is one that can do the patient some good and that is true; this also holds for what can be considered a correct treatment. In scientific gambling, then, we seek not only the good outcome that the horseplayer or casino patron seeks; we also seek truth. Nor are the two easily separated. In the experimentation practiced under the Probabilistic Paradigm, one way of finding out is by taking action, which in turn can affect what is learned.

Treatment can lead to diagnosis, while diagnosis affects the course of treatment.

A type of gambling in which the true and the good are sought differs from the competitive gambling in which one person must lose for another to win. In competitive gambling a group of friends may arrange a card game or football pool in which there is a "pot"—a fixed pool of goods—that changes hands in the course of the game. Some players win, others lose, but the total amount won equals the total amount lost. This is called a "zero-sum game" (a term used in Chapter 4 to describe family relationships based on the principle of exchange). A casino or racetrack operates in the same way, although here the "house" sets the odds so as to skim off a small percentage of the total amount exchanged by the players. In a zero-sum game the doctor and the patient would be gambling against each other—hardly an attractive model for the doctor-patient relationship. However, the scientific gambling that we are applying to medicine more closely resembles another kind of gamble, one in which all the players can win or lose together.

Such cooperative gambling can be illustrated by a party game. Several cone-shaped objects are placed in a large, narrow-necked bottle. Each player holds a string attached to one of the cones. Only one cone at a time can be drawn out of the neck of the bottle. When the players are rewarded individually for the speed with which they get their cones out, they all tend to pull on their strings at the same time. The cones bunch up inside the neck of the bottle, and a traffic jam ensues. When the players are rewarded for teamwork, they cooperate by pulling out their cones one at a time.

Gambling in science takes this cooperative form because there is no fixed pool of winnings. Goods are not simply exchanged, but produced, in the form of knowledge that can be shared. This gambling differs from recreational gambling in that it not only draws upon all our knowledge and experience, but also contributes to it. The stakes are indefinite not only on the losing side, but on the winning side as well. For example, a physician and family who gamble well in their handling of a death can create a positive, nourishing experience even in the face of a large loss. A physician and family who are insensitive in their handling of a birth can rob it of some joy and so suffer loss even when the birth has a "successful" outcome.

Cooperative gambling proceeds according to the principles that govern scientific investigation under the Probabilistic Paradigm. Guided by these principles, one does not gamble in the unprincipled manner of the recreational or acquisitive gambler. Rather, one gambles with an attitude of critical trust toward the operation of cause and chance in the world, toward the gambling strategies with which one seeks to understand cause and chance, toward oneself as a gambler, and toward those with whom one is gambling. In each instance one has some doubt, but one also extends the benefit of the doubt. These principles make it possible for people gambling together (such as a patient, family, and doctor) to make the best of uncertain situations. They make it advantageous, therefore, to face uncertainty and gamble consciously rather than unconsciously.

Unfortunately, this model of cooperative, principled gambling is not always followed in medical practice. This is not surprising, since people are still guided more by the Mechanistic Paradigm than by the Probabilistic. The following case, which S. observed when he was an intern, shows how people sometimes gamble against rather than with each other in difficult medical situations. S., although he had not yet made a habit of thinking of medical decisions as gambles, sensed that there might have been another way to go in this case, a way that might have lessened the family's and the physicians' suffering. The case is a study of unconscious and conscious gambling.

A Double-Edged Gamble

A three-day-old baby looked as if she might have two severe medical problems. For one thing, she "looked funny." Her features were distorted in a way that suggested Down's syndrome, a genetic disease characterized by chromosomal abnormality.

Down's syndrome is commonly known in America as mongolism. Having Down's syndrome would mean being physically and mentally retarded for life. As if this weren't bad enough, the baby looked blue and had difficulty breathing—signs which pointed to heart trouble. In addition to doing a chromosome typing test for Down's syndrome, the family and the hospital staff considered the choice of whether or not to diagnose the heart trouble by catheterization. If a surgically remediable heart condition were found, they would then face the choice of whether to operate.

Both parents were in their mid-thirties. They had two other children. The father found it natural to do most of the talking, and the doctors found it natural to talk mostly with the father. The mother participated in the decision-making by speaking privately with her husband. This role was most comfortable for her because it was her customary role within the family, as well as because she was still exhausted from giving birth. Since it was the father who articulated the family's concerns, the doctors could not tell to what extent his wife agreed with his decisions. This would not have concerned them if he had agreed with *their* decisions. As it turned out, however, serious differences arose.

The father, whose primary concern was with whether the child had any prospect of a normal life, chose to test for Down's syndrome. He did not want to do anything about the heart condition until he had the result of the chromosome analysis, which would take a minimum of three days. Under pressure from the hospital staff he did agree to have the baby catheterized. However, he refused to sign an operative permit, which would have authorized the doctors to operate immediately if they found something they could operate on.

Catheterization revealed "critical aortic stenosis," a marked narrowing of the main artery through which blood is pumped from the heart to the rest of the body. The effects of this condition can be minimized for a few days by carefully administering cardiac drugs and regulating fluid intake. However it is best operated on quickly. Since the father refused permission to operate until the Down's test result was known, the baby was placed on medication to keep up her blood pressure. The catheterization had been a useful procedure, since it established the probabilities on which further action (or nonaction) could be based. And yet the doctors had almost refused to do this procedure without having an operative consent form signed in advance, since for them the only reason for catheterizing was to be able to operate. For them, that is, diagnostic information was meant to be used not only to inform the choice, but to dictate the choice. They wanted the decision to operate to be predetermined. It did not occur to them that it might be better to wait and then evaluate that particular gamble in the context in which it arose—the context of the baby's condition and the parents' feelings at the time.

"It's all so clear and simple," said the senior resident. "You just do the operation." But it was not so clear and simple. The operation promised only to relieve, not cure, the condition. By a senior clinician's rough estimate it might increase the odds from two out of ten to three out of ten that the child would survive and have a chance at normal development. Nobody told the parents this, however. They told them only that the baby would surely die without the operation, but that with it she might have a chance to live. Nonetheless, the father had a pretty realistic understanding of the situation. He sensed that this was not, and would not be, a normal child. He was aware that (1) she might have Down's syndrome; (2) the operation, even if successfully performed, might leave her with a serious heart condition; and (3) even if the operation could give her a normal heart, she might already have suffered brain damage.

The next couple of days were a very difficult time for the baby's parents. Now that an operable condition had been discovered, the doctors stepped up the pressure on the father to operate. With the nurses, like a chorus in the background, chanting, "Don't just stand there; *do* something," the doctors confronted the father: "You mean you're not willing to do anything to save the baby's life?" Driving a wedge of shame through the distressed family, they asked him whether he thought his wife incapable of raising a disabled child. They threatened to take him to court and get an injunction forcing him to let them operate. Warning that the baby would likely die while the father was waiting for the Down's test result, they threatened not to revive her if her heart stopped. In this way, they insinuated, the father would be responsible for his child's death.

It is easy to imagine a reasonable way in which the last threat might have been worded. The doctors might have said, "Well, if that's the way you feel, then we don't see any reason to take extraordinary measures to save the baby if she arrests." And it is easy to see how the doctors would not have wanted to fight a battle with one hand tied behind their backs. Still, by being unwilling to give the father the benefit of the doubt (i.e., to assume until shown otherwise that he was a reasonable person to gamble with), they made it almost impossible for him to gamble reasonably with them. Indeed they made it a matter of reproach that he was gambling at all! Apparently they were unaware that they, in doing what they thought was the "safe" thing, were gambling, too.

As is often the case, the reproach served to bring the father into line. He could not easily bear so many accusations, insinuations, and threatened complications of his family life from respected authority figures. While he may have felt that it was best for the baby to die, he could not accept that prospect in such concrete and immediate form. At that point, however, S., who was one of several interns assigned to the case, promised to resuscitate the child if necessary, so that the father could get the information he wanted before deciding to act. By sharing the gamble with the father, S. sought to make it possible for him to gamble consciously.

The father was trying to find out the odds that the child would have Down's syndrome. But none of the doctors knew. "We don't know what the statistics are," they all said. Some of them offered optimistic predictions on the basis that Down's syndrome occurs more commonly in conjunction with heart lesions other than critical aortic stenosis. These considerations, in fact, had little bearing on the case, since the question at hand was not "What is the likelihood that a newborn child with Down's syndrome will have critical aortic stenosis?" but "What is the likelihood that a newborn child with critical aortic stenosis will have Down's syndrome?" Finally the father decided that since three out of four doctors thought the child would turn out to have Down's syndrome, the probability was therefore seventy-five percent. About the only conclusions that can be drawn from this exchange of misinformation are these:

1. Most doctors are not comfortable making subjective probability estimates in the absence of "objective" relative-frequency data.
2. The idea of probability is sufficiently complex and ill-understood that it can easily be distorted into an instrument of confusion, manipulation, and control.
3. When denied access to reasonable probability estimates or a reliable basis for making them, people will make their own estimates, however ill-founded.

After two days the father, who previously had said only that if the Down's test came back positive he would refuse to operate, announced his intention not to act to save the baby's life even if she did *not* have Down's syndrome, since she clearly had a very limited life ahead of her. The sudden revelation angered the only doctor besides S. who had supported the father all along. This doctor, a young cardiologist, *had* given the father the benefit of the doubt. Now he felt that the father had shown himself to be unworthy of his trust. He didn't take into account the conditions that made it difficult for the father to act reasonably and consistently. Concluding that he could no longer give him the benefit of the doubt, this doctor joined the others who were trying to shame the father into accepting surgery.

The father, capitulating to the pressure, then consented to the operation, which was performed immediately. The next day the test result came back negative for Down's syndrome, but by then the baby had died. "If only your husband had agreed to operate earlier . . ." wailed the nurses to the mother. (Again, the delay probably only slightly diminished the child's already unfavorable prospects for survival.) The father was left with feelings of shame; the mother was left questioning her husband's judgment at a deeply serious moment in their life together. It was, in a sense, a broken family.

Afterward, as a way of quantifying the biases of the physicians (including his own), S. made up a quick version of decision analysis for the young cardiologist, to see how sensitive the decision would have been to different probabilities: "Taking the probability that this child would be capable of normal development as ninety, seventy, fifty, thirty, or ten percent, which of the following options would you choose?"

1. Obtain a court injunction authorizing surgery.
2. Manipulate feelings of shame to induce the father to operate.
3. Adopt a neutral position.
4. Support the father if he decides not to operate.
5. Manipulate feelings of shame to induce the father not to operate.

The heart specialist chose options 1 and 2 at fifty percent and above, 3 at thirty percent, and 4 at ten percent. S. chose options 1 and 2 at ninety percent, 3 at seventy percent, and 4 at fifty percent and below. Although no "official" estimate of this baby's chance for survival and normal development had been made, in retrospect the senior cardiologist's best guess was that it was not better than thirty percent. The younger heart specialist was left feeling that he should have adopted a neutral position, while S. felt that he ought to have supported the father's decision more publicly.

As this case was actually handled, it seems fair to say that human feelings, family prerogatives, and medical realities were violated by those whose responsibility it was to respect them. Shame is a dangerous drug, with severe side effects and high costs attendant upon its use. This does not mean that it should never be used (there are such things as child neglect and wife beating), but that, like other dangerous drugs, it should not be used indiscriminately.

How might S. have used a gambling model to define the alternatives more clearly for this family, and to make the physicians more sensitive to the family's needs and priorities? First, he might have laid out the decisions that were required in the form of a bet or a series of bets. When one bets on a coin flip, the outcomes look like this:

OUTCOME

		Heads	Tails
BET	Heads	**Win**	**Lose**
	Tails	**Lose**	**Win**

Here the value of the available choices was similarly affected by the contingencies of the outcome:

CONDITION

ACTION		Down's	Not Down's
	Operate	**Worse**	**Best** (if operation works)
	Not Operate	**Better**	**Worst**

There were two possible bets here. The surgeons, by choosing to operate, were betting that the child did not have Down's syndrome. The father, by choosing not to have the operation done, was betting that the child did have Down's. This is an oversimplification, since the doctors stood to gain by operating (by their values) whether or not Down's syndrome turned out to be present. The father, on the other hand, had reasons not to operate even if Down's was not present, since he was also concerned with the possibility that the heart operation might not prevent a cardiac-related disability comparable in severity to the retardation produced by Down's syndrome.

The father and the doctors chose different bets for one or both of the following reasons: (1) they evaluated the probabilities differently, or else just paid attention to different possibilities, the father being more concerned with the Down's contingency, the doctors with the Not Down's contingency (cf. Kahneman and Tversky, 1973); (2) they had different values. The doctors were most concerned to save a life (and exercise their skills) while the question of the quality of the life saved did not stand out in their minds. The father was most concerned about the costs of raising a child with a serious disability (of whatever origin). The doctors also felt that failing to save a life by not operating was far more reprehensible than taking a life by having the child die right after the operation, as in fact she did. Or as one senior surgeon put it, "Sometimes we have to be executioners" (that being, at least, a skill). The father, on the other hand, did not see letting a baby with severe defects die as a reprehensible act.

The feelings of the doctors and the father might be paraphrased as follows (although it is highly unlikely that either side articulated what is written here, even to themselves): One of the surgeons might have thought, "If I let this child die, then in the future I am committed to letting other children die. This would be a precedent. I find it all very painful. Though I could stand the pain of letting this one child die, I could not do the same thing again and again and again. That's just too painful for me. So I'll draw the line right here. I'll commit myself to operating to try to save this child, because that's the only policy I can imagine following consistently." The father might have said to himself, "This is the only time I'll ever have to decide whether or not to let a child die. Though I can stand the pain once, I couldn't stand having over and over again the pain of letting her live, which I would have to if it's going to be matter of repeated operations. Therefore I'll accept the pain I can more easily endure—that of letting the child die once."

Conceiving of the choice as a gamble would not have provided an "answer" to this dilemma. What it *would* have done was to reveal plainly that there *were* value differences involved, and that these needed to be addressed by all concerned. Once these differences had been brought into the open, the family's values would likely have been honored, provided that these did not violate societal values protecting infants from indifferent or malevolent parents. In this instance society's values would have left considerable leeway for responsible people to make different decisions.

The use of the gambling model also would have made clear

that probability estimates were required for making those decisions, and that the family needed to be better informed about
the probabilities than they were in the actual case, where they
were left in near-complete uncertainty about the likely outcomes of actions that were presented to them as moral impera-
tives. On the basis of the probabilities and values, the father's
gamble could have been seen in a clearer light. The doctors and
nurses who thought him callous and inhuman might have understood that three days and a small reduction (from thirty
percent to twenty percent) of the baby's chances for a healthy
existence were a painful price that he was willing to pay for
more information and some time to make up his mind.

Once the gamble had been analyzed, S. might have sat down
with the husband and wife and said, "We all have mixed feelings about what to do. Can we come up with a course of action
that will incorporate all those feelings? If not, can we set some
priorities and agree to leave some differences unresolved?
Whatever happens, it won't be that one of us was right and the
others wrong. Some gambles are reasonable; others are not. In
many situations it would not be reasonable not to try to save a
baby's life. In this case, although there are differences among
us, we all have good reasons for making certain choices. It may
be right to operate immediately and have a child with Down's
syndrome. It may be right to wait, even if we find out only after
the child has died that she did not have Down's. The main thing
is to know what is we are gambling for; and why."

Gambling and the Unconscious

The doctors in the Down's syndrome case gambled unconsciously, in the sense that they did not admit to themselves that
they were gambling. They also gambled badly, both in that they
did not work together in a trusting way with the family with
whom they shared the gamble, and in that their choice of gam-

bles (whether right or wrong) was not justified by their stated reasons for choosing it.

We can also imagine other ways of gambling badly. Suppose the baby's father had said (as he did not) that he and his wife preferred not to have the baby operated on because, having already reconciled themselves to the baby's death, they did not want to open themselves up again to the possibility of disappointment. They would rather just accept their "fate." Hope brings anxiety in its wake, and disappointed hope makes a bad outcome worse, so why not just accept the worst? This choice, absurd on the face of it, makes a kind of sense if one cannot bear anxiety and possible disappointment as costs of trying to better one's condition.

People differ in the degree of anxiety that uncertainty arouses in them. They also differ in their ability to bear the anxiety they experience. If, for example, you give children a basketball and watch them take their shots, you will find that some stand so close to the basket that they almost always get the ball in, while others stand so far back that they almost never get it in. Still others stand at an intermediate distance, where they have a reasonable, but by no means certain chance to score (McClelland, 1958). Presumably, as they practice and improve, they step back farther from the basket, where they can continue to face a challenge. These individuals either feel less anxiety or are better able to bear it. Those who choose either the safe situation or the impossibly difficult one are trying to get away from anxiety by moving to a situation of very low or very high risk.

When people are made anxious by uncertainty and also do not tolerate anxiety well, they will be more likely to gamble unconsciously and, in so doing, to choose certain kinds of gambles (Fuller, 1975). Moreover, anxiety about uncertainty is characteristic of the unconscious, so that anyone, regardless of personality, who is gambling unconsciously is likely to be in full flight from uncertainty. Unconscious thinking (in particular, what in the psychoanalytic literature is called "primary process" or "id" thinking) tends to take the form of mechanistic thinking. The unconscious polarizes the world into yes or no,

all or none, good or bad, rather seeing it in more subtle degrees
of probability or value. It assumes one's own values to be universal. Its causal explanations (as noted in Chapter 4) are unicausal and primitive: "I am the cause" (narcissistic) or "the
Other is the cause" (paranoid). Either "I cause everything," or
"I cause nothing."

The narcissism of the unconscious is expressed in the belief
that the outcome hinges solely on the application of skill, as by
a physician: "I can be the cause of all. If I take over, it will turn
out right." It also is expressed in the gambling error of paying
attention only to one's own wins or losses instead of to the
actual probabilities (e.g., the number of "tens" remaining in
the blackjack deck). This error can take the form of what is
called the postmortem fallacy ("if I have been losing, I must be
doing something wrong") or the gambler's fallacy ("if I have
been losing, perhaps now I'll win"). Either way it reflects the
egocentric assumption that all that matters in the world is what
happens to oneself; there lies the cause of it all. This kind of
mechanistic thinking, which assumes that the future will be
like the past, can result in actions that make this a self-fulfilling prophecy. In contrast, probabilistic gambling also relies on
past experience, but only if understood critically, i.e., in terms
of the variables that actually influence the probabilities, including (but not confined to) those that engage the emotions of
the gambler. The critical gambler is one whose hopes and fears
are tempered by realistic expectations.

Just as unconscious thinking considers only one cause at a
time, so it considers only one outcome at a time. The outcome
it tends to focus on is the most extreme, so in the unconscious
all consequences resolve themselves into either life or death.
Every choice is one of "to be or not to be." The unconscious does
not weigh costs and benefits or hold various outcomes in some
kind of emotional balance. Instead it responds to the stimulus
most immediately at hand, to whatever possible outcome is
most salient emotionally. Thus instead of an expected-value
strategy for gambling (which entails weighing costs and benefits, probabilities and values), the unconscious follows what in
game theory is called a *minimax* decision strategy, which

seeks to minimize the maximum possible loss. A minimax strategy ignores probability and is concerned with only one outcome, the worst, which it seeks to avoid. (In medicine, as in the unconscious, the worst outcome is death.) As such it is appropriate not for a probabilistic universe, but for a completely uncertain universe (where probability is useless) or a completely certain universe (where probability is unnecessary). The world of the unconscious is the world of the primitive, oscillating between these extreme states of total understanding and control (self as omnipotent cause) and no understanding and control (other as cause, self as impotent).

This fear of maximum loss, together with the anxiety about uncertainty that is strongly felt under the Mechanistic Paradigm, leads to the avoidance of risk, since risk involves both uncertainty and the possibility of maximum loss. The risk that is most to be avoided, according to this logic of the unconscious, is that of death, for death in the savage universe of the unconscious is maximum loss and maximum uncertainty (no one knows what it really is). Death is the ultimate fear that lies behind the minimax strategy. It is also what some doctors and hospitals, in the K. and Down's syndrome cases and throughout contemporary practice, have shown themselves to be quite literally preoccupied with, sometimes to the exclusion of other values. Doctors often speak of what they do as "saving lives," although few medical situations involve life-or-death issues. Behind the choices of gambles that doctors make (such as the choice in the case of K. to avoid the worst outcome at all costs) there lurks the fear of death.

In the cautious, insecure world of minimax strategy a sharp line is drawn to separate the permissible from the unthinkable. Beyond this line gradations of value cannot be entertained, since all possibilities are regarded as intolerable. For example, given these choices:

a) to kill a patient
b) not to do anything for a patient, who then dies
c) not to try very hard for a patient, who then dies
d) not to do everything for a patient, who then dies
e) to lose a patient while doing one's best

the last is the only acceptable outcome for many doctors. All five of these outcomes involve cost for the patient (death), but the first four also involve cost for the doctor—the cost of believing and having it believed that one did not do everything to prevent the patient's death. The problem with this bias is that, while (e) is best for the doctor, (d) may in some instances be best for the patient.

This, then, is how the Mechanistic Paradigm and the use of unconscious processes reinforce each other. When one's thinking is guided by the Mechanistic Paradigm, with its unattainable standard of certainty, one becomes anxious when one sees that one is taking chances. Since one cannot avoid taking chances, one seeks to avoid the anxiety by closing one's eyes to the fact that one is taking chances. What one sees with one's eyes closed is the possibility of death. With this fearsome prospect in view one understandably seeks the assurances that the Mechanistic Paradigm offers: certainty (Criterion #1), control (Criterion #2), and objective knowledge (Criterion #3). The more one shuts one's eyes, the more difficult it is to open them again.

The Probabilistic Paradigm offers a way to break this vicious circle by reducing some of the emotional costs of gambling. Since certainty is not set up as the standard for knowledge under the Probabilistic Paradigm, people do not feel (on top of the anxiety inherent in uncertain situations) the added anxiety of trying to make these situations certain. The Probabilistic Paradigm enables people to acknowledge their values, including the value of reducing anxiety, and to act consciously to reduce anxiety if that is a desired end. It enables people to cope with the anxiety associated with risk by seeing the feared outcome not as certain to occur (as the unconscious would have it), but as having a probability of occurrence that can be estimated and lived with. Even death can be contemplated in a more realistic, less overwhelmingly frightening way. Because gambling under the Probabilistic Paradigm is not as scary as under the Mechanistic, it can more easily be done consciously. And consciousness in turn makes it possible to gamble according to scientific principles.

How do we break out of the mechanistic cycle and initiate the

probabilistic one? We can't gain control of our gambling without understanding the factors, internal and external, that cus-
tomarily exert control over the gambles we take. When we
gamble unconsciously, we aren't really making our own
choices. In part it is the unconscious that exerts control. But
there are other controlling factors as well, and these lie outside
ourselves.

Who Controls the Game?

Just as people individually feel more or less anxious about uncertainty, people together find themselves in—and create—
situations where such anxiety is felt and heeded to a greater or
lesser degree. It has been observed, for example, that surgeons,
in the aftermath of an unexpected death on the operating table,
prefer to operate on hopeless cases. The reason they usually
give for doing this is that they wish to practice their technique.
What they are also doing is choosing a low-anxiety task in a
situation where their anxiety level has been temporarily
raised. Just as anxious people avoid middle-range risks (high
uncertainty) in favor of high risks (almost certain failure) and
low risks (almost certain success), nearly anyone may do so in
anxiety-provoking situations. Just as people who seek the approval of others tailor their gambling strategies to gain that
approval, nearly anyone may do so in situations where the approval of others is crucial.

People are sensitized to how others take risks. If someone
does so in an unusual manner, he is identified as a gambler, and
his risk-taking is thereby considered excessive. Since anxiety
can be caused just by seeing others take what appear to be
unacceptable risks, people often seek to limit the amount of
risk-taking that others do. In situations that bring out such
concerns, people are put under considerable pressure to avoid
dreaded consequences by gambling as everyone else does. For

example, the father in the Down's syndrome case, who on his own was able to respond reasonably to uncertainty and risk, was reduced to confusion and inconsistency in the stressful situation created by the hospital staff.

Unfortunately most of us spend much of our lives in similarly stressful situations. The world described in Chapter 4—a world of "exchange" relationships and zero-sum games in the family, the workplace, and the marketplace—is guided by the workings of the unconscious and by the Mechanistic Paradigm. In the absence of trusting relationships in which the emotional burdens of uncertainty can be shared (indeed, in the presence of relationships that generate suspicion and self-seeking behavior), we find ourselves much of the time on guard. After all, someone else's gain is likely to be our loss. We react to uncertainty with fear, and we react to fear with self-protective strategies. For example, when we have to do our jobs under the threat (explicit or implicit) of being fired for departing from ritual, or for thinking critically, we will tend to make a habit of thinking mechanistically. Our gambling will be furtive, our strategies automatic. Such gambling resembles the gambling that is done at the casino and the racetrack, not in the scientist's laboratory.

All this does not magically change when we walk into a doctor's office. On the contrary, the threats are more severe, the risks even less acceptable in a setting where life as well as livelihood is at stake. Here even people who elsewhere in life gamble consciously and cooperatively may slip back into fear and ritual.

Medicine is not only a science; it is also a social institution. To be a science today medicine needs to follow the Probabilistic Paradigm. To be a social institution today, it can only follow the Mechanistic Paradigm. As in other workplaces and marketplaces, people who gamble unconsciously have their choices of gambles controlled by corporations intent on profit. A Las Vegas hospital created an unwitting parody of the kind of gambling that goes on in medicine today when it established a lottery to pull in the customers on weekends (when people usually don't go into the hospital unless they have to). Anyone who checks in on a Friday or Saturday (usually for nonemergency surgery) automatically is entered in the sweepstakes. The winner gets a four-thousand-dollar vacation trip, or (for those too ill to travel) the equivalent in cash. And if you die while you're in the hospital, your winnings go to your estate. Of course, the "house" gets its cut too.

Medicine, like many activities that people engage in together, is a mixture of cooperative and competitive (zero-sum) gambling. The patient and the doctor (and the hospital if one is involved) are gambling together for the patient's health. The doctor also is gambling for experience, the satisfaction of exercising skill, and a professional reputation. The doctor and the hospital are gambling to make money, and the patient (when not completely covered by insurance) is gambling not to lose money. Finally, all three parties are gambling for control. To the extent that they can control the gamble, they are all better able to win the stakes they are gambling for. But control is itself part of the stakes, since people—and institutions—get satisfaction from exercising control. Control would not be an issue if medicine were a cooperative gamble guided by scientific principles. The fact that it is an issue points to the zero-sum aspect of gambling in medicine.

In commercial gambling establishments the "house" controls important elements of the game. In medicine the doctor's office or hospital is the house. Here the house does not control the odds as a casino does, but it does control information about the odds. Whereas in gambling under the Probabilistic Paradigm information is produced in order to be shared, in the zero-sum gambling of the casino (and the hospital when it acts like a casino) information is hoarded so that it can be selectively shared and withheld. For example, in Mrs. Pinelli's case the hospital personnel freely shared information with the patient about how much an arteriogram might reveal, but failed to mention that the data thus revealed were not likely to be useful.

By knowingly or unknowingly giving the gambler a false impression of the odds, the house can influence the gambler's choice, as when the house staff exaggerates the dangers of a condition to ensure a patient's cooperation. The most extreme bias in the presentation of odds is the claim that one course of action is a gamble (a matter of probability) while another is not a gamble (a matter of certainty). When a doctor tells a patient, "You're taking a chance by taking care of this condition at home rather than in the hospital," without adding that it is also taking a chance to go into the hospital, the doctor, though not intentionally deceiving the patient, is simply thinking in the way that comes naturally—i.e., in terms of the Mechanistic Paradigm. The doctor, too, is gambling unconsciously, but in such a way as to control the patient's gamble on behalf of the hospital.

Along with information the house controls contingencies that affect the outcome for the gambler. In the Down's syndrome case, for example, the doctors pressured the father to sign an operative consent form by threatening to withhold life-saving efforts that might later be required. In everyday medical situations the threat is neither so explicit nor so drastic; it can simply take the form of the selective withdrawal of the acceptance, approval, and affection that many people seek from a doctor. Through these means of control, doctors and hospitals (often out of a sincere desire to do what is good for the patient) induce patients not only to stay in the "game" longer than they need to, but to raise the ante by betting on what are probably unnecessary technical procedures. Patients, like tourists in Las Vegas, can get swept up into the game, staking more than they initially intended.

It isn't only patients, though, whose gambling is controlled by the corporate interests that constitute the "house." Doctors who gamble unconsciously are also susceptible to such control. A doctor's effectiveness is always on public trial, with judgment being rendered by patients, peers, and the courts. Doctors are afraid to be called gamblers. They are afraid of being singled out as unorthodox for failing to participate in the rituals of defensive medicine, rituals that grow out of a fear of failure and a preoccupation with the approval of others. The day-to-day reliance on "safe" procedures alternates with the daring emergency operation where the doctor becomes a hero by succeeding but has nothing to lose by failing.

S. found that the setting mattered too. He gambled differently with his patients in the office, the home, and the hospital. In his office, where he was the "house," he tried to share the control with patients as much as he could (though he didn't flatter himself that he was completely successful). In a patient's home the family was in a sense the house, although S.'s medical knowledge and authority gave him some control as well; there, too, a cooperative spirit prevailed. When the hospital was the house, however, S. sometimes felt as if he and the patient were gambling together *against* the house. The physicians in training known as house officers (as S. well knew from having been one, as well as from his later dealings with them) were like casino employees, running the tables by the rules of the house. S., on the other hand, as a private "attending" physician, felt more like a tipster, picking up inside information that might help the patient and family turn the odds in their favor, but unable to influence the outcome as much as he would like.

S. concluded that he and his patients would be able to take control of their gambling decisions only by learning to gamble consciously—by taking the gamble, as it were, of thinking of themselves as gamblers and learning the skills needed to be scientific gamblers. As S. was to learn, gambling skills are equally useful whether one is gambling with the house in a spirit of cooperation or against the house in a tense adversarial atmosphere. Perhaps most important, they can provide a way of getting from the latter state to the former.

Skill and Chance

To gamble is to acknowledge the part that chance plays in all events. And yet gambling is itself a skill, the skill of dealing with chance. In order to gamble consciously and effectively we need to distinguish between situations that are largely governed by chance and situations in which skill can be decisive (Langer, 1975). We can then turn what we might call "chance situations" into "skill situations" by applying the skills of gambling.

By "chance" situations we mean those where nature must take its course; by "skill" situations we mean those where human action can influence the outcome. Thus when we speak here of "skill" versus "chance," we are talking not about the degree of predictability that a situation exhibits, but about the degree of control that one may exert over it through the exercise of skill. One can almost always predict the course of a common cold, but one cannot change it. We therefore consider a case of the common cold to be a predominantly chance situation, different in degree, not in kind, from a roll of the dice. The probabilities of the outcomes are different, but the two situations are equally uncontrollable.

Skill situations satisfy our natural urge to *do* something, to be in control. On the other hand, there are times when we would just as soon put down the burden of responsibility and leave things to chance. Thus two common errors in gambling (including medical gambling) are to interpret chance situations as skill situations and to interpret skill situations as chance situations. A gambler who tries to "psych out" the roll of the dice is trying to apply skill to a chance situation. A gambler who sits at the blackjack table and plays without keeping track of the cards that come up is leaving a skill situation to chance. In medicine to disregard chance and use skill inappropriately is a form of defensive medicine. To neglect necessary skills and rely inappropriately on chance is a form of malpractice. Ironically, the wish to control, like the wish to relinquish control, leaves us open to having our choices controlled by the unconscious or by others who are gambling against us.

A third error is to treat the "skill versus chance" distinction as an all-or-none thing. In situations where skill is found, so is chance, and vice versa. Skill and chance situations can be thought of as existing on a continuum, both in actuality and in people's perceptions of them, as illustrated in Figure 7-1. At all points on the diagonal running through the box, the degree of skill, as opposed to chance, that people choose to apply matches exactly the degree of skill, as opposed to chance, that is required by the situation. Appropriate responses to situations are those that fall on this line. The dots appearing elsewhere in the box represent instances in which people's perceptions of a situ-

The Skill-Chance Continuum

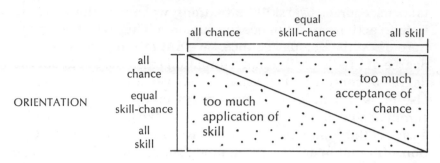

FIGURE 7-1

ation do not match the actuality. The greater the distance between a dot and the line, the less appropriate the response.

For the sake of simplicity it is useful to think of situations as involving *predominantly* either chance or skill. In a predominantly chance situation a chance orientation is appropriate, a skill orientation inappropriate. The reverse is true in a predominantly skill situation.

The trick is to identify the skill and chance aspects of the situation. Suppose, for example, that a woman in her late sixties is dying of bowel cancer. Nothing can be done to save her life. If we are looking at the life-or-death outcome, then by our definition this is a chance situation. (The cards have already been dealt.) If, on the other hand, we are looking at the possibility of making the woman more comfortable with loving care and supportive treatment (caring and supporting being skills), then this is a skill situation. (There is still an opportunity to bid on the cards that have been dealt.) To try to alter the course of the patient's condition by performing investigative procedures would be to treat a chance situation as if it were a skill situation. To say that nothing can be done to make the patient feel better as she is dying would be to treat a skill situation as if it were a chance situation.

Figure 7-2 shows that this one case can illustrate an appropriate acceptance of chance (1); an inappropriate acceptance of chance (2); an inappropriate application of skill (3); and an appropriate application of skill (4). (In this and subsequent diagrams, the inappropriate choices will be shaded.)

Leaving aside the issue of nurturant care (important as it can be, not only for a dying patient but for any patient), we can use two other cases to illustrate the skill-chance distinction with regard to "purely medical" outcomes, as shown in Figure 7-3. A child has a runny nose and sore throat. A common cold is diagnosed and left to run its course, although medication may be given to ease symptomatic discomfort. That is a predominantly chance situation. Another child comes in with severe ankle pain. X rays are taken so that a possible fracture can be identified and, if present, treated. That is a skill situation. But if viral cultures are taken to isolate the specific organism causing the common cold (even though there are no antibiotics to kill such a virus), or if the child with ankle pain is simply sent home without being examined and told, "It will get better in a few days," then we have again confused chance with skill, or skill with chance.

It is unlikely that any reputable doctor would make either of these elementary mistakes when dealing with a common cold or a possible broken ankle. But in the case of K. (Chapter 1), physicians with the best training and the best intentions made *both* mistakes. They inappropriately exercised the skill of diagnostic testing, when the precise identity of K.'s condition

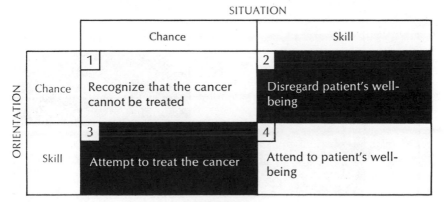

Skill and Chance: Terminal Cancer

FIGURE 7-2

Skill and Chance: Common Cold and Ankle Pain

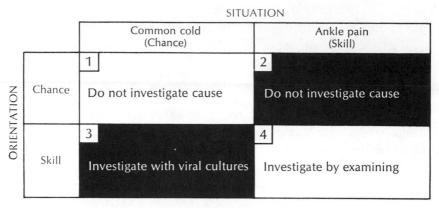

SITUATION

		Common cold (Chance)	Ankle pain (Skill)
ORIENTATION	Chance	**1** Do not investigate cause	**2** Do not investigate cause
	Skill	**3** Investigate with viral cultures	**4** Investigate by examining

FIGURE 7-3

could, after a while, have been left in the realm of chance, and they failed to exercise fully the skills of feeding and nurturing, which might have benefited K. Dr. S., who held different views about which skills would influence the outcome, did not make these mistakes here (which is not to say that he never made them). Note that this case, as represented in Figure 7-4, differs from that of the dying cancer patient, where neither kind of skill could have affected the medical outcome. In K.'s case the use of inappropriate skills may have hastened the patient's death, while the use of appropriate skills might have saved the patient's life.

Skill and Chance: The Case of K.

SITUATION

		Chance	Skill
ORIENTATION	Chance	**1** Dr. S: do not investigate cause beyond a certain point	**2** Hospital physicians: do not concentrate on feeding and nurturing
	Skill	**3** Hospital physicians: investigate cause without limit	**4** Dr. S: feed and nurture

FIGURE 7-4

Overdiagnosing and undernourishing are errors made commonly under the Mechanistic Paradigm, which does not acknowledge (as the Probabilistic Paradigm does) that even the exercise of skill is always a gamble. The Mechanistic Paradigm places emphasis on skills that can be exercised with an appearance of precision, such as diagnostic testing and technically oriented treatment. More subtle skills, such as diagnostic "watching and waiting" and nurturant treatment (food, love, comfort), it abandons to chance. "That's not science," it says. But the Probabilistic Paradigm makes possible a science of chance, which in turn changes the nature of skill as well as the relationship between skill and chance. The fact that the effects of nourishing a child are difficult to measure, and obviously involve a large element of chance, no longer justifies disregarding them or the skills they entail.

The inappropriate use of skill in chance situations is one of the rituals by which people, including doctors, cope with the anxiety aroused by uncertainty. A better way of coping, one that answers the same emotional needs without denying reality, is by using the skills of gambling. These include assessing causes and effects probabilistically, estimating probabilities and values, understanding the effects of time and social context on gambling decisions, dealing with the emotions that arise in the course of gambling, and recognizing and avoiding the common errors of gambling. Most of all, gambling under the Probabilistic Paradigm means being able to do all of these things with other people in a relationship where uncertainty is shared. In this kind of gambling the doctor, patient, and family ideally can work together with the openness and mutual respect of fellow scientists.

S. encouraged patients to be his partners in gambling, as we see in the following case:

A seventy-year-old man had a feeling of tightness and discomfort in his legs whenever he climbed stairs or walked a short distance. On examination Dr. S. found weak pulses in the thighs and below. S. diagnosed a reduced blood flow to the legs—insufficient for exercising—caused by clogged blood vessels. He said to the patient, "I have no way of treating your condition medically. If you want to do something about it, you will need to go to a specialist to see if it can be treated surgically. Surgery helps some people, but it also involves risks. At your age you may prefer to accept the restrictions this condition places on your life. Or you may accept the risks of surgery in an effort to improve it. If it gets worse, and the circulation is blocked off completely, you may eventually be forced to do something about it. In any case you should get more information from a specialist to help you decide whether you want to have surgery now. If you don't have surgery, that's a decision, just as it is if you do. You know how the racetrack works. If you bet on a race, you want to know the odds on each horse before you bet, and you may want to hedge your bet. It wouldn't make sense to bet on one of the horses, or not to bet on any of them, without knowing the odds."

Here S. was sharing his perspective on reality so that he and the patient could engage in common action. Working with patients in this way made S. feel as if some of the load had been lifted from his shoulders. It's not that he was "punting," or passing the buck of responsibility to ill patients who may just have wanted to be taken care of. Rather, instead of taking full responsibility to impose order on an uncertain world, he was sharing responsibility with patients and with chance.

What patients gain from such an exchange is a chance to learn some of the doctor's detachment. A doctor has less to win or lose on each gamble than a patient does. Doctors also get more practice in gambling, more experience in winning and losing. The doctors who gamble best for their patients are those who can, when needed, take a certain emotional distance from their gambling, though not to the point of losing empathy and gambling recklessly "for the fun of it." Patients who gamble with a doctor like S. not only can learn to achieve better outcomes, but also can gain some perspective on the wins and the losses. They can take responsibility for choosing reasonable gambles, but still be able to live with themselves—and with uncertainty—if they lose. Thus when doctors and patients gamble together, both can learn not only to see each gamble from up close, as a patient feels it, or from a distance, as a doctor approaches it, but to move back and forth between the two points of view (Havens, 1976).

Since gambling, with its characteristic skills and attitudes, acts as an analgesic for anxiety in cases of uncertainty, it is not surprising that it, like other analgesics, can be overused. A harried doctor may try to shed too much responsibility by habitually turning skill situations into chance situations, i.e., "punting." It is nice to be able to blame one's failures on chance. Given human nature and the conditions under which doctors must work, some doctors will use the notion of gambling to let them off the hook in difficult situations, just as few doctors today, in comparable situations, go to the narcotic cabinet. If doctors, who are gambling only for their reputation, time, and the feelings they share with patients, feel a need to escape, then it is not surprising that patients, who are gambling for life and health, will also seek relief. There will be some who will say, "It's all up to chance," and continue smoking or, like Mrs. Pinelli, stop taking their medications.

Although gambling is open to abuse, the primary effect is to enable patients as well as doctors to use skill to live with their anxiety rather than to allow anxiety to reduce their skill. Through the experience of gambling, patients will gain a better sense of the probabilities, that is, of which contingencies are controllable and which are not. They will then be able to make better choices in the future. Beyond this, the very act of making an informed choice can give a patient a sense of being in control, which in itself may reduce the stress of illness and with it the physical as well as emotional damage suffered by the patient. In keeping with the second criterion of the Probabilistic Paradigm, both the consequences of particular choices and the habit of making choices have an impact on one's experience, capacities, and character. A habit of making choices consciously, and recognizing a degree of uncertainty in one's choices, can produce a stronger, wiser self.

8

GAMBLING SKILLS
FOR MEDICINE

Once he realized that one could not avoid gambling, S. set out
to learn to gamble well. If he were going to have to gamble
anyway, he ought to be able to tell the difference between a
good gamble and a bad gamble and act on the good one. This
skill, he reflected, was the same as the scientist's skill of choosing the hypotheses most likely to yield true and good outcomes.
It was as important for his patients as it was for him. Patients
sought the good, in that they wanted to get well. They sought
the true, in that they wanted to understand why they were sick
and how they might get well. Understanding was what gave
patients a sense of control—and some real control—over their
fate. As S. came to see, though, it would have to be an understanding of gambling as well as of medicine.

Gambling strategies are heuristics, or rules of thumb for solving problems. As we saw in Chapter 7, people generally gamble
according to unconscious heuristics. By gambling unconsciously, they don't have a chance to learn from experience,
correct gambling errors, and exercise gambling skills.

As S. became a more conscious gambler, he began to look
critically at two types of heuristics: (1) preferences for one type
of gamble over another; and (2) patterns of gambling decisions

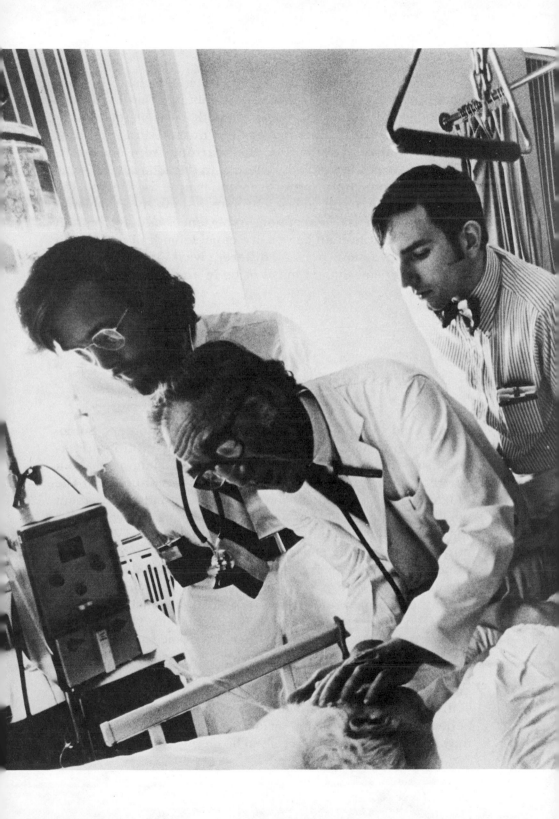

over time. In the course of his clinical practice S. asked himself what kinds of gambles he favored and under what conditions he changed his gambling choices. In both areas he found himself making what he later judged to be mistakes. In gambling, however, unlike decision analysis, learning from one's mistakes is part of the method. Whereas in decision analysis the "irrational" human factor tends to undermine the method, the gambling approach involves a human rationality incorporating common sense, perception, experience, and feelings. It recognizes that human beings are capable both of acting and of evaluating actions in many different ways, and that what is a mistake in one context may not be in another.

Gambling Preferences

People tend to prefer some type of gambles to others. Sometimes it is reasonable to act on a particular gambling preference; sometimes it is not. One must make a judgment about whether an act is reasonable in a given situation. Like the judgments that scientists make, this is a judgment about whether acting on a given preference is consistent with what we know to be true and what we know to be good. Thus the purpose of gambling consciously is not to learn to gamble in some ideal way, but to understand how we do gamble so that we can decide whether or not we are gambling reasonably.

A few gambling preferences are logically inconsistent, as we have seen in the so-called Dutch Book situation. These preferences can be called mistakes. Other preferences are specious, in that they do not serve the gambler's interest in the way the gambler imagines they do. A gambler may, for example, habitually seek what seem to be skill situations in the belief that his skill can almost always overcome chance. Another gambler, believing that he is "lucky" or lacking confidence in his skills, may habitually seek what seem to be chance situations. These preferences are specious if they are maintained without regard to the contexts in which the gambles are chosen. As we have seen, the preference for either skill or chance situations can be a reasonable one, but only when applied in an appropriate context.

As S. began to watch how he and others gambled, these were some of the common gambling preferences that he observed:

1. Preference to avoid gambling.   In a society that understands itself and its environment in terms of the Mechanistic Paradigm, the uncertainty of gambling makes people anxious. People who don't want to gamble choose gambles that don't look like gambles at all. For example, they may go into the hospital (or, as doctors, bring patients into the hospital) in the belief that the hospital is a "safe" environment whereas taking care of the condition at home would be "taking a chance."

When people who don't want to gamble *are* aware that they are gambling, they prefer to have a "sure thing"—a gamble they can't lose. Suppose someone is given the choice of these two gambles:

> Gamble A: 90% chance of winning $10
> 10% chance of losing $1
>
> Gamble B: 50% chance of winning $2
> 50% chance of winning $1

Gamble A has the higher expected value, by far. One would almost surely win more by choosing it over a series of trials, and would probably win more by choosing it once. Yet some people would choose Gamble B, simply because they wouldn't want to risk losing anything. And this would be the right choice for a person who wandered into the casino without having any money to pay off a loss. In the never-never casino that offered such bets, this gambler could build up a small bankroll by betting Gamble B the first few times, and then switch to Gamble A.

Gamble B likewise may have been the right choice for Dr. S.

in the case of K. Faced with a starving child who had no resources of physical or emotional strength, he could not risk
depleting the child's strength further by testing (losing one
dollar) to try to gain a definite diagnosis (winning ten dollars).
Actually the odds on his winning that bet were more like ninety
percent against than ninety percent for. So instead he chose the
conservative option of feeding and emotionally supporting K.,
which might more or less benefit him (winning two dollars or
one dollar), but would be unlikely to hurt him. Once K. had
built up some reserve strength for surviving traumatic investigations, Dr. S. could reevaluate the option of going for the jack-
pot (the ten-dollar diagnosis).

Of course, the odds were not quite so favorable for Dr. S. as
Gamble B indicates, since K. stood some chance of dying of an
undiagnosed infection while he was being nurtured back to
health. Real life seldom offers us gambles that we can't lose.
When we think we have found such a gamble, it is usually
because we deny the possibility of losing and imagine that a
loss would be really just the same as maintaining the status
quo. In choosing Gamble A, the doctors who treated K. didn't
take into account the possibility that the tests were contributing to the deterioration of K.'s condition. To the extent that they
even saw themselves as taking a gamble, they thought they
were betting to win ten dollars (by finding the diagnosis) or *lose
nothing.* For them (though not for K.) the gamble came free of
charge.

When the possibility of losing cannot be avoided, those who
prefer not to gamble choose gambles in which there is little
difference between winning and losing (i.e., where there isn't
much to lose). When given a chance to remain at status quo or
risk an equal chance of gaining or losing an equal amount,
people tend to prefer to stay where they are. In a "double or
nothing" game, where the choice is between a sure five dollars
and an equal chance of having ten dollars or nothing, "gamblers" will take the bet, but our culture encourages the conservative choice of keeping what one already has. For example, a
disease is controlled at a tolerable, though moderately disabling level by medication. Radical surgery offers the chance
for a dramatic improvement or complete health, though at

some risk of greater disability or death. A person who prefers gambles with less variance of outcome will stick to the medication. On the other hand, a surgeon trained to regard any condition of less than perfect health as unacceptable, or a patient whose self-esteem is tied to the notion of perfect health, may well choose the gamble with greater variance.

This and other preferences can be illustrated with a probability distribution curve, where the possible outcomes are laid out from left to right in order of ascending value, and the probability of each outcome is represented by the height of the curve at that point. For the sake of simplicity the expected value (probability multiplied by value) of the gambles represented in the graphs equals zero. (In other words, if one took any of these gambles many, many times, one would expect to come out with neither a gain nor a loss.) As shown in Figure 8–1, a gamble with little variance of outcomes is the next "best" thing to no gamble at all.

Probability Distribution Curve:
Gambles with Lesser and Greater Variance

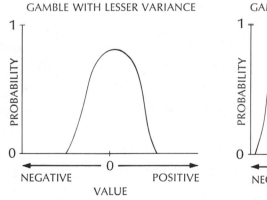

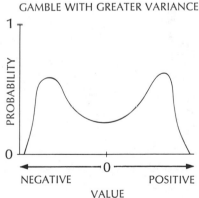

FIGURE 8-1

2. Preference for gambles with positive skew. The term *skew* describes an uneven distribution of probabilities along the value continuum. As shown in Figure 8-2, a positive skew involves a small chance of a large gain, and a large chance of a small loss. A negative skew involves a small chance of a large loss, and a large chance of a small gain.

With a positively skewed gamble there may be a greater overall chance of a negative than a positive outcome, while there may be a greater chance of a positive outcome with a negatively skewed gamble. What attracts people to the positively skewed gamble is the hope of a big payoff. What scares people away from the negatively skewed gamble is the dread of a big loss. In both cases considerations of probability take second place to the hope or dread in question.

The case of K. illustrates positive and negative skew. The physicians who ordered all the tests accepted the small, highly probable incremental losses from testing in order to play for the long-shot win of a definite diagnosis. Their gamble was a positively skewed one. They saw it as a highly responsible gam-

Probability Distribution Curve:
Gambles with Positive and Negative Skew

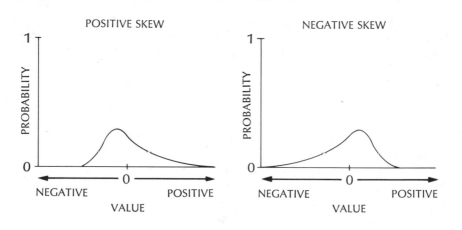

FIGURE 8-2

ble—not a gamble at all, really—because it avoided the risk of a major defeat (failure to diagnose a treatable condition). A negatively skewed gamble was unacceptable to them because it involved that risk (as well as the risk of being sued). Dr. S., on the other hand, accepted that low-probability risk in return for the small, highly probable incremental gains to be derived from good care and nutrition. He reasoned that, rather than leading to either a breakthrough or catastrophe, a sustained investment in one treatment strategy or the other would result in an accumulation of minor gains or losses. These, he thought, would ultimately decide the issue. As S. saw, by repeatedly using negatively skewed gambles one can build up a bankroll that eventually will support positively skewed gambles.

A preference for positive skew reflects a focusing of attention on the most extreme possible outcomes. A big gain surely is better than a big loss. But this strategy, pushed to its extreme, ignores all the outcomes in between and their likelihood of occurrence. It is, in effect, a concentration on values, together with an indifference to probabilities. In the context of complete certainty or complete uncertainty it would make sense, but our world is generally somewhere in between.

3. Inconsistent preferences: the Preference Reversal Phenomenon.
In evaluating a gamble, one may attend primarily to the values at stake, as in the preference for positive skew, or to the probabilities of the outcomes, as in the preference for negative skew. When there are two gambles, one of which offers a higher payoff, the other a higher probability of winning, a person who is asked to choose between them will often choose the one with the more favorable odds. But when the same person is asked how high a price he or she is willing to pay for a "ticket" to make the bet, his or her attention is focused on the payoffs, and he or she will often name a higher price for the gamble with the higher payoff. Thus when the gamble is presented in one or another way, inconsistent responses can occur. This is called the Preference Reversal Phenomenon (Lichtenstein and Slovic, 1971). Although it is something that people commonly do, it represents a logically inconsistent set

of preferences, for which a Dutch Book can be made against the gambler.

In the case of the infant with the heart disorder who was suspected of having Down's syndrome, the father at first paid more attention to probability (the probability that the child would not have a normal life). Later he reversed himself and went along with the doctors, who paid more attention to value (the value of saving a life, and particularly that of saving the life of a normal child, even if there was a very low probability of the latter). The father's change of heart can be understood in terms of the different ways in which he was led to see the gamble. He initially believed that the decision was his to make. What he heard the doctors telling him was "It's your choice." Under those conditions he focused (as most people would) on the probabilities. The doctors, displeased by the choice he made, then let him know that he would suffer the consequences of having made it. "You'll pay for it" was the message he now got from them. Looking at the gamble in this new way, he chose (again as most people would) on the basis of the values.

4. Preference for gambles about which there is information. People usually prefer gambles where they know something about the odds, whether or not the odds are actually better. This preference is illustrated by the Ellsberg paradox, which was devised by Daniel Ellsberg (1961), later to be known for his prodigious feats of photocopying. To take a hypothetical example from medicine, suppose someone in your family has leukemia, which leaves patients particularly susceptible to infections that tend to be fatal if not treated. Two drugs have been developed for treating these infections, but their effects are different for each of the three major types of leukemia: t-cell, b-cell, and null-cell. Drug X cures infections in patients with t-cell leukemia, but not b-cell. Drug Y does just the opposite. Neither drug is effective in cases of null-cell leukemia. The two drugs cannot be used together; a choice must be made.

Suppose further that at this stage of the disease tests can show only that this patient has a 33.3 percent probability of having t-cell leukemia. The tests cannot distinguish between the b-cell and null-cell variants, and thus the probabilities of these remain unspecified. Given the following possible outcomes (where + stands for survival and 0 stands for death), which drug would you choose?

Case I

OUTCOME

CHOICE		T-cell (33.3% chance)	B-cell (0–66.7% chance)	Null-cell (0–66.7% chance)
	Drug X	+	0	0
	Drug Y	0	+	0

Now consider a different case in which drugs X and Y are both *effective* against null-cell leukemia (all other conditions remaining the same). Now your choices look like this:

Case II

OUTCOME

CHOICE		T-cell (33.3% chance)	B cell (0–66.7% chance)	Null-cell (0–66.7% chance)
	Drug X	+	0	+
	Drug Y	0	+	+

In the first case most people choose drug X. They are more comfortable with a known probability of one third than with a probability that may be anywhere from zero to two thirds. In the second case many of the very same people choose Drug Y. They prefer a known two-thirds probability to a probability that may be anywhere from one third to one. The paradox, as a quick look at the diagram makes clear, is that the two cases offer the same choice. (Drug X helps patients with t-cell, while

Drug Y helps patients with b-cell.) Why, then, do people change their preference so as to get the known odds in each case? One reason is that they prefer certainty to ambiguity—to know for sure what the odds are. Another reason may be that most people, when dealing with life and death, expect the worst. So, although there is no reason to believe that the odds in the indefinite condition are closer to, say, 0 than 66.7 percent, one's instinct is to believe that this is the case.

People prefer to have information about the odds even when the information is known to be unreliable. Take, for example, the standard medical practice of taking six blood cultures to compensate for false negative results (i.e., where the test fails to record something that is there). A blood culture is a test performed to determine whether or not bacteria are present in the blood. If they are (i.e., if there is a true positive culture), it means that they are being carried throughout the body, posing the threat of infection wherever they might lodge. K. had over forty blood cultures, with the consequences we have seen. To take six, on the other hand, is normal practice in many instances. In fact, the accuracy of the test does improve (say, from seventy percent to eighty-five percent) by taking three cultures rather than one. From then on not only are there diminishing returns (in true positive results) from taking additional cultures, but there is an increase in false positive results (where the test records something that is not there) from contamination, to say nothing of the trauma and blood loss.

Most people would argue that the costs of a false positive blood culture are less than those of a false negative. The latter might mean a patient's death. Sooner or later, though, the costs of false positive blood cultures add up: the financial and social costs of treating patients who should not be treated, the side effects of such treatment, the occasional failure to diagnose a treatable condition in a patient for whom initiating antibiotic treatment on the basis of a false positive blood culture shuts off further investigation. Pushed to its extreme, the standard medical preference for avoiding false negative cultures exemplifies the preference for information, however inaccurate. One prefers to have something to believe which isn't true than to have nothing to believe at all.

5. Preference for gambles with a higher expected value.   In saying that other gambling preferences lead people to make choices that are against their own interests, our standard of comparison has been the preference for gambles which have a higher expected value. This is a reasonable standard. Other things being equal, the gamble with the higher expected value is the better gamble. But when are "other things" (e.g., the values of all the people affected by a decision, the consequences that a decision will have at different times) equal? As we saw in our discussion of decision analysis (Chapter 6), there isn't any single numerical scale on which the satisfactions of different individuals—or of the same individual at different times, in different situations, or in different moods—can be measured.

In the case of decisions in which, say, immediate human wants are weighed against the welfare of future generations, the health and safety of individuals against productive activity benefiting large numbers of people, the calculation of expected values cannot possibly encompass the many values, interests, and points of view that are involved. The same is true for what are thought of as purely individual decisions. As Mrs. Pinelli's case illustrates, people experience mixed feelings, unconscious motives, changes of mind. People gamble differently, depending on whether they are alone or with other people, whether they are taking the same gamble many times or just once, and whether they are focusing on long-range or short-range consequences.

A person will assign one expected value to the gamble of eating a hamburger when in the presence of a freshly cooked hamburger, another when in the presence of a bathroom scale. Which expected value is the correct one? Each is correct in its own context. True, in the presence of the hamburger one may try to calculate its expected value as if one were in the presence of the scale, so as to resist temptation. But that is a choice, made on the principle that the consideration of long-range consequences provides a better context for decision-making than the consideration of short-range consequences. Expected values take on meaning from the principles by which one gambles.

Such principles are in turn established in the process of making choices—of gambling. Simply in the course of living, people develop their own repertoires of intuitive decision-making methods that take into account the various contexts in which the consequences of decisions are experienced. One way of making decisions is to calculate expected values mathematically. But when one lets the number that represents expected value dictate the decision, rather than keeping it in mind as information that may be further qualified by thoughts, feelings, and experiences, one may be avoiding the responsibility of considering the contexts in which one gambles. By making one's gambles one's own through exercising one's capacity to reason, one strengthens that capacity by establishing principles and strategies for future gambles. Being able to say why one chooses something involves both self-definition and insight. In the long run, being able to say "this is who I am" may be more important than making the choice with the highest expected value.

Gambling Over Time

When he laid out medical decisions as gambles—and as choices between gambles—S. focused on some of the same issues as he did when he was doing decision analysis. Here, too, he was concerned with probability and value. Here, too, he was making choices on the basis of at least an informal estimate of the expected values of possible outcomes. "How likely is this to happen? How good or bad would it be if it did happen?" These questions, he found, were as central to the gambling method as to decision analysis.

But he learned that there were differences as well. He discovered that one of the strengths of the gambling model is its sensitivity to time. When he thought of his decisions as gambles, he found it natural to think in terms of the Probabilistic Paradigm. As a scientific gambler he acknowledged that the world changes (Criterion #1) and that the relationship between the world and the decision-maker changes (Criterion #2). Time, together with the feelings of the people involved in the decision (Criterion #3), creates a fluid context in which decision-making occurs. As time passes, probabilities change; values change; information changes; feelings change. The results of one gamble affect the next. Time also gives people who have an interest in the outcome a chance to influence the gambler's decision. The gambling framework, by incorporating the context of time, enables people to make decisions that are suitably sensitive to a complex and changing environment.

Even in what we ordinarily think of as gambling, the effects of time can be observed as people place their bets and wait for the outcome to be decided. At the racetrack a collective anxiety can be sensed as the odds fluctuate during the half hour prior to each race. As the clock runs down to post time, spectators agonize over whether to bolt from their seats and place a last-minute bet, perhaps "hedging" a bet they have previously made on a different horse. In medicine a treatment plan is decided upon, and the doctor and patient wait to see how well it is working. They, too, may have to decide whether to change horses in midstream.

Once the bet is won or lost, the gambler must interpret the results. Future gambles will be based not simply on the results of previous gambles, but on the gambler's interpretation of the results. In this sense gambling closely resembles scientific experimentation under the Probabilistic Paradigm, where the data, rather than dictating the conclusions, must be interpreted by the experimenter. When a doctor prescribes a treatment for strep throat, inflammation of the intestine, athlete's foot, or hypertension, the doctor must evaluate the results when deciding whether to follow the same treatment strategy, either in continuing to treat the same patient or in treating future cases of the same disease. Perhaps the strategy was wrong in the first place; perhaps it has been made obsolete by changing conditions; perhaps it is appropriate for some cases but not for others. Perhaps it was the right strategy but simply hasn't been given enough time to work.

There is, unfortunately, no simple way of interpreting the results of past actions for the benefit of future decisions. In fact, people often misunderstand and misapply such information, either because they don't perceive the situation correctly or because they don't think clearly about it. Like preferences for individual gambles, patterns of gambling over time may be based on specious assumptions. People may habitually react in ways that do not in fact lead to better gambling decisions and better results. Two of the most common misinterpretations are referred to as "postmortem hindsight" and "the gambler's fallacy." S. knew them both well from his own experience. He knew that he had to be as conscious of his long-range gambling strategies as he was of his individual gambles.

Postmortem Hindsight

It seems natural to assume that a gamble won was a good gamble, and that a gamble lost was a bad gamble. People almost inevitably change their probability estimates from hindsight (Fischhoff, 1975). They underestimate the degree of uncertainty that existed before the outcome became known, and revise their probability estimates upward or downward depending on whether the event in question did or did not occur. The fallacy in this is that a gamble would not be a gamble if chance did not intervene. A gamble would not be a gamble if the best decision always led to the best outcome. Sometimes a wise strategy does not win. Sometimes a foolish strategy does win. One win or one loss in and of itself says little about the probability of winning or losing, or about one's skill in choosing a gamble. Yet people commonly take pride in a win or blame themselves for a loss, as if the outcome really had been a matter of only skill rather than of skill plus chance. People sometimes give up a good gambling strategy, just because of one bad outcome, and switch to one that has less chance of winning.

In order to avoid this error, it helps to remember that past decisions were based on estimates of an uncertain situation, and that these estimates must be evaluated not only on the basis of what is known after the fact, but on the basis of what was known—and not known—before the fact. A technique that

S. found useful was to record his probability estimates before the outcome became known. Such written information, he found, can correct the bias of memory and act as a check against later overreactions.

A *series* of wins or losses, on the other hand, may provide real information about probable outcomes, and one may appropriately revise one's probability estimates—and subsequent actions—on the basis of this information. In this way one may profit from one's mistakes. To do so, however, one needs to have the attitude of critical trust that the scientist employs when testing hypotheses and accumulating data. A gambler who does not doubt himself will be unable to question what appears, on the basis of one lucky shot, to be a winning strategy. A gambler who does not give himself the benefit of the doubt will be unable after an initial setback to pursue what might ultimately be a winning strategy.

Translated into gambling terms, the scientific principle of critical trust tells the gambler that it doesn't pay to take the outcome of most individual moves in a game too seriously. But it does pay to try to understand how the game works and to develop a strategy for making one's moves accordingly. The sense that one is following a sound strategy can bolster the gambler against the disappointment that arises from individual losses—and the temptation to react with rash shifts in strategy. When it becomes clear, however, that a strategy isn't paying off—that the outcomes are going against the probability estimates on which the strategy is based—then it is time for a new strategy. And even if a run of losses is due only to bad luck, one may have to revise a sound strategy and bet more cautiously in order to avoid losing all of one's resources.

The "Gambler's Fallacy"

If a fair coin comes up heads three times in a row, what are the odds that it will come up tails the next time? The correct answer is one out of two, but many people will say the odds heavily favor tails. This is called the "gambler's fallacy." Coins do not have memories, and their behavior when thrown up in the air is not affected by their past history. Yet many people assume that there is some pressure on the coin—or dice—to even out the odds on the next throw. This assumption is based on a misinterpretation of probability. Chance outcomes do tend to even out according to probability, but only over the long haul. It is true that the odds that a coin will come up heads four times in a row are only one out of sixteen. So are the odds on any specified sequence of four coin flips, such as heads-tails-heads-tails. But these low odds are for the *combined* outcome of four coin flips, not for the fourth alone. Once the coin has come up heads the first three times (an event with a probability of one out of eight), the odds on the next throw are just the usual one out of two. A person who walked into the room without knowing about the first three flips would correctly assume these odds, and such a person would, after all, be observing the same outcome as the people who have been in the room all along. On the other hand, if a coin keeps coming up heads, maybe it is a trick coin. In that case it is appropriate to revise one's probability estimate on the basis of this new information. The revised estimate, however, would be in the opposite direction from that predicted by the gambler's fallacy.

If, in the case of the child K., the doctors who did all the tests were to justify their actions by saying, "We've had such a long run of negative test results, we're bound to get a positive one soon," they would be committing the gambler's fallacy. As in this instance, the gambler's fallacy can encourage the gambler to stick to a losing strategy in the belief that his luck is about to change, while the fallacy of postmortem hindsight (which says that a lost gamble was an unwise gamble) can lead the gambler to give up too quickly on a strategy that appears to be losing. Let's say a medication is prescribed which may or may not alleviate a given condition. If the medication did not work immediately, a doctor working from postmortem hindsight might give up on it, ascribing the result to insufficient skill ("I prescribed the wrong thing"). A doctor who believed in the gambler's fallacy might keep trying the medication long after its inadequacy was demonstrated, in the hope that luck would change.

The gambler's fallacy combines with postmortem hindsight in a way that makes gambling-house owners happy—and rich. People have a tendency to attribute their wins to skill and their losses to chance. It is in the interest of the house to encourage this way of thinking, because it leads the customers to stay in the game whether they are winning or losing. The gambler on a winning streak wants to "keep doing what works" (assumption of skill). The gambler on a losing streak invokes the gambler's fallacy, with its promise of a reversal of fortune (assumption of chance). Both believe that future prospects will be favorable. Partly on account of these inconsistent interpretations, people tend to take more risks when they are winning big or losing big. Another reason is that as the game goes on and the winnings or losses mount, each dollar (proportionately and psychologically) means less than the one before.

Unconscious, emotionally driven gambling can be costly enough in the casino. It can be even more costly when it is applied to real-life gambling, as in medicine. Suppose a husband and wife are concerned that a hereditary condition that one of them has, such as club feet, may be passed on to their children. If they have a child who does not have the condition, they may think it that much less likely that the next child will inherit it (postpartum hindsight). If they have a child who does have the condition, they may think that the odds will be that much better for having a normal child the next time (gambler's fallacy). The probabilities do not justify either of these inferences.

Commitment Strategies

Readers of the Sunday newspaper in a large metropolitan area learned of the "million-dollar baby," a two-and-one-half-year-old boy in a local hospital who had been resuscitated fifty times in his short lifetime. These recurrent life-or-death sieges had left him with permanent brain damage. His body riddled with needles and tubes, he led a miserable life. The newspaper article, which commemorated the first million dollars spent by the child's family and by society to keep the child alive, praised the hospital's heroic effort. But someone with different values (someone who valued the common good or the quality of life as well as the survival of an individual) might have regarded this heroism as a perverse commitment to a lost cause.

How does one decide when to stick to a gambling strategy and when to abandon it? Would the doctors of the "certainty" school who treated K. ever have reached a point where they would have stopped testing? And if Dr. S. had remained in charge of the case, might he have had to rethink his own strategy if K.'s course had turned downhill despite all the food and love he was getting? How does one maintain a valid strategy when there is pressure (from oneself and others) to change it? How does one discover that one's commitment to a given course of action is irrational or unnecessary and that reevaluation is in order?

Changes in strategy can, of course, be built into a plan of action, as demonstrated by Dr. S. in the following case. A two-year-old boy had had a birth defect which had caused food to pass from his stomach into his lungs, sometimes causing pneumonia. Even after the problem was corrected, the boy continued to struggle when he was fed, because he associated food with pain and illness. Since he was seriously undernourished and underweight, S. decided to feed him only through a gastric tube going directly into his stomach, thus removing a major source of irritation and conflict while he nurtured him in other ways. The treatment plan called for feeding the boy by mouth again when he reached a certain weight, for at that point feeding would no longer be a life-or-death issue. This is an example of a planned change in strategy. In devising a plan of action, it makes sense to allow for anticipated change. But in an uncertain world one cannot allow for every possible change.

In the face of setbacks and unexpected developments people feel a need to maintain a commitment to a course of action— a commitment that is sometimes justified and sometimes not. It is a question of when it is worthwhile to pay the "retooling costs" that a change in policy entails—a question (to cite again the scientist's principle of critical trust) of when to doubt one's gambling strategy and when to give it the benefit of the doubt. Sometimes a commitment to a strategy is a commitment of principle; sometimes it is a commitment of fear and rigidity. To the extent that K.'s doctors felt "If we stop testing now, then all the tests we've done will go to waste," or "We've invested so much in testing that we can't switch now," they were showing a rigid commitment to their strategy and a reluctance to abandon "sunk costs" and incur "retooling costs." Sometimes, by a psychological process called "cognitive dissonance," people show a greater commitment to a strategy that doesn't appear to be working than to one that does, as if the lack of apparent benefit from pursuing the strategy necessitated a greater resolve in defending it, perhaps to prevent embarrassment. In the case of K., doctors invested their honor in sticking to a strategy in the hope that it would eventually work, as if the acceptance of new information constituted a damaging admission of error.

People have strategies for maintaining consistent behavior, as well as for maintaining the flexibility needed to change, when faced with doubts raised by themselves or by others. The same commitment strategies that bolster a "bullheaded" stubbornness can also defend commitments to principle or to sound policy. Whether the strategies are being used constructively in a given instance depends on the value of the commitment itself.

Psychiatrist George Ainslie (1975) has analyzed the ways in which people question their commitments and the strategies they use to reaffirm them. People reconsider their strategies for a number of reasons, such as internal conflict about the rightness of a decision (conflict which may have existed before the decision was made), fluctuations of mood, and conflict with other people. A major threat to consistency comes from what Ainslie calls specious preferences. A person embarked upon a course of action aimed at achieving a highly valued long-range outcome may be tempted off course by a more immediately attractive alternative. This dilemma is expressed by the Greek myth of the Sirens, who lured sailors to death by overriding with the beauty of their singing the sailors' long-range preference for living. Odysseus wanted to hear the Sirens, yet be able to resist them. He accomplished this by having himself tied to the deck while stuffing the ears of his crew with wax and instructing them to continue past the Sirens regardless of how he struggled and pleaded. In other words, he suppressed the crew's capacity for perception and his own capacity for action.

People's capacities for perception and action are routinely suppressed when they are sedated before surgery. This is done in part because many people who decide weeks in advance that an operation is in their best interest become anxious about the pain and risks as the hour of the operation draws near. The same sort of anxiety is known to affect couples who are about to get married. Many more people would call off their weddings during the final days before the ceremony were it not for the fact that by then society has taken the matter out of the couple's hands by interposing elaborate arrangements that would be embarrassing, inconvenient, and costly for the couple to cancel.

Ainslie calls these additional contingencies "side bets," in that they do not affect the probabilities on which the original gamble hinges, but simply change the value of the overall outcome by adding new outcomes to the equation. A person can make these additional rewards contingent on doing what will be rewarding in the long run (or punishments contingent on not doing so), so as to compensate for the specious reward that comes from deviating from that strategy. Since the appeal of the specious reward is usually that it is immediately gratifying, the same should be true of the payoff from the side bet. Giving a patient a tranquilizer before an operation changes the immediate value of having the operation (by making it more comfortable). Side bets can also involve financial costs and benefits. For example, a dentist or a psychiatrist may stipulate that patients will still have to pay for appointments that are canceled within twenty-four hours of the scheduled time. That will make a person think twice about canceling an appointment out of last-minute fear. Or a side bet may be based on psychic costs and benefits. One can strengthen one's commitment to a course of action by affirming the commitment publicly. If you tell enough people, including your family, that you're going to get married, then you'll look like a fool if you don't.

Side bets are one method by which people make themselves act in a manner consistent with long-range goals and policies. Another is simply to give more attention to the anticipated outcomes whose value reinforces the original decision. For example, one can deliberately think about the benefits of surgery and not think about the discomfort and risk. That most people find this mental discipline difficult to achieve is illustrated by the modern medical versions of the Sirens' song—smoking and overeating. One may "know" that one will benefit in the long run by not smoking or overeating, but that distant reward is hard to keep vividly in view when the immediate pleasure or emotional relief of the cigarette or the dessert is at hand. The longer projected life span that the nonsmoker enjoys is not a very tangible value at any given moment; likewise, the increased personal attractiveness that comes from losing weight is not yet evident when a person is just beginning to eat less. Some people can substitute for those delayed rewards a sense of increased self-respect from doing the right thing. This subjective self-rewarding is a kind of private side bet: a person who fails to do the right thing loses self-respect. If a person needs more tangible rewards and punishments to make the consequences of smoking or overeating sufficiently salient, the person can create them through side bets as in behavior-modification techniques.

Commitment in the
Face of Opposition

Not only do people themselves have mixed feelings about carrying out the decisions they have made, but others may disagree with those decisions. They may estimate the probabilities differently, or they may value the outcomes differently. Even when those others are not betting directly against the person making the decision, as in a competitive game, their interests may conflict with those of the decision-maker. For example, what is good for the patient may not be good for the doctor or for other members of the patient's family. All are affected by whatever action is taken, and yet only one action can be chosen.

The opposition of other interested parties is thus another

important source of conflict for the decision-maker. There are several ways in which other people can try to reverse a person's decision. They can make it physically impossible for the person to carry out the decision, as by putting him under anesthesia or declaring him mentally incompetent and institutionalizing him. They can call attention to implications of the decision, and of other possible decisions, that the person had not considered seriously enough (such as other outcomes, other probabilities, other values). Finally they can set up side bets, just as the decision-maker can. They can raise the ante by adding unpleasant contingencies which make it more costly for the decision-maker to stick to a bet, or they can tempt the decision-maker with positive rewards for switching.

All of these avenues of influence are illustrated by the case of the baby whose father refused permission to operate on her heart condition until he learned whether or not she had Down's syndrome. The doctors who disagreed with this decision threatened the father with a court injunction which would have taken decision-making power away from him. They called attention to the negative consequences that they thought his decision would have on the infant's chances for survival. Mainly, though, they put him under various kinds of pressure which increased the costs of maintaining his position. They insinuated that, as an added outcome of his choice, he would be regarded—and would have to regard himself—as a bad father and a bad husband. As yet another outcome, they implied that they would not resuscitate the child if an emergency occurred. The man's wife (perhaps influenced by the doctors) added a contingency of her own—that if his decision proved wrong she would not forgive him. The doctors and the wife were serving notice that they would blame the man for losing a gamble they disapproved of, but would not blame him if he lost a gamble that was acceptable to them. No wonder the man broke down after two days!

It is appropriate that people sometimes can change each other's minds, since decisions can be wrong, and the interests of others may legitimately overrule the decision-maker's own. On the other hand, since this is not always the case, it is also useful that people have commitment strategies by which to stay firm in their decisions when pressured by others. These strategies are the same as those used when the questioning of one's purpose comes from within oneself: side bets, selective attention, and even, as in the case of Odysseus, the relinquishing of one's physical capacity to change one's decision.

When people use such commitment strategies, when people make choices about where, when, and how long to apply such strategies, they are doing more than simply influencing a single decision or set of decisions. To establish a policy and stick with it in the face of initial failure or disappointment is to build character. Indeed, to do so inflexibly is to build a character armor which in the process of protecting the self can also serve as its prison. But to do so consciously, on principle, with an awareness of the risks and a readiness to change when change becomes advisable is to educate oneself about probability and strengthen one's capacity to cope with uncertainty. By the second criterion of the Probabilistic Paradigm, the making of a decision changes the decision-maker. The effect of making one choice may not be noticeable, but as making choices consciously becomes a habit, its impact on character is cumulative. By taking responsibility for one's choices and their consequences, one trains oneself to make further choices—to be a full participant in a difficult but not entirely unknowable or uncontrollable world.

Gambling in Practice

The following four cases from S.'s practice demonstrate ways in which the gambling approach to probabilistic thinking can be used beneficially by doctors and patients. The first case, incidentally, is one in which the hospital setting, instead of frustrating gambling with institutional conservatism, made it easier to gamble:

A baby born two weeks after his expected birth date had some initial difficulties in maintaining a constant body temperature and was taken to the intensive-care unit for observation. Dr. S. encouraged the baby's father to feed him two hours after birth; immediately thereafter, the baby stopped breathing and had to be resuscitated. Initial tests, including a complete blood count, did not suggest a possible infection. To explore whether there might nonetheless be an infection, more invasive procedures such as a lumbar puncture (spinal tap) and blood culture would be required. S. decided to forgo the tests for the time being. Other doctors questioned his decision, saying, "Why do we have the baby in the intensive-care unit, if not to perform tests?" He replied, "That's just it. If the baby were not under such constant observation, we might play it safe, do the tests, and wait for the results before treating. But here, where we can test immediately if something goes wrong, we don't need to test unless something goes wrong. Meanwhile, we can begin treatment and see how that works." Under this regime the child thrived and was spared not only the tests, but the three days of penicillin and kanamycin that are routinely given after the tests. In this case S. made two gambles on the patient's behalf. He gambled on an early feeding, and lost. But since he had gambled consciously, he could interpret the results realistically, instead of imagining more drastic reasons for the baby's breathing failure. He gambled on not testing, and won. Both, however, were good gambles, since they were made under conditions where the consequences of losing could be limited and where there was a good probability of recouping a loss.

A young woman's transplanted kidney began to fail while she was pregnant with twins. Since the pregnancy contributed to the strain on the kidney, S. considered it necessary to deliver the twins early. But as the woman's family doctor, taking into account such issues as her desire to have children and his own commitment to saving the babies if possible, he did not want to deliver them so early that they would have little chance to survive. A minimax strategy would dictate delivering the twins at the earliest possible time so as to avoid the death of the mother. The expected value strategy which S. and the woman actually adopted, however, entailed weighing the probabilities of survival for the mother and babies given the time chosen for delivery, along with the value of the mother's and babies' lives. The twins were delivered after thirty-two weeks of pregnancy, when both they and the mother would have a good chance to live.

A twenty-year-old woman had a sore throat which gave the appearance of strep throat, along with headache and swollen lymph nodes. S. had the choice of waiting one to two days for the results of a throat culture, which would confirm or disconfirm the diagnosis of strep throat, or treating with penicillin immediately, either with one injection or a ten-day supply of pills. If the woman did have strep throat, immediate treatment would relieve her symptoms without the need for a return visit, and would almost surely prevent complications (as would, in all likelihood, delayed treatment). On the other hand, the costs of using penicillin included the possibility of an allergic reaction to the drug, resulting in the patient's being denied a useful treatment when she might really need it on some later occasion. If she did not now have strep throat, this cost would be incurred without benefit. S. estimated the probability that the woman had strep throat at fifty percent. Given the estimate, he felt that the decision should hinge on the patient's values. Explaining the costs and benefits to the patient, he asked her to take her own gamble. She chose the penicillin shot, which he administered. He also took a throat culture for the purpose of educating his clinical judgment.

An elderly woman presented symptoms suggesting a diagnosis of arthritis of the neck. S. told her, "I'm ninety to ninety-five percent sure that that's what you have, and I'm willing to treat you now on the basis of that estimate. If treatment works, fine. If it's still bothering you in a couple of weeks, we can look at it again. On the other hand, if you want to spend a hundred dollars on tests, we can narrow down the area of doubt and come close to a hundred percent assurance. But I should warn you that the conditions that make up the other five or ten percent are not easily treatable anyway. It's your choice. I'll go either way with you on it." The patient asked, "What do we have to lose by treating for arthritis if that's not what I have?" S. replied that there was not a great deal to lose in terms of side effects or lost time and expense, and the patient agreed to begin treatment.

The gambling approach illustrated in these four cases presents options, probabilities, and values so that people can see them all together as part of a larger picture. When S. and his patients made decisions in this manner, they had a sense of greater control; they also felt the personal responsibility that went with that control. The language of gambling is not a panacea, a flight from responsibility. It is, rather, a constant reminder that there is no panacea. It is a language of responsibility in an uncertain world.

When S. and his patients gambled consciously together, they created their own categories for decision-making as they went along. Working in the contexts of everyday living, they could change their categories as the contexts changed. Among the most important contexts were the relationships patients had with their families, with the people they worked with (or worked for), and with S. as their doctor. People didn't make decisions as an abstract exercise; rather, they were influenced by the feelings they shared with others. If S. was going to help people make better decisions, he would have to understand those feelings. His own relationships with patients and families would have to be the kind of relationships that would foster wiser gambling.

PART III

RELATIONSHIPS

9

A FAMILY

If any one case taught S. that scientific gambling was more than an intellectual exercise, it was that of Rose Heifetz. Confronted with breast cancer that was well advanced before it was diagnosed, Rose had to gamble on a choice of treatments, as well as on how to face the possibility of death. Rose did not face these gambles alone. Her family and even S. himself shared the gambles with her. Yet this family still had much to learn about what it meant to share a gamble, and as a result Rose was not able to gamble as effectively as she might otherwise have done. As for S., he was learning even as he was teaching.

The irony was that the Heifetzes wanted to gamble consciously and, on the strength of their medical backgrounds, were well equipped to do so. Rose, a psychiatric social worker in her early fifties, knew about all the latest "holistic" therapies in psychology and medicine. Her husband, Herb, a statistician on the editorial staff of a medical journal, was conversant with the language of the physicians with whom he was in contact. Together they were prepared to consider carefully a wide range of options in cancer treatment. But they were less prepared to

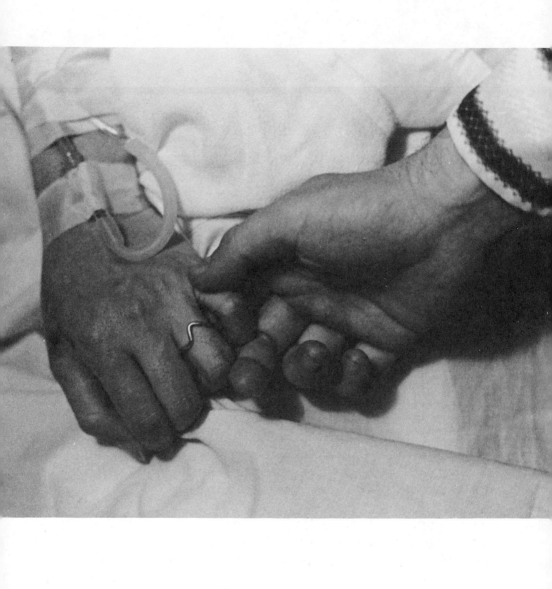

share the feelings that would arise in a situation of great uncertainty, where life itself was at stake.

Rose and Herb had been living apart for almost a year; that had something to do with it. However, they still saw each other frequently, in the company of their two grown children and three grandchildren, and continued to support each other in their respective careers. With all the estrangement that has come to exist among families who live under one roof, the Heifetzes' situation was in some ways a common variation of normal family life. Illness strikes families in good times and bad; it struck the Heifetzes at an awkward, unsettled moment in their life as a family. Still, it was as a family—with all the complications thereof—that they responded.

By the time Rose went to a doctor to confirm that she had breast cancer, it had already grown to be a massive tumor that had spread to the lymph nodes in her armpits. The odds on her ultimate recovery could scarcely have been worse. But if anyone could beat the odds, Rose thought, it was she. She believed that she formed a special category of patient to whom the statistical probabilities did not apply. After all, they were just "averages," and she was not average.

In many ways Rose *was* special. In addition to being very knowledgeable in medical matters, she had the strength of will to undergo a year-long "detoxification" program (a diet aimed at removing the "poisons" that had accumulated after a lifetime of bad eating habits) under the supervision of a nutritional consultant. This regime had left her clear-skinned and thirty pounds lighter. No longer troubled by frequent colds, she was more attractive and energetic than she had been in years.

On the other hand, in spite of her professional experience with breast cancer and her observations of the way women whom she had counseled had reacted with denial (such as by refusing to believe that they had cancer or were at risk of death), her own initial reaction was similar. In fact, even when the lump had become too noticeable to ignore, it had taken her a few weeks to pick up the phone and call a doctor. In part, this was because she needed some time to get used to the prospect of dying. In addition, her holistic approach to her health, much as it strengthened her in other ways, may have contributed to her reluctance to acknowledge that she was seriously ill.

One might wonder—as S. did, for instance—why this medically sophisticated woman had not had annual breast examinations or done monthly self-examinations, which might have revealed the presence of the tumor at an earlier stage. Perhaps she would have if breast examinations had been associated with the alternative health movement rather than with the medical profession. As it was, she seemed to feel that if she just ate right, lived right, and felt right, she wouldn't get sick; so why bother with examinations? By the same logic, however, if she did get sick, she might well wonder whether she had lived right after all. Hard as it was for Rose to face the fact that she might have cancer, it was even harder when she feared that she was the cause of it. When there was hope of a good outcome, the belief in oneself as the cause of one's health and illness could lead a person to gain knowledge and thereby gain control. The same belief, when there was fear of a bad outcome, could lead a person to avoid knowledge and thereby give up control.

Rose might have taken even longer to look into her condition had she not been able to call upon Herb for support. When she told him of her condition, Herb offered to accompany her to the doctor's office and to help her gather and interpret medical information and make the necessary decisions. Rose cried and accepted the offer. Herb was, as he put it, "able to be helpful in the way I had always been helpful. An intellectual role was the most comfortable one for me to play." He knew that Rose had wanted more from him emotionally than he had given during their years of marriage. If he could not or would not be her husband, he could at least be an involved, responsible friend and researcher.

What Rose was later to call her "odyssey through medicineland" did not begin, as it would have for many people, with a visit to a family doctor. Although she had met S. at a professional meeting and formed a favorable impression of him, she did not think first of him when she became ill. Thus S. was not involved in the early stages of her care, and he only knew about her initial decisions and experiences from what she and Herb told him later.

The doctor Rose called was an oncologist (cancer specialist), who did a biopsy (i.e., excised a piece of the breast mass for analysis) to verify the diagnosis of cancer that his examination of the lymph nodes indicated. Given Herb's connections, Rose found it natural to go first to a specialist. She chose this one in particular because he had a reputation for not sugar-coating the truth. Indeed, when she returned with Herb to see the oncologist along with a radiotherapist, she found them positively grim. "Look," she finally told them, "when you're with me, it's okay to smile."

In these physicians' opinion the treatment of choice was radiation plus drug therapy. Although no treatment could guarantee that a cancer which had already spread would not remain in her system and subsequently recur, nonsurgical treatment seemed a better bet than mastectomy (surgical removal of part or all of the breast) to arrest the tumor's growth and reduce its size. The particular type of drug therapy chosen was based on the knowledge that a lack of estrogen (female hormone) inhibits the growth of some forms of breast cancer. In order to see whether Rose's tumor was sensitive to the drug Tomaxifen, which neutralizes estrogen, the oncologist ordered additional tests performed on a tissue sample that had been preserved from the biopsy.

At the end of the session the oncologist and the radiotherapist answered Rose and Herb's questions and told them to feel free to call if anything further needed to be clarified. Some questions did arise when the couple discussed the visit that weekend, and Herb called the hospital on Monday to relay them to the doctors. But it happened that this was the first week in August, and he was told that both doctors had gone off on two-week vacations that day. Was anybody covering? Yes, but these doctors would need to familiarize themselves with the case. Frustrated as they were by what they experienced as abandonment, the Heifetzes nevertheless decided to wait for the oncologist to return rather than involve another doctor. Besides, under the circumstances it was easier to wait a little longer for the bad news.

When he got back from vacation, the oncologist reassured Herb that "a week or two doesn't matter anyway." This reassurance was immediately undermined when he couldn't locate the Tomaxifen test results. With a sinking feeling Herb wondered whether the lab work had been done at all and whether (as a result of tissue spoilage) Rose might have to go through another biopsy. Several days later the results were located: Tomaxifen could be expected to retard the growth of Rose's cancer. Rose and Herb were relieved, but the delays and mixups had shaken their trust in physicians.

Herb began to accumulate a thick file folder full of information about various treatment programs. He made it his task to evaluate the claims of numerous variations of conventional and holistic therapy (some of which invoked widely differing criteria of evaluation). He reviewed published research and consulted with people he trusted, and still there were no sure answers.

The first question to be resolved was whether to go along with Rose's wishes and the oncologist's recommendation and refrain from surgery. Rose and Herb decided against surgery for the following reasons: (1) The statistics on outcomes of surgery for Rose's sort of advanced breast cancer were not as encouraging as those for the combined radiation-drug therapy treatment. (2) Even the surgeon they consulted did not recommend surgery for cancer this advanced, since he felt it might interfere with the body's capacity to resist the spread of the disease. "When the *surgeons* say don't do surgery," said Herb, "when they're telling you not to come to them and do their thing, it's hard not to listen." (3) Rose had a general philosophical bias favoring "natural" remedies, those that interfered as little as possible with bodily functioning. Though drugs and radiation were objectionable to her, surgery was even less acceptable to this woman who didn't smoke and would not take aspirin for headaches. Besides, she was confident that she was in such good overall health that she could lick this illness without surgery. (4) Surgery would involve a difficult convalescence and would have residual effects on Rose's chest and arm areas. (5) Rose would not choose to be disfigured unless she absolutely had to. "It might be different if I had a loving husband who'd be there whatever I looked like," she explained, "but now that I'm on the market again my breasts are important to me." Later she added, referring to the breakup of her marriage as well as to her mother's having committed suicide while she was still a young child, "I've lost enough in my life. I'm not about to lose my breasts too."

Rose made these remarks some weeks later when she brought S. up to date on how she had dealt with her illness before he was involved. They were part of her interpretation of cancer as "a disease of separation and loss" and of herself as a "cancer-prone personality." With her mother's suicide she suffered emotional deprivation at an early age. Then she led an isolated life until she married Herb and began to raise a family. When she lost that bond too, she became, by her account, psychologically vulnerable to cancer.

Rose's life history and emotional state may well have been contributing causes of her illness. In proposing them as the only causes, however, she appeared to S. to be falling back on mechanistic thinking, as surely as if she had been giving an account more compatible with the standard medical model's search for a causative agent such as a virus. S. could see how, both despite and because of the Heifetzes' familiarity with scientific methods, their thinking was so strongly influenced by the Mechanistic Paradigm. Here was a couple who felt a lot of mistrust toward each other in the aftermath of their recent separation. They had lost some vital parts of their family relationship, the parts that went with living together. Without the support that they might have given each other in better times, they didn't have the emotional freedom to think critically about life-and-death matters. What they did have was a way of thinking and feeling urged on them by their upbringing, education, and unconscious promptings, a way that enabled (or compelled) them to blame themselves and each other for a misfortune that had many causes, some of them unknown.

Rose was in no position to think critically when she felt alone and abandoned. Living on her own, uncomfortable about calling on her family for support, and unsure about how much support there was to call upon, she had little choice but to deny the terrifying prospect of disabling illness and death. When she decided early on that the statistics on mortality from breast cancer were insufficiently refined to fit her special case, she

was, on the one hand, quite reasonably making a subjective
probability estimate that took into account her special capacity
to respond to the illness knowledgeably and effectively. On the
other hand, by refusing even to incorporate the available statistics into her subjective estimate, she was seeing herself as
entirely special, or unique, i.e., not subject to the same uncertainties that other people were. "Think of all the anxiety I'd
have if I believed the statistics!" she explained. She couldn't
bear the anxiety because she felt she had no one with whom to
share it.

So she imagined herself the all-powerful cause of her condition, and when she wasn't feeling so powerful, she imagined her
family to be the cause. In citing the breakup of her marriage as
the final "separation" or "loss" that left her susceptible to cancer, she seemed by implication to be pointing the finger at Herb.
And when she suggested that she had decided against surgery in
part because she no longer had "a loving husband," she was
assigning to Herb a lion's share of responsibility for that choice
(a choice that might have life-or-death consequences).

After he got to know the family, S. wondered whether Rose
was blaming Herb as a way of holding on to what was left of
their relationship. The relationship, at least as she saw it, no
longer existed as a full communal bond, by which Herb would
feel an unconditional commitment to help care for Rose. Perhaps, though, she could still keep it going as an exchange relationship by saying to him, in effect, "Since you caused this pain, I
have a right to ask you for help." In fact, Rose may not have
needed to remind Herb what he "owed" her. He may well have
felt committed to supporting her, as he said he did, simply
because she was the person with whom he had shared so much
of his life. In fact he invited her to move back in with the family,
but she declined to do so. She may not have been quite sure of his
devotion. Now that they were living apart, she may not have
trusted him to be at her side when she needed him. And in a
world of isolation and loneliness, a relationship held together by
guilt or blame would be better than no relationship at all.

For whatever complex reasons, Herb committed himself to
sharing the gamble with Rose. He was involved, not only with

his mind and his expertise, but with his feelings. He had loved Rose for too long to accept easily the prospect of her dying. He may indeed have felt guilty about having put her "out on the market" where the loss of her breasts would be a disadvantage to her. And he may not have completely given up on the possibility of a reconciliation with her.

Herb and Rose did not, however, acknowledge all the different feelings they had toward each other. Instead they settled back into their old, comfortable roles. Rose expressed some of her feelings by ascribing magical causative or curative powers to them, while Herb played what he described as a "detached" scientist gathering "hard data" and hoping that the data would make his decisions for him. He became the professional patient advocate—a role originally modeled after that of a concerned family member—in a family where concern could be expressed only in the language of mechanistic science. The Heifetzes tended to speak of "data" on the one hand and "feelings" on the other. Yet feelings, along with data, entered into every decision they made.

The big decision, they felt, was to go with a combination of nonsurgical treatments. As Rose later told S., "I put together my own package—a piece here, a piece there—out of the best of both traditional and alternative medicine." The "traditional" part of the package was the relatively noninvasive form of medical intervention represented by the radiation and drug therapy. The main issue here was that of sequence. Tomaxifen originally had been used to shrink tumors before applying radiation, so that less radiation would be necessary. Recent studies, however, had shown that Tomaxifen interferes with the effects of radiation (but not vice versa). Rose's doctors therefore decided to go ahead with radiation first. Herb objected that since radiation only works at the site of the tumor at which it is directed, while Tomaxifen affects cancer cells throughout the body, it might be of more urgent importance to retard the spread of the cancer with the drug than to attack the tumor with radiation. It was a choice between gambles.

After weighing the priorities, Herb and Rose went along with the doctors' choice. Rose began a four-month course of escalating doses of radiation for which she had to go to the hospital daily—an exhausting, dispiriting procedure. Tracing the extent of the tumor with a dye, the radiotherapist precisely mapped out the area to be irradiated on a grid. At one point Rose was hospitalized for radiation implants. Filaments were placed directly into the tumor and then removed several days later.

Meanwhile she continued to see the nutritionist who had prescribed her "detoxification" program, a person in whom she placed a good deal of trust. Her anticancer diet consisted of dietary restrictions together with vitamin supplements and enzymes that the nutritionist believed would break down cancer cells by making them more permeable to outside agents. (The vitamins and enzymes sometimes numbered a dozen in a single meal.) The diet was based on a little that is known and much that is guessed about the relationship between cancer and nutrition. Among the nutritionist's recommendations were the following: Cancer patients suffer an extreme deficit of Vitamin A, so add Vitamin A. A fatty diet is associated with breast cancer, so cut out fat. The liver, which must eliminate the toxins produced by cancer and cancer treatment, can be strained by having large amounts of carbohydrates to convert into sugar, so limit carbohydrate intake. Cultivation of cancer cells in the laboratory requires a saline solution, so no salt. Actually, *all* living cells are cultured in saline solution, which as a culture medium has a different function from salt in one's diet. A person would die without body salt. Other aspects of this diet were equally debatable. Much indeed is known about variations in the incidence of various cancers in regions with different diets, but the curative value of dietary modification has not been established. Still, Herb went along with Rose's view that any treatment should be tried in the absence of evidence that it was incompatible with another treatment or otherwise harmful. If it might do some good, why not?

On this principle Rose went to a number of different practitioners simultaneously. Along with regular visits to the oncologist, radiotherapist, and her nutritionist, she undertook a program of "visual healing imagery" (Simonton *et al,* 1978; Fiore, 1979), which sought to mobilize her body's defenses against malignancy by having her visualize them in action, and saw a conventional psychotherapist to deal with her anxiety about death. If nothing else, drawing upon varied specialists gave her a feeling of having a support system and being actively engaged in her own care. A firm believer in "mind as healer, mind as slayer" (Pelletier, 1977), she was determined to work up some positive emotional energy to combat the illness that emotional stress had, she felt, in part caused.

For Herb, though, this meant more far-out approaches and extravagant claims to investigate. The file folder grew thicker and thicker. Finally he threw up his hands and cried, "No more!" He was having his troubles with "establishment" medicine as well. The oncologist and radiotherapist were only infrequently in touch with each other, let alone with the nutritionist. The resulting duplication of effort was sometimes harmful to Rose, as when she took the same blood tests two weeks in a row because each doctor didn't know what the other was doing.

Herb, along with Rose, experienced considerable stress in dealing with doctors and medical facilities. When Rose was hospitalized to have the radiation implants removed, Herb thought it would be nice to celebrate by picking her up afterward and taking her out to dinner. (She had been told that she would be able to leave the hospital a few hours after the procedure.) Upon arrival Herb was greeted by a security officer, who told him that he had five minutes to bring Rose down before his car would be towed. As Herb remembered it, up on the ward he found Rose walking around in a stupor. She was pale, lethargic, and irritable. "Are you sure you're okay?" he asked. "Maybe we'd better ask the nurse." While Rose stood by mumbling, the nurse reassured Herb that a doctor had said that his wife was able to go home. The next day Rose couldn't remember anything that had happened. Herb hypothesized that she had had to be anesthetized more heavily than expected for the implant removal, but that the staff, once assured that she had survived the procedure, had not checked up on her afterward. As in the case of the child K., the hospital personnel appeared not to be concerned with smaller, subtler gains and losses. Later Herb regretted that he had not questioned the judgment of the absent doctors when his own eyes had made another judgment.

When the radiation treatments were over, Rose did her own

version of the *experimentum crucis* by temporarily discontinuing her vitamin and enzyme supplements. "Within two days I was miserably sick," she reported. "That experiment was one hundred percent evidence of the value of my diet. I didn't need any more evidence." In her confidence that the only cause of her symptoms was the cause that she manipulated (her diet), Rose ignored evidence of other possible causes—in this case, the fact that people who have radiation treatment almost always feel as she did forty-eight hours after the treatment is stopped.

Herb, meanwhile, was finding it increasingly difficult to apply the *experimentum crucis* model to the situation at hand. He was beginning to realize that he was facing decisions he couldn't make by using what he had been taught was the scientific method. How was he to apply research data from mice to human beings? How much credence could he give to the words of a true believer? He was an old hand at collecting "hard data," but was much less confident when the need for subjective judgment in decision-making became inescapable.

He also was learning that he wasn't able to be as objective as he had hoped in conveying information to Rose. In trying to provide the "facts" she needed while also giving her reason to hope, he was treading a thin line—especially since he was not comfortable thinking about facts and hope together. In his concern over Rose's reaction to potentially devastating information he found himself unable to be a detached observer. "My mind played tricks with me," he later recalled to S. "I wouldn't hear things, or I would unconsciously distort them. The facts would get transformed in my head." He was coming face to face with the second criterion of the Probabilistic Paradigm. He had been trying to live up to the idealized conception of a mechanistic scientist that he had formed in the course of working for a scientific journal. Every time he rationalized, made unwarranted inferences, and evaded the worst possibilities, he learned how an observer creates the data as he interprets it. But what he considered a failure on his part was really a kind of growth. Herb was beginning to realize that even in science one could not deny feelings.

In any case, he wanted help. He felt out of his depth in a sea of data and conflicting claims. It was then that Rose mentioned the family doctor whose name she had been keeping in the back of her mind in case she ever needed him. "You need him now," Herb told her.

S., too, remembered his earlier meeting with Rose Heifetz. It felt odd to have as a patient someone whom he had met as a fellow professional. Seeing Rose as someone like himself, he felt closer to her and to her illness than he would have liked. Even more than usual he wanted to be of help.

At first, though, with Rose's treatments well under way, he wondered how he could be of help. It wasn't (as he originally hoped) by working directly with the various practitioners who were treating Rose. Some of these practitioners, being outside the medical system he represented, had no reason to honor his position or his authority. And the ones who *were* part of the system seemed too intent on protecting their turf to yield any of it to him. Or else they were too busy, and so was he. He never once met the oncologist or radiotherapist.

Not that it mattered to Rose. She was glad enough just to have someone to go to when she didn't feel well and wanted to know whether her symptoms were related to the cancer and its treatment. For example, when she had mucus and a metallic taste in her mouth, was this from the radiation? But perhaps the most important thing she and Herb got from S. was a sense that here was a doctor who cared. He arranged to speak with them at least once a week, and if they didn't call him, he called them. "I've got a doctor who calls *me!*" announced Rose to her friends.

S.'s contribution was to support the Heifetzes both intellectually and emotionally in the decision-making process. Much of what they wanted him to look into was completely new to him. He couldn't do the legwork himself; he didn't have the time, and no insurance plan would pay for it. So he simply read the materials Herb collected and reacted to them on the basis of his clinical experience. As he did so, he saw that Herb had a point of view, however much he claimed otherwise. Herb's bias was to give too much credence, to take too seriously the claims of various therapies. In the delicate balance between doubt and trust that every scientist (or scientific gambler) must strike for himself, Herb erred on the side of giving too many approaches the benefit of the doubt. He did this not only with the materials he researched, but also in interpreting what S. said to him. When S. tried to level with Herb about the odds against survival for a woman whose breast cancer was as far advanced as Rose's was, Herb understood the message as something less grim. S., however, did not yet feel comfortable about pressing the point.

Among the various treatments that Rose and Herb presented for his consideration, some struck S. as potentially helpful, some as useless or even harmful. When he spoke on the phone with the nutritionist, for example, S. was angered by her claim (with no evidence to substantiate it) that her diet could serve as a primary treatment for cancer, as well as by her marketing with great fanfare what he thought of as standard principles of good nutrition. Still, a good diet (along with medical treatment) might well contribute to a favorable outcome.

S. granted that, although some of the measures that they tried were of dubious rationale, the Heifetzes' energetic efforts may have helped Rose avoid the depression that can accompany a grim diagnosis. By being active in her own care, by busying herself with many small decisions, Rose gained a sense of accomplishment and hope which made her feel better and may have helped keep up her physical strength. Still, there was a substantial likelihood that the eventual outcome would not be favorable. Even if the unlikely came to pass and things turned out well, many of the choices Rose and Herb made would nonetheless be far from having been scientific gambles. S. wondered whether Rose and Herb were maintaining a frenetic pace of activity so as not to have to acknowledge the large role that chance, rather than their own skill, would play in the outcome. He could hardly blame them if they were.

It occurred to him that he might be patronizing this family by encouraging the hope they placed in long-shot cures. But on the whole he felt that he was building trust so that they could learn to estimate the probabilities more realistically. By his willingness to entertain new approaches, by his implicit and explicit assurances that he didn't consider the Heifetzes crackpots for looking into remedies that he could not endorse, he extended to them a trust that they could then reciprocate. He let them know that he trusted their judgment, and they in turn came to trust his. To Rose it meant a great deal that she had a doctor who kept in touch with her, who was considerate of her feelings, and who respected her thinking. The more certainty she felt about her relationship with her doctor, the more uncertainty she could accept about her illness and its treatment. Now she could keep a more open mind, acknowledging that orthodox medical approaches had some benefits and unorthodox ones some disadvantages.

Not that she hadn't thought critically before meeting S. She had accepted radiation treatment (which some of her colleagues were as much opposed to as Herb's were opposed to megavitamins and psychic healing) and rejected such all-or-none schemes as residential care in a Mexican natural-healing retreat. But it was S. who supported her growing willingness to look critically at the "natural" remedies that she was predisposed to favor, such as Laetrile, the controversial apricot-pit extract that is illegal as a cancer treatment in the United States. S. said, "I do not find any evidence that Laetrile works, and therefore I see no rational basis for using it. But I can understand your reasons for wanting to try anything, and it certainly won't get in the way of my being your doctor if you do want to use it." This advice gave Rose and Herb the emotional space they needed to make a rational decision. Herb had accumulated a vast file of sometimes contradictory findings on Laetrile, some of the positive results having seemed sufficiently credible to warrant further investigation. But in the end he and Rose passed up the Laetrile program.

In making it possible for the Heifetzes to be more rational in their choice of options, S. became perhaps a little less rational both in what he said and what he thought about the overall prognosis. In the relationship of trust which he established with the family, he was coming to feel like "one of the family" himself. He liked Rose, and he didn't want to see her suffer. It wasn't any easier for S. than it was for the Heifetzes to admit that skill might be powerless to overcome all the effects of chance. He shared this feeling with the Heifetzes so that they might understand why other doctors sometimes came across as grim, especially when confronted with cancer. They responded by telling him that they were comfortable with his saying, "I don't know." Indeed, his willingness to say "I don't know" was what enabled them to trust him as much as they did.

The problem was that he did know more than he felt able to say. In their readiness to accept "I don't know" as an answer, the Heifetzes were treating the unspeakable as merely uncertain. It would be necessary at some point to turn uncertainty into probability, but this they were not yet ready to do. S. somehow felt that he did not have their permission to speak about death, that Rose would regard the mention of death as an intrusion, or perhaps even as a cause of the very possibility of death that S. wished they could all look at together. On S.'s side, if one of his principles was to honor the truth, another was not to impose it. In order for him to be able to present the gamble to the Heifetzes as it really was, they would have to participate in creating the categories of the gamble. They, and not S. alone, would have to be able to acknowledge the possibility of death. It would take more time and more trust before they would be ready to hear the unwelcome message.

Under the circumstances, then, S. let himself be carried along, half consciously and half unconsciously, by the Heifetzes' energy and by their hope. It wasn't that he told them anything that wasn't true. But when they would make a remark that might have struck him as a denial of the probability of death, he would let it pass. He stretched to the limit to give the benefit of the doubt to the things they said. In the presence of such a compelling, strong-willed woman as Rose, S. almost became a believer. On some level he shared her feeling that, yes, she *had* lost enough; why should she lose her life too? With any patient he would hope for the best; with this patient he was persuaded to expect the best. He did not want to dampen Rose's fighting spirit. He wanted to support her determination not to give in to the illness, and yet he felt that sooner or later she would want to face the truth of her prognosis.

After six months of radiation and Tomaxifen, Rose went to the oncologist for a routine checkup. She looked so healthy that the doctor almost didn't recognize her when she walked into the office. To his surprise (since he had hoped to shrink the tumor in a year) there was no tumor left, either in the breast or in the lymph nodes to which it had spread. Finding on examination no evidence for even identifying Rose as a cancer patient, he told her that he had no basis for estimating the probability of recurrence. Actually such remissions are common after the first course of treatment for breast cancer. Even a complete remission did not alter the fact that Rose had had advanced breast cancer. But the oncologist found it all too natural to join in Rose's relief and delight. "Just keep on doing whatever you've been doing," he told her—which meant continuing the Tomaxifen for a few months as a precautionary measure and staying indefinitely on a moderate, "maintenance" version of her diet.

When these results were relayed to the radiotherapist, he jumped up with excitement. Previously so pessimistic, he, like the oncologist, reacted with unguarded joy. It was as if Rose's unexpected reprieve was a reprieve for all concerned. Indeed, the Heifetzes became the toast of the medical community, in which they already were well regarded. Each of the practitioners Rose had consulted, "establishment" and otherwise, regarded her apparent success as a personal vindication. She soon received a number of invitations to do taped and filmed interviews and speak before self-care and holistic health groups as model patient.

S., too, joined in the general optimism. While Rose had been fighting her desperate battle with cancer, he had accepted her treating the situation as one of complete uncertainty ("I don't know"). Now that she was in remission, he accepted her treating it as one of complete certainty. When she spoke of her illness, it was in the past tense. "For a while I wanted to die," she told S., "but when my body called my bluff I realized I didn't want to. I made myself better. I did it, and it makes me feel so powerful, as if I can do anything and don't need anybody to help me. I have every intention of not getting this cancer again." Her fear that she had been the cause of the cancer had been translated into a belief that she had been its cure. Behind her bravado there lay a concern about who really would help take care of her if she became ill again. But S. couldn't quite get down to that level with her. "Okay," he would say to himself, "we'll talk about it the next time she comes in." But each time there were so many other things to talk about that they just didn't get around to it.

What they talked about instead (besides issues that came up in the course of the medical checkups) was a recapitulation of the successful experience they had had together. Rose included S. prominently among the practitioners to whom she liberally gave credit for her recovery, and S. showed an understandable disinclination to interrupt such praise by bringing up disturbing complexities. Rose also was more than happy to honor S.'s way of thinking. "When people ask me to what I attribute my recovery," she said, "I tell them I really can't say that any one ingredient 'did it.' But I know from the reactions of all those doctors that by doing all those things together I came out a lot better than chance." S. assented to this multicausal stochastic explanation. "Your approach didn't focus on a single cause, or even one cause at a time, but on many different causes working together in ways that you and your doctors couldn't understand and that might have changed over time. It wasn't as if you could say, 'We'll add the diet to the radiation treatment and increase our chances of success by twenty percent.' Who knows how the diet may have interacted, for better or worse, with the radiation or the drug therapy? It was more a case of 'Here we've done all these things, and together they've worked so far.' "

Talking about the Probabilistic Paradigm is not the same thing as practicing it. Sometimes talking about it can be a way to avoid practicing it. Yet in Rose and S.'s case the very act of talking in terms of the Probabilistic Paradigm, even in a defensive way, seemed to remind them of its implications. Perhaps by reviewing a successful experience in dealing with one kind of uncertainty, they became comfortable enough to look at other uncertainties. Perhaps they were building up an additional fund of trust with all the praise and encouragement they gave each other. In any case, Rose finally began to raise, or give S. permission to raise, some issues that were of vital importance to her.

As she spoke of the support Herb had given her during her illness, Rose began to voice other concerns. Yes, Herb had been a big help, and she was grateful for that. But what about the time he disappeared for two weeks on a research project while she was home convalescing? Herb was accessible by phone, like a doctor, but he was not accessible in the heart. He was a man of honorable words, sensitive words, but where were the feelings? Herb had never been a man of feeling.

S. asked Rose how much support she had had from her children. "They were too busy to be bothered," she said. "Living alone like I do, there have been times when I've really needed bodies around to help me, like when I've been too tired to prepare a meal. It would have been marvelous to have someone come around to my apartment and help with the housework or simply visit me when I didn't have the energy to go out and socialize. My daughter thought she was being supportive by helping Herb with all the reading, which was really supporting *him;* I'd rather have had her come over and watch TV with me. And did my family take me out for a big celebration at the end?"

S. felt uneasy when she said "the end." Again she was talking as if the ordeal was over and she was cured.

Rose answered her own question. "Not on your life. You should have seen how blasé they all were about it. The only one who showed any emotion was my four-year-old grandson, for God's sake! And if I bring any of this up, they tell me I'm laying a guilt trip on them. My daughter says to me, 'You act as if you were always hungry. Whatever we gave you would never be enough!' And now they tell me I didn't let them have enough candy when they were kids!"

S. reflected that this was indeed a family of the mechanistic era, fighting over food and other forms of nurturance. It was a case of people starving one another, perhaps beginning with Rose's mother, who hadn't cared to live long enough to give Rose a good start in life.

"Well," Rose concluded, "I've never been celebrated in my family, so what else is new? I survived this time by my own strength, and I'll go on surviving alone."

"I get the feeling," S. ventured, "that deep down you feel uncertain about who's going to take care of you if you ever relapse."

"Uncertain is right!" Rose exclaimed, becoming suddenly

agitated. "That's why I'm so determined that I won't get sick again. I can't afford to be sick. What would I do? Where would I go? Who could I count on? Why, I have friends who are more like family to me than my family."

"They may have to become your family," said S.

After a brief silence Rose mused, "The only way this cancer will ever come back is if I again let myself sink into despair."

S. could understand how he and Herb had both kept silent about some of the grimmer possibilities. Neither of them wanted to be the bearer of bad tidings who would lead Rose into despair. If that was what Rose thought could bring back the cancer, who, after all, would want to be the guilty party? S. was relieved, therefore, when Rose told him that she and Herb wanted to have a series of family-counseling sessions with him. Having been forced together by illness after they had decided to live apart, they saw how their feelings toward each other were both keeping them together and keeping them apart. Perhaps S. could help them better understand these feelings.

Their view of the family, like much else in their lives, was colored by professional jargon. "The family doctor," pronounced Rose, "is in a perfect position system-wise to help structure the management of the family. He also is there to help family members with their feelings about what it's like to have Mama as a patient." Her first sentence might be said to represent the chaff, her second the wheat, of contemporary therapeutic approaches to the family—and of S.'s family practice. What S. found encouraging, however, was the Heifetzes' realization that they would need to understand themselves as a family so that they could understand Rose's illness and the way they thought, felt, and acted with regard to it.

By now S. had a clear sense that he had been colluding with Rose and Herb in excluding one of the possible outcomes—death—from the gamble that they were consciously making together. Now that Rose was in remission, now that the three of them had some trust and some experience in working together, he felt both compelled and permitted to share with Rose and Herb his concern that this outcome was a real (perhaps even a large) possibility. In making the choice to do so, he realized that he was taking a chance. For he was acting against one of the messages he had been getting from the couple: "Don't rock the boat when things are going so well." But there was clearly another side of the Heifetzes that wanted to gamble consciously even where death was concerned. After all, these were people who placed considerable stock in learning, knowledge, and truth. So was he. It thus would have been out of character for all three of them just to sit back, let nature take its course, and enjoy what would probably be only the temporary success of the treatment. Rose's taking the initiative concerning family counseling strengthened S.'s belief that she and Herb held it as a principle, as he did, to gamble as honestly, as scientifically as they could. The side of them that wanted to know the truth had come to the fore.

The family-counseling sessions began where Rose's previous conversation with S. left off—with the stalemate she had reached with her children. "I don't complain anymore." She shrugged. "They don't want to hear it. I got the message, and I comply with it." To say that one complies with a one-way message, rather than that one interprets and thereby helps create it, is mechanistic in the sense that one does not acknowledge one's own part in the interchange that produces the message. Rose had, after all, helped produce the family that was giving her this message. But it was less painful to think of herself as complying—to think of her family as an external force acting upon her.

Still, in a family where no one wanted to hear anyone complaining, things were difficult enough in times of health and good fortune. When serious illness presented itself, the simplest way to make life bearable was to deny the possibility of death. Everyone participated in the denial—Rose by imagining that she alone among women with advanced breast cancer could give herself a favorable prognosis, Herb by being a data-gatherer, and the children by assuming an even greater distance than usual from their mother. For Rose the unpalatable choice was to deny her feelings and the reality behind them or to use guilt ("You caused it") to make her family listen.

One night, after a difficult evening with Herb at his house, their daughter had come back with Rose to her apartment because Rose appeared to be so upset. In an attempt to be reassuring her daughter had said, "Look, I'd do this for anyone." Rose was not reassured. The remark touched off her fear that even to her family she was no different from "anyone." Rose hastened to add that her upset on that occasion had been "purely emotional, nothing to do with my daughter or my illness"—as if "subjective" emotions could be separated from their "objective" context. Again, fear was driving Rose back to mechanistic thinking. She was living in too cramped an emotional space to think freely.

The same was true for Herb, who during the initial counseling sessions was silent much of the time. In an effort to break through the wall of guardedness and mutual suspicion and get Rose and Herb talking to each other, S. began making provocative paraphrases and interpretations of what they were saying. ("So Herb is not to be trusted? How does it feel not to be trusted, Herb?") He hoped that, in reacting to these statements, they would start responding to each other's feelings.

What emerged was that Rose and Herb, like Rose and the children, were at a standoff. Rose could trust Herb, as she put it, "not to let me starve in the gutter," to support her in professional and medical matters, and to be, by his lights, fair and dutiful. But she could not trust him to be available to her in a fuller sense. For his part Herb saw no reason why he couldn't be "very close friends" with Rose. She, on the other hand, still hadn't given up on him as a husband. She wanted him "to be a companion, a playmate, a lover, a comforter; to be honest and not run away when I'm upset." Those were the things she had wanted all along, although she had been the one to move out once the situation had come to seem hopeless. "For God's sake, Herb!" she exclaimed, turning to face him for the first time. "You think I feel welcome in your home when I know that I'll hardly be cold in the ground before you'll find a replacement?"

S. was beginning to see how little choice Rose had. A person who felt herself to be interchangeable to her husband and "just anyone" to her children might well seek whatever immortality was to be gained from the approbation of a retinue of health professionals. Through them, if not through her family, she could keep alive a record of the good she had done in the world.

Without the consolation of being able to leave behind such a record death could only mean (as it does when it is experienced in the unconscious) total separation, the annihilation of the self.

What makes death a gentler prospect is the conscious awareness that one's memory will be carried on in the lives of others. As the dying Socrates in *Phaedo* was internalized by Plato, all of us hope to be internalized by our families. But in the atomized, dog-eat-dog world of today, that hope cannot always be convincingly maintained. Rose Heifetz was an assimilated Jew who did not see her memory surviving in a community and a tradition. She feared death as much as she did because the structure of her family (and of the society of which her family was a part) did not allow her to glimpse a connection between herself and those who would come after her. Once she died, the connection would be broken (Lifton, 1979).

S. found it so hard to confront her about her evasive strategies because he saw that there was little else she could do. She was living her life under the conditions that her life had established for her. By now he could understand what Mrs. Pinelli, the thirty-five-year-old woman with hypertension, had meant when she said that she didn't care if she lived beyond fifty as long as she lived to see her children grown. What was it to be fifty and unconnected? But if up to that point you had lived for your children, perhaps your memory could continue to live in and through them after your death.

"So now you two have split up for good," S. said to Rose and Herb, wondering what kind of response he would get. Rose answered by saying that she didn't think she could trust Herb. S. wondered how easily she could trust anyone after her mother had died while she was still a child. "Could you learn to trust him short of being husband and wife—say, just at the level of his taking care of you when you're ill?" Could she assume a flexible distance toward her husband and trust him about one thing if not another—trust him, that is, critically instead of blindly? Rose didn't think she could. "I guess that's my *schtick,*" she said. "That's just how I feel." She was declaring her feelings, but in a way that defined for herself an area of subjectivity where she could not be challenged. It was as if to say, "I am the

only cause of 'my *schtick,*' which I know you won't accept, but
which you can't take away from me, either."

Herb, meanwhile, had "issues of my own" that he was exploring through the separation and that kept him from making the
commitment Rose wanted from him. Both of them were working on an individual level, clinging to "issues" that they saw as
subjective, private, and not subject to reason. S. did not think
that any movement would be possible that way. Not that he was
trying to bring about their reconciliation as a couple. It was just
that, simply from their past relationship, their "issues" concerned each other. They needed to work them out with each
other rather than with the fantasy images of each other that
arose when they tried to work them out alone.

At this time, though, there did not seem to be enough trust
between them. Whenever the counseling sessions became too
tense or reached a standstill, S. let the couple withdraw from
their intense emotional currents and remind themselves how
well they had cooperated with each other during Rose's illness.
S. hoped that they might learn to gamble with each other in
everyday life as they had gambled with each other—and with
him—in an emergency. Having learned to trust a doctor who
sometimes said "I don't know," perhaps they could learn to
trust each other when they said "I don't know" about their
feelings toward each other.

Where Rose's prognosis was concerned, however, it was time
to go beyond "I don't know." By this point, S. thought, the Heifetzes would not be able to deal realistically with their family
relationships unless they faced the reality of Rose's illness. If
he let them go on talking complacently about Rose's "self-
cure," he would not be doing what deep down they wanted him
to do.

To get to the probabilities, he began by pointing gently to the
uncertainty. "It would be nice to be out of the woods with this
cancer."

Rose looked at him. She appeared both hurt and angry. "Why
talk about that now? For now I am out of the woods—what else
is there to say?"

"I know you've heard this said before," said S.

Rose swallowed hard. "Not lately, it seems. I guess the idea of an uncertain future looked a lot better when things were going badly. But when you talk about it now, it's almost as if you don't want me to stay well." She paused. "But of course you do. I know that."

"We all want that very much," Herb added.

"So much so," S. went on, "that we find it hard to talk about the possibility that you may not stay well. We have to remember that the odds aren't what we'd like them to be."

Rose shook her head sadly. "As hard as we've all worked . . ."

". . . some things can't be changed." Herb had finished the sentence for her.

S. sensed that he was not the only one who felt relieved.

Once Rose and Herb found that they could accept the possibility (and perhaps the probability) of a recurrence of Rose's cancer, they were able to talk more openly about its real and imagined causes. In subsequent sessions they began to be relaxed enough to talk to each other about themselves as a family. They could open up and express greater honesty, greater humor, and less simple meanings.

Here S. gambled again in order to show the Heifetzes a mirror of the mechanistic thinking that they were outgrowing. Again he made their implicit beliefs and feelings explicit, thereby exposing them to critical rationality, as when he said to Rose, "You wouldn't blame Herb for your cancer," or to Herb, "How does it feel to be a cause of your wife's cancer? How would you feel if she died of it?" Of course, he did not intend these remarks and questions literally. Rather he was bringing to the surface long-held irrational attitudes in the hope that these could then be acknowledged and repudiated. This process was especially valuable for Rose, who in her irritation with S. ended up defending Herb as *not* having been the cause of the illness.

S. now explored Rose's fantasy that she had called the cancer into being to show that she needed Herb and then vanquished it to show that she didn't need him. It was with considerable satisfaction that S. heard her enunciate a multicausal stochastic explanation of the cancer: there were many causes, and Herb was in a sense a cause and in a sense not a cause. Perhaps

now she could give up the all-or-none attitude toward Herb by
which she insisted on trusting him blindly and then was disappointed. Perhaps she could consider whether she wanted to
have him as a friend. She admitted, at least, that she did not
know him as well as she thought she had.

As Rose inched away from her blind trust in Herb, he showed
signs of giving up his blind acceptance of himself. Perhaps he
did not have to be the emotionally evasive intellectual he had
always been. As he put it, he was, at any rate, learning:

> I've always played the rescuer without realizing how I
> wasn't responding to Rose's emotional needs. My way has
> been to solve problems; if there wasn't a problem to solve
> here and now, I felt I couldn't be of use. This recent experi-
> ence has enabled me to hear better when Rose is upset. My
> eyes were opened when I learned that I could just listen to
> her, hear her, support her, and that that would be helpful,
> even if I didn't solve any specific problem.

If Herb had been more in the habit of giving himself due credit,
he would have realized that, in alleviating Rose's loneliness, he
was "solving a specific problem."

Perhaps it was not as easy as he thought to be "just very good
friends" with someone with whom he had been intimate for
twenty-five years. In one of the last sessions with S., Herb spoke
in probabilistic terms about the past, present, and future:

> Being alone has given me the time and the freedom to
> explore the issues that are important to me. I had blamed
> Rose for a lot of what had gone wrong between us, but as
> I saw myself re-create the same patterns in other relation-
> ships, I realized that some of these barriers were of my own
> making. I saw that I, too, was a cause. And I saw that I
> couldn't erase all the years of our relationship and all the
> good things about it, even if I was not ready to get back into
> it. Then Rose's cancer took me away from my own preoccu-
> pations and showed me that I don't have forever to deal
> with them. Time is a thief; it won't stand still while I ex-
> plore other sides of myself. Right now I am still very unset-

tled. I still want very much to be good friends with Rose, but I don't know how easy that will be. I know that we will be better friends if I can respond to her more spontaneously and sensitively and can let her know when I need her.

S. more than once acknowledged the courage Rose and Herb showed in coming in for family counseling. They would not have taken that gamble, he said, if there had not been a great deal between them. Nor would their relationship have lasted as long as it had if it had been all bad. Wherever there were strong feelings, there were always mixed feelings. In their efforts to resolve their relationship with a clear hello or a clear good-bye, Rose and Herb had lost touch with their mixed feelings and thereby further confused matters. They could achieve some degree of clarity if they accepted their mixed feelings, either by getting back together and accepting that there would be conflict or by separating and accepting that there would be grief.

S. hoped that they would be able to make this choice, either on their own or through further counseling. Again, however, time proved a thief. S.'s counseling sessions with the Heifetzes ended when Rose was hospitalized after complaining of swelling in her abdomen. Although Rose and Herb would not believe it at first, S. gently made clear to them that the cancer had reappeared, only now in a part of the body that was inaccessible to the treatments that had eliminated the tumor in her breast. Once the effects of the illness began to make themselves felt in her daily life, Rose gave up her apartment and accepted Herb's invitation to move back into her old home with him and their daughter. Her spirit and determination not to give in to the illness, not to "go gentle into that good night," had had a chance to steel itself through a shared understanding of the prospect of death. When death came, as it did before long, it came to a troubled family, but a family nonetheless.

10

TRUST

If Dr. S.'s patients found it hard to reconcile his concern with gambling with his interest in being a scientific practitioner, they were even more puzzled about what either of these ideas had to do with trust, which he spoke of in the same breath. Trust seemed too "soft" a notion for the precise language of science. And where was there less trust than in gambling? At least in the image of gambling that most people carried away from film Westerns, where the card sharks would sit around the table, each with one hand poised at his waist, ready to come up shooting at the first hint that one of the others (always it was one of the others) was cheating.

On S.'s side, he was as concerned as any of his colleagues were with what was now commonly referred to as the "doctor-patient relationship," but he felt that to talk about that relationship chiefly in terms of "rights" and "powers," as most of the books currently written either for patients and doctors were doing, missed the point. As he practiced, and as he shared his thoughts and feelings with his patients, he and they came to see that trust was at the center of probabilistic medical practice. Only when trust was established did it make sense to start thinking about "rights" and "powers," and when trust was es-

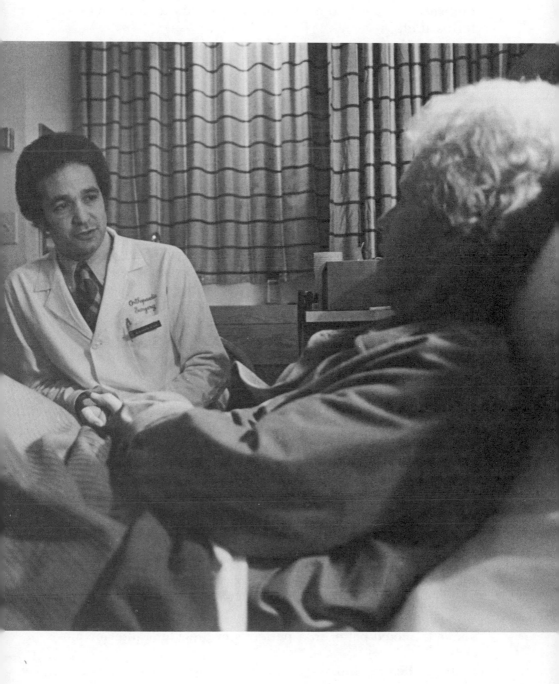

tablished, it was often no longer so necessary to think in those terms at all.

From sad experience he knew what trust was like under the Mechanistic Paradigm. For the patient, at one extreme, it came down to "You're the doctor. I'm putting myself in your hands. Whatever you say goes." But how easily blind trust turned to its opposite, blind mistrust, when things did not work out, or when he had to tell the patient something that the patient did not want to hear. Then, too, some of the very people whose fathers and mothers had blindly trusted their family doctors would approach S. full of suspicion: "Watch out, he's in it for himself. Either he'll say I need more time with him so he can charge me more money, or he'll rush me out the door so he can make money on other patients." This fluctuation between blind trust and wariness was not confined to patients. S. would assume that patients automatically took prescribed medications and, when they didn't, would feel rejected by this "noncompliance." "How can I go on being your doctor?" he would think. It was also easy to be cynical from the start. "What's he here for?" he would catch himself thinking. "What's his hidden agenda? I'll bet he's here just to get a drug prescription out of me."

Both absolute trust and absolute mistrust are intertwined with the Mechanistic Paradigm's denial of uncertainty. To accept a person at face value and not look any further is to deny the possible existence of other, unseen causes that may sometimes influence the person's actions. However, to disregard completely what is on the surface and only to look beneath it for a "hidden agenda" that represents "the" cause of a person's actions is equally mechanistic. Either you see the cause of something, in which case you trust it completely and have absolute trust that a good outcome will follow; or you don't see it, in which case there is no sense of understanding and control, and you have no trust at all. This is the "show me" attitude of the *experimentum crucis,* where the "facts," bereft of understanding, reveal the determining cause with certainty. With blind mistrust, on the other hand, no facts are sufficient to shake the fixed belief in a patient's or a doctor's ulterior motives.

Under the Probabilistic Paradigm scientists do not draw conclusions directly from the evidence; nor, of course, do they disregard the evidence. Scientists (including physicians) who work within this paradigm recognize that evidence takes time to appear, that it requires interpretation, that it is never complete, and that it can never ensure complete control over the outcome. Instead of performing an *experimentum crucis* to settle the issue once and for all, the scientist may take provisional action that leaves room for further evidence to reveal itself. Under the Probabilistic Paradigm trust (like other "soft," subjective factors) becomes a part of science itself. This is not blind trust, however, but a kind of reasoned faith that must be critically reevaluated as new evidence emerges.

When we recognize that even in science the evidence is not immediately apparent, that even science requires a degree of trust in uncertain findings, it becomes easier for us to be trusting in our relationships with people, including the doctor-patient relationship. Doctors and patients who are mindful of the Probabilistic Paradigm do not decide all at once whether they find each other trustworthy. Rather they begin by accepting each other, make an initial estimate of how far to extend their trust, and then keep an open mind.

At any point along the way deciding to what extent to trust someone is a gamble. It is a decision like any other, one made on the basis of probabilities, values, and principles. Without a willingness to gamble, without the recognition that in an uncertain world one must always gamble, there can be no trust.

Without trust, on the other hand, the encounter between doctor and patient can take the form of a competitive, zero-sum gamble. When doctor and patient see each other as adversaries, and thereby as untrustworthy, they may tend to be shortsighted and to engage in the kind of actions whereby one cuts off one's own nose to spite one's opponent's face (e.g., by withholding cooperation so that one can later say, "I told you so!"). It is then that the patient and doctor are gambling against rather than with each other.

Trust allows for a different type of gamble, a cooperative gamble, in which doctor and patient share a time perspective that allows them to keep playing instead of folding up their game (and maybe drawing their guns) after a single loss. Trust allows time for both parties to evaluate critically whether a given diagnosis is a reasonable basis on which to proceed, whether a given treatment has had a chance to work, or whether a given doctor can work well with a given patient. Trust allows doctor and patient to stick with a decision long enough to assess its long-range as well as immediate outcomes; it also gives them time to change their minds and recoup their losses. Conversely, time is what builds trust—especially when it is time spent gambling consciously together.

Engendering Trust

S. often wished that he could trust his patients more. Having been "burned," however, by missed appointments and broken agreements (especially when it came to taking medications), he found this difficult to do. He could simply have gone on reflecting, with some sadness and anger, on how untrustworthy his patients were. But his growing understanding of the Probabilistic Paradigm, together with his willingness to listen to what his patients were telling him, led him to realize that his patients weren't the only ones who might not be able to be trusted. Before he could think about trusting them, he would have to consider his own causal role. He would have to become trustworthy.

There were several ways in which S. learned to gain the trust of his patients. One of the most effective was just by being with them for a long time. When people get to know each other over a period of time, they reveal themselves to each other as trustworthy or untrustworthy in large and small ways. Sometimes, of course, what is revealed makes people turn away from each other. In most cases, however, increased familiarity builds increased trust. It was important to S. that what he communicated about himself should make his patients more comfortable with him and more willing to gamble with him.

S. worked for trust between his patients and himself by acknowledging uncertainty, by not trying to make things seem more certain than they were, by making clear that he and his patients were gambling and that he was willing to learn whatever he could to gamble with them more effectively. To avoid the disillusionment so often brought about by doctors who seek to gain absolute trust by encouraging in the patient a sense of absolute certainty about what outcome follows what course of action, he spoke in terms of probabilities and admitted when he reached a point where he did not know or where no one could know. Uncertainty did not mean, however, that any one course of action was as good as any other. Acknowledging his own causal role as an active observer, S. articulated his values so that his patients would know where he stood.

It wasn't enough that they know that he knew the "facts" and that he would tell them when he didn't know. They also needed to know how he selected and interpreted the facts so that they could work with him in thinking critically about the decisions they needed to make together. He found that while people often started out trusting him on the basis of external indicators of his expertise (his various degrees), they ended up trusting him by seeing what his biases were and how he obtained working knowledge on a day-to-day basis.

S. also inspired trust by being available to his patients (within reasonable limits) where and when they needed him. For instance, he went to people's homes to attend births and to visit those who were bedridden or who could not easily get around. Much to his surprise, he had to emphasize to patients his nighttime and weekend availability (in rotation with his partners). He found this out when someone would call him in the morning after having been ill during the night, in the belief that he could not be reached except during his normal office hours. Sometimes family members would even take the sick person to a hospital emergency room, thinking that this was the only alternative to going without medical attention until morning. "We didn't know we could call you," they would say. To S. it was a sad thing that people could no longer trust doctors to be available when they needed them. He had to tell people that if he was to be their doctor, he would be their doctor even at 2 A.M.

S.'s on-call availability was an important ingredient in establishing trust. Though he was quick to acknowledge his resentment at being awakened, he appreciated the opportunity that the after-hours calls represented. For one thing there were occasions when those phone calls allowed him to follow up observations made during a prior contact. Moreover, it was by being close to people at moments of crisis that he really became their family doctor. It was a rare chance to get to know a family. "I think it's important that you would get up at this hour to take care of your sick child (or parent)," he would tell them. "If you can be awake, I can be awake." By putting himself on the line for people at such moments, he built up a reservoir of trust that carried over to the times when he was not physically with them. Once they knew that he would come when they needed him, they could believe him when he reassured them that they didn't need him. Even when he answered a late-night call by saying, "You can stick this one out yourselves and call me in the morning," the family could feel that he was, in a real sense, there with them as their doctor.

S. found that people who might at the drop of a hat call upon the hospital emergency room or the night shift of alert strangers at a prepaid health-care facility did not presume upon his availability. They knew that he had human needs that were not to be lightly overridden. This was a good thing, for there was a danger that his willingness to serve might become a tool to make people dependent on him. S. and his patients fashioned guidelines to help them decide when they needed him (a crucial gamble that everyone faced once in a while). "Knowing when to call a doctor isn't always easy," he would tell them, "but I know you wouldn't call unless you felt it was important. You wouldn't call in the middle of the night just for a cold, but severe pain that you can't relieve on your own is another matter." In this way he let people know that it was as important for him to be able to trust them as for them to be able to trust him. Dependency there was, as there always is in relationships between people. But in a trusting relationship the dependency is mutual.

S. learned from his patients that small gestures could make a big difference when it came to establishing trust. A patient of his who was concerned with women's perspectives on medical care suggested that he should do more than just set up a screen for women to use when changing their clothes in the gynecological exam room. Since then he made a point of leaving the examination room so that the woman could have the room entirely to herself while she undressed. Instead of dividing the territory with her, he tried to say by his actions, "Just as you're important enough for me to answer your calls at night and come to your home, so you're important enough for me to inconvenience myself by leaving the room so that you can have some privacy."

Patients told him the same thing in their own ways. When a couple planning a home birth asked S., "Is there something *you* like to eat that you'd like us to have in the house?" they were telling him that they wanted to break bread with him, to establish a relationship of mutual respect and trust. A week after he had made a home visit to a sixty-seven-year-old woman who was nearly incapacitated with a pulled muscle in her upper back, the woman's daughter called to tell him that the anti-inflammatory drug, local heat, and massage he had prescribed had worked very well. When she told him, "I had my doubts about it," it was as if she were also telling him, ". . . and I trust you enough to tell you about them." To S. the call would have been useful whether or not the treatment had worked. These follow-up reports, which made it possible for him to learn from his successes and failures and from his patients' beliefs and doubts, were a way in which his patients took steps toward building mutual trust.

It wasn't always easy for S. to acknowledge uncertainty and share it with his patients. Some people were surprised and unsettled when he admitted that there were things he did not know. In retrospect many of them appreciated his extending them this trust, but at first they felt, in the words of one expectant father, that he had "thrown us a curve." Patients who were used to doctors handing out orders with crisp authority tended to react to S. in one of two ways. Some thought him wishy-washy and ill-informed. Even though he was as sure of his facts as he could reasonably be, a doctor who spoke of gambles could not inspire confidence in these patients. Others were so used to an authoritarian approach that they didn't even hear that S. was saying anything different. They simply assimilated what he said into their own framework. For example, he might tell the parents of a child with a fever, "Right now it looks like just a virus cold—annoying, not dangerous, and, frustrating as it is, not curable by any means now available. If he develops any complications such as labored breathing, drowsiness, or crying as though in pain, call me back so that we can take another look." In the few cases where the child took a turn for the worse, some parents judged S. to be a poor doctor, as if he had not qualified his initial assessment. Yes, it was risky to practice probabilistic medicine.

On the other hand, the patients who came to S.'s practice asking to be actively involved in the decision-making process were the ones who were most enthusiastic about learning scientific gambling. They were the ones who most readily adopted the principles of critical doubt and critical trust from the Probabilistic Paradigm. When it came to initiating a trusting relationship, these patients were S.'s teachers.

Initiating the Gamble

Both the doctor and the patient can take the risks and initiate the gambles that make for a trusting relationship. In the most trusting, most satisfying relationships both sides do some of the initiating. Initiating such a gamble feels different from reciprocating it, and there is something to be learned from both. Given the way doctor and patient roles have been defined in our society, S. as the doctor often found himself doing most of the initiating. But there were some patients who came prepared to take the lead.

Charlotte Martin, a thirty-nine-year-old divorcee who had had her first child a dozen years before, was an unusual prenatal patient for S. to be seeing, in that she was not now married and was of advanced age for childbearing. She knew that she faced a difficult decision about whether to continue with the pregnancy, and she wanted a doctor who would not pressure her to make the decision and who would be supportive whichever path she chose. She began by letting S. know that she was willing to trust him enough to share the preconceptions she had formed about him. "A friend of mine recommended you as being 'dry'—that's how she put it. She said that while you're slow to warm up, you're a very warm person. I guess that's what I'm comfortable with, what with my WASP upbringing. I may come across as cold at first too."

S. stiffened. In his mind he had a commitment to openness of communication, but in his heart he was embarrassed to find himself out on the table for review. At first trying to evade the issue, he replied woodenly about the importance of feeling comfortable with a person one chose to work with. Somewhere in his upbringing and professional education he had decided that being himself—acknowledging his feelings—was unbecoming to him as a person and a physician.

After speaking for a while in generalities about trust, he felt safe enough to answer Ms. Martin directly. "I guess I am a bit dry," he remarked, "and I hope you will find me warm deep down. I've heard enough people have that reaction to me to believe that it must be true. And I've actually changed so as to reveal such warmth as I do have. But seeing myself as others see me is not easy. It has been a blind spot for me, as it is for most of us. Had I not been practicing medicine in this context where I couldn't ignore or deny the way I was coming across to people, I might never have had the chance to change."

This relationship got off to a good start in part because Ms. Martin gambled on sharing with S. the feelings she had about him, and in part because S. gambled on revealing to her his feelings about himself. Both learned something by playing out of character instead of automatically assuming the attitudes that have become hardened into so-called doctor-patient roles. Not only did the patient initiate, but it was the doctor who was being "examined." Patients show trust each time they stand still while being examined by the doctor. That trust is enhanced when the patient sees that the doctor, too, is willing to stand still for examination. On the doctor's side it helps to feel what it's like to be a patient once in a while. A taste of the vulnerability that patients feel all the time can help close the emotional gap that inhibits trust.

It is easy to talk about gambling; it is not so easy to gamble when you have a lot at stake. Some patients are initially hesitant to accept the gambling approach, and with good reason. The kinds of gambles that one takes with one's health are different from those in a "game." When gambling is presented with glib confidence by a doctor who can afford to feel detached from the outcomes of the "game," the patient is quick to realize that it is not the doctor's body, the doctor's pain, the doctor's life, that are at stake. The doctor takes risks, too, but these risks are much smaller, and thus the doctor stands at a greater psychological distance from the gamble.

Because he did not want to fall into glib detachment about the feelings of the people he was treating, S. was willing to be, like his patients, sometimes even an object of observation—to be "objective" about himself and to have others be objective about him. If his relationship with a patient could not be equal in terms of magnitude of risk, it would be equal in that the patient's feelings about him would be as important as his feelings about the patient. Recognizing his own reluctance to gamble with his self-esteem (as when he asked his patients for comments, positive and negative, on the care he was providing), he came to understand how courageous it was for patients to initiate the sort of trusting relationship that made principled gambling possible. His appreciation grew for patients such as Charlotte Martin who took the initiative in getting involved in the decision-making under conditions where there was some uncertainty.

When a patient initiated, S. was ready to reciprocate. After two months of prenatal visits a couple who were planning a home birth told him that they were now confident that he could handle their delivery. S. replied that he now had confidence in them too. At first they were slightly taken aback; this was not something they would expect to hear from a doctor. But they were intrigued as well, and they pursued the subject until S.'s meaning became clear. He was telling them that not only did they depend on him, but he depended on them. This was not the supermarket, where "home delivery" was a service performed for the consumer. It was, rather, a relationship of mutual reliance.

Another couple, after extensive consultation with S., decided that they could not have a child at the present time and reluctantly chose to have an abortion. In the course of the discussions they asked S. whether the procedure was a difficult thing for him to do. He replied that he had doubts and sadness whenever he performed an abortion, even though, on balance, it could be an important contribution to a family. A week later the woman sent him a letter that said:

> I appreciated your honesty in expressing the difficulty you felt in carrying out what we had agreed upon. You walked well the delicate line between being open and passing judgment. In sharing your feelings you made it so much easier for us to acknowledge our own mixed feelings, which below the surface are very much there. Thank you.

What S. in effect had said was, "I'm strong enough to do this without denying the sadness and doubt that come with it. You don't have to pretend to me that you are happy about this in order to go through with it." He trusted this couple enough to share with them his sadness and doubt, and they in turn trusted him enough to let him share theirs.

Sharing the Gamble

For S. trust began with his getting clear on the difference between sharing and shirking the gamble. As he shared responsibility—which he did as much as possible for each patient—he felt himself becoming more rather than less responsible. He also saw that patients who wanted to be actively involved in the

decision-making process were increasing rather than detract-
ing from his responsibility. By trusting him, yet doing so critically, these patients were seeing him as he was, rather than as
some paternalistic fantasy figure that a doctor so easily evoked.
They trusted him and themselves enough so that they did not
have to hide behind an illusion that he could never live up to.

Soon he felt it his responsibility to act in such a manner that,
even when he was dealing with a frightened child, there could
be some sharing of the choices and uncertainties of the gamble.
Even a routine procedure like taking a child's throat culture
was transformed when it was seen as an opportunity to involve
the patient in the decision. A throat culture is useful for distinguishing a bacterial (streptococcal) infection, which can be
treated with penicillin, from a viral infection, for which only
symptomatic treatment and "watchful waiting" are available.
Even for an adult it is uncomfortable to have the cotton tip of
the culture stick touch the back of the throat. For a child the
discomfort is compounded by fantasy. Thus when six-year-old
Lena had to have a throat culture taken, S. carefully explained
the procedure and its purpose to Lena as well as to her mother.
His next step normally was to tell the mother to hold the child
on her lap, securing her arms, legs, and head so that she
couldn't jump when the stick was inserted.

Then Lena's mother stopped him. "Look," she said, "I remember that when I had to have a throat culture done, you
asked me to hold still. At least you can ask Lena whether she
wants to give it a try to hold still by herself."

Of course, S. had already involved Lena in the gamble of
taking the culture; why not involve her in the gamble of restraining her from hurting herself? The procedure would be
more acceptable to her and would mean more to her if he didn't
simply talk over her head to her mother. So he turned to Lena
and said, "Even though this test is only painful for a second, it's
scary when it's happening. When the cotton touches someone's
throat, the person often jumps back without thinking, like
this." Lena laughed as S. jerked his head and shoulders back
and his arms up and out. "When someone with a stick in her
mouth jumps like that—and it's hard not to—she can really get
hurt. So that you don't hurt yourself that way, I can ask your

mother to hold you tight. Or you can give it a try by yourself."
Lena answered, "I want my mother to hold me." "Okay," said
S., "but after it's over I want you to tell me how it felt and
whether what I'm telling you turned out to be right."

After the procedure S. congratulated Lena for being brave
and for helping him find out whether she needed medicine for
her sore throat. "And your mom had the chance to show how
much she cares about you by not letting you get hurt," he added.
Then he showed her the office laboratory where the germs
would be grown in a culture medium. She watched the technician plant her culture and put it in the incubator. Later that
week her mother told S., "Lena really got a kick out of that
throat culture. She didn't stop talking about it all evening."

S. learned that he could gamble directly with a child of
Lena's age as well as with her family. In the case of eleven-
month-old Toby he could not gamble with the patient. Instead
he gambled with the family as a means of establishing the
conditions that made trust possible.

Toby had been running a high fever. S. checked him over,
saving for last the examination of the ears, which would be
most upsetting to the child. But wax filled both canals, blocking
the view.

There were many reasons why ear wax was called the bane
of a pediatrician's life. S. had memories of being drained physically (he had to stoop down over the table to align himself with
the tiny ear canals); of falling behind on his schedule (it often
took an extra ten minutes to do the job properly); of the sight
of bleeding from the canal that sometimes was induced by the
metal curette used for wax removal; of parents upset over a
crying, bleeding child ("What a butcher!" their faces, if not
their words, seemed to say); of screaming, frightened babies
with God knows what perception. It was with such experiences,
perhaps, that bad feelings toward doctors began.

Heretofore S. had assumed that there was no alternative to
cleaning out the ears—unless one wanted to do nothing about
a possible ear infection. But when the wax was particularly
resistant and there was a high probability of an ear infection,
his experience in structuring decisions as gambles led him to
see another option—that of beginning antibiotics along with

ear drops to dissolve the wax. In a day, with the wax gone, the antibiotics could be discontinued if an infection was not found. This gamble, which would involve another visit, entailed all the usual costs of using antibiotics without what was called a "definite diagnosis," together with the benefits of avoiding the horror show of wax removal while still treating the infection (if one was actually present). With this alternative in mind the standard procedure of ear cleaning could become a choice instead of a necessity.

S. shared the gamble with Toby's parents. "Even though I've been removing wax from children's ears for years and am good at it, I sometimes nick the ear canal with my instrument. Then there is bleeding, and no one likes to see blood. You get upset, I get upset, the baby gets upset. Not that it's dangerous. It's like a nosebleed, and it will heal in a few days. I'd say it happens to me about once in twenty tries. But you ought to know about it so that you can decide whether or not to go ahead."

Toby's parents decided to go ahead. By having an explanation of the choices, they were prepared to participate not only in making the decision, but in doing the procedure and living with the risks it entailed. They continued to be involved as the three of them huddled over Toby on the table, father holding his legs, mother his arms, and S. at his head. "The procedure, so far as I can tell, shouldn't be painful unless the canal is nicked. He'll be screaming mainly out of fear and resistance to being immobilized," S. told the parents as they took up their battle positions. First S. used the otoscope to see the wax. He formed a mental image of it, removed the otoscope, and then went after it with a curette.

Throughout the procedure the distraught baby was soothed by his mother. "Good Toby. The doctor is just trying to help you. You'll be okay." Although Toby was too young to understand the words, S. thought that he was likely picking up their tone and intent.

When enough wax had come out for S. to say with reasonable assurance that the left ear was normal, he suggested that all four of them "come up for air" before getting down to the right ear. After taking a few deep breaths, they resumed their positions around the table. Once exposed to view, the bulging drum of the right ear offered convincing evidence of infection. The procedure had been accomplished without any bleeding. Had this not been the case, S. felt that Toby's parents would have understood and felt themselves to be part of what had happened. They all could share in the responsibility.

"One small child and three grown-ups to handle him!" the father exclaimed. They all smiled.

Mistrust in the Family

Sometimes the trust S. showed in patients came as a surprise to them because they were not used to being trusted in their families. In such cases S. worked to establish trust between himself and the family. This would sometimes reawaken trust in those families where it was dormant.

Fourteen-year-old Rodrigo Santos sat in sullen silence while his mother told S. about the earache that had kept him awake the previous night. "It seems," said S., "that you don't want to be here at all."

"I feel better now," Rodrigo finally said, "so why bother coming?"

"You and your mother don't seem to be in agreement about this," S. persisted. Instead of minimizing the disagreement and getting down to treating the earache, S. articulated the mother's and son's conflicting positions so that both could be honored in making a decision—a necessary prelude to trust.

"Listen, Doctor, when I was a child in the Islands," said Mrs. Santos, referring to the Portuguese Azores, "I once had a terrible earache. There was no doctor, and I suffered for three days. That's why I want to have my children's ears checked."

"So ear pain has a special meaning for you," S. commented.

"I never heard that story," said Rodrigo.

"If you listen long enough," thought S., "there is always a 'story' that helps explain the other person's feelings and actions." S. went on to explain that, in the case of an earache, the possibility of ear infection made it prudent to check with a doctor even if the pain went away. He encouraged Rodrigo and his mother to make such important decisions together and reminded them that they could include him even in their emergency health decisions by calling him at night, if necessary, instead of waiting until the next day.

There were more extreme, troubling instances of mistrust in the family. Dolores Clayton was a woman in her thirties who complained of pain in her ribs. Recently she had been hospitalized because a small bone near her eye had been fractured. How had this happened? Actually her husband had beaten her, but in the hospital emergency room where her ribs had been X-rayed (revealing no fracture), she had said that she had "fallen." In the emergency room, where there isn't enough time to build trust, patients give expedient answers which an overworked staff is all too happy to accept. Dolores had also lied to her employer about why she had had to stay home from work. It was clear that she had mixed feelings. She was ashamed of the truth, and she was ashamed of lying. She didn't want her husband to be put in jail, but she was about ready to leave him.

She had to have some initial trust in S. even to admit that she had been beaten, and he did not want to presume upon that trust. "So this is the first time he's ever beaten you," he said. No, she replied, he had done it several times. S. did not want to make her feel cornered by bombarding her with questions. He listened, and she was able to volunteer that her husband was beating her because she couldn't stop gambling her money away.

They proceeded in the same conversational mode, which gave the patient room to express her viewpoint without having to align herself on the "yes" or "no" side of a question. Dolores was able to fill in the background of her story. Brutally beaten by her father, sometimes for no reason at all, she had as a child found an escape in gambling, where at least she had some notion of what the rules were. Once married, she had not gambled again until her husband had left her, briefly, a couple of years earlier. When asked whether she was winning much money, she said she always lost; the game was probably rigged.

S. tried to express his own values without passing judgment on either her or her husband. Her husband's beating her, he suggested, wasn't doing either her or her husband any good. Dolores stated that her husband was now ashamed of his act and concerned about her. He had offered to drive her to S.'s office.

After listening to her breathing to check that her lungs were normal (a broken rib might puncture a lung), S. presented the "gamble" of doing another X ray versus prescribing pain medication. Dolores smiled when he mentioned gambling. "This isn't like the gambling you've been doing," S. told her. "It's not a game, and so far as I know, it's not rigged. But you should keep a sharp eye out anyway." S. didn't see much payoff from another X ray, so the choice came down to a weak pain medication versus a strong one such as codeine, along with a binder to restrict chest movements. "I can give you some medication that won't take all the pain away, but it will take away some of the pain, and the chances of your getting hooked on it are less." Drug addiction, he felt, was something to watch out for in a person addicted to gambling.

He concluded by stressing that this was a serious and a sad thing that had happened. He gave her the name and address of a shelter for battered women, and she took the responsibility of deciding whether and when to report the beatings. When he suggested contacting a therapy group, she replied that she would probably leave her husband instead. "Then he doesn't care for you?" S. asked. No, she told him, her husband did care for her and was in most respects a good husband and father. He did not beat their children. "Well, maybe you should leave him, but keep an open mind," said S. in parting.

The next week she called and said that the pain was worse and that she needed stronger medication. Now the odds had changed. A new X ray, which she and S. agreed was called for, revealed a fractured rib. The fracture, too small to show up on the original X ray, probably had been made worse by strain. This meant revising the gamble on the pain medication as well. "I think I can avoid getting hooked on the codeine," Dolores told S. "What do you think?" S., too, thought that she was ready to use the drug responsibly. He prescribed codeine along with the

weaker medication so that she could choose which to take depending on the severity of the pain at any given moment.

"Maybe the pain is all in my head," said Dolores. "Well, there
is a broken rib there," S. reminded her. "On the other hand, the
way you perceive the pain depends on whatever else is going
on with you. And drugs alone won't help you with that. Speaking of which, now that we know that your rib has been broken,
maybe it's time for me to see your husband." He gave her a note
informing her employer (and her husband) that she needed to
stay home from work with a rib fracture.

Upon reading the note, her husband agreed to come in with
her to see S. the following week. At that time she reported that
she had needed the codeine only twice during the week. S. and
Dolores's gamble that she could bear the responsibility of making that choice had paid off. In a mistrustful world in which she
had had no control over her life (as when her father had beaten
her), she had sought the illusion of control over uncertainty in
pathological gambling—where, however, she always lost, so
that she still had no control. S. was showing her that she might
gain some control even by choosing between two bottles of pills.
Here she could gamble and sometimes win.

In order to remove some of the strain of her family situation
S. was establishing a mild therapeutic dependency in Dolores.
They discussed it and agreed that (again remembering her
potential for addiction) they did not want to let it go too far.
Before meeting with her and her husband, he told her that as
a physician he would not be doing family counseling with them
on a continuing basis. They would have to learn to talk to each
other directly, not just through him. Not surprisingly, though,
he found himself doing a considerable amount of relaying and
transmitting as their joint session began. He began by telling
Charles Clayton that he knew that he had broken his wife's rib.
"She beats me verbally," Charles countered. "Maybe that's so,"
said S., "but that's still a broken rib."

The broken rib was real, and so was the verbal abuse. S.
noticed that whenever Charles started to speak, his wife cut in
and caused him to stop talking. S. unobtrusively encouraged
Charles to continue by keeping his eyes focused on him while
he was talking, even after Dolores interrupted. After that the

husband and wife started talking to each other. S. supported them in doing so by emphasizing the courage it took for them to come in together and talk things over. "Maybe I'm wrong," he told them, "but the two of you wouldn't be here if it were all bad between you."

Charles's side of the story was that, having had to keep several younger brothers in a fatherless family away from the temptations of the street, he lost his head whenever he saw his wife gambling. "You sound as if you don't trust gambling very much," S. remarked. "Maybe you're not that comfortable being here, which is certainly a gamble." Indeed he was not. "And the only way you can stop your wife from gambling is by beating her." S. was articulating Charles's thought processes so that he could examine these critically and make his unconscious choices conscious. After all, S. reminded him, Dolores had been gambling a lot more since he had started beating her.

With all his distaste for gambling, Charles was taking a big gamble. He was showing considerable courage and involvement in his marriage by speaking openly to a doctor, an authority figure who might be taking evidence against him. S. returned his trust, and his wife's, by assuring them that everything they said would be held in confidence. He showed them the chart where he had written only the words, "Family seen for family counseling." "I'm gambling too," he added. "If things get worse between you and the law is called in, I could be charged with not reporting a crime." Since they were taking the risk of meeting with him, he would take this risk, given Charles's agreement not to beat Dolores again. Although he urged the couple not to discount the healthy commitment they had to each other, further commitment on Dolores's part would not be healthy if the beatings continued.

S. agreed to see the couple one more time. After exploring their mixed feelings about making contact with a social-service agency to begin family therapy, both Dolores and Charles felt that it would be easier for them to do so if they knew that they could share with S. their initial experience with the agency. It would still take courage to go to the agency. S. suggested that Dolores make the call to set up the appointment with her husband listening in—a precaution that was needed at this early stage to nurture the small amount of trust remaining between them. In letting his own availability be tied to their taking this step to further their own well-being, S. was willing to have his own presence be at stake in a side bet. The Claytons did see him for a final visit after contacting the family therapist.

S. made it possible for this couple to gain some control over uncertainty in their relationship with him, in the hope that this control would carry over to their relationship with each other. He had shown them how to create ground rules for a trusting relationship, and he believed that by taking the additional gamble of family therapy, they would be able to go on from there.

Gambling Against the Odds

It was particularly difficult to overcome the odds against critical trust when a patient wasn't sure if anyone, including herself, could be trusted. This was the case with Barbara Reilly, who came to S. for the first time with a complaint of back pain. Her first baby had been a "crib death" casualty five years earlier. At that time her husband had shown the first signs of the muscular dystrophy that had since confined him to a wheelchair. Two weeks before her visit to S. she had had a second child, whom she brought with her to the doctor's office. "You might say," she joked bitterly, "that my husband is my first child."

During her pregnancy Barbara had strained her back while helping her husband out of bed. A doctor had prescribed Percodan (a mild opiate), which she had continued to use after her back problem had cleared up. Now she told S. that she had reinjured her back and needed more Percodan.

S. wasn't so sure. He did not like to prescribe a drug with the addictive potential of Percodan before he knew the patient well enough to trust her when she said she needed it. "That's quite some baby you've got there. Look how she looks up into your eyes. You must have your hands full, what with your husband and this little one as well. No wonder you are in pain."

Barbara Reilly began to cry. "I'm sorry," she said.

S. didn't think she had to apologize. "Maybe there is a better way to express the sadness you feel, but crying is certainly one good way to do it, and it sounds like you have lots to feel sad about. What a beautiful baby—bundles of joy, people call them. People must think you're the happiest woman in the world. They forget that even beautiful babies can make you angry! Everyone is cooing over the baby, but you're the one who has to change her diapers."

"Sometimes it can drive me crazy," she said. She soon made clear to S. that her need for Percodan was caused as much by the strain of being alone in taking care of the baby and her husband as by her back pain. She felt burdened by both her husband and baby and may have blamed herself for the death of her first child. With so little going for her she may have seen doctors as opponents whom she needed to outwit in order to win the one thing that eased her pain.

This was one of those situations of mutual mistrust where each party was trying to get an "angle" on the other. "What's she after?" S. found himself thinking. "Is she just giving me a story so she can get a prescription?" And on her side, "How can I 'reach' this guy? What story do I have to tell him to make him give me the pills?" Each of them had a hidden agenda. The question was how to bring it out into the open.

How could S. gain this patient's trust without prescribing the Percodan? He thought that here it would have to be him who took the initiative. Should he hedge his bet by giving her what she wanted in the hope that she would stick with him long enough to learn to gamble with rather than against him? Or would giving in to her demands only inspire a superficial, cynical form of trust? There was just one gamble that he felt right about taking, a gamble that he chose on principle even though it meant he would risk losing her at the outset.

"Listen to that!" he said, calling attention to the baby's cries for food. "When this baby wants something, she really wants

something. She won't give you a chance! It's good to know that
ten years from now she won't need you quite so much. But she'll
still need you, and you'll have to think about how you can best
take care of yourself so that you can give her what she needs
through the coming years."

It wasn't only the baby who wanted something right away. S.
dramatized the baby's demands in order to mirror what the
mother herself was doing. At the same time, he held up an
image of the mother as different from the baby—as an adult
who, being responsible for others, could not give way to immediate impulse. The image also had in it a time perspective, a
reminder that decisions could change with time and that decisions made now would influence decisions made later. S.
wanted to help Barbara Reilly be aware and unashamed of her
mixed feelings toward the baby and her husband so that she
could accept and live with these feelings. If she was going to be
making the important decision about using a highly addictive
drug, then it ought to reflect both the joys and anger in her life
—both, rather than whichever one was uppermost at the moment.

Regarding that decision, S. gently reminded Barbara that
there was more than one cause of her pain. Percodan would
remove one of those causes, but it would reinforce others. For
a person who did not have much control over her life, giving up
responsibility for her life to an addictive drug would in the long
run only make things worse. S. felt uncomfortable telling someone what to do, but he would not practice "consumer medicine"
in the sense of giving the patient whatever she wanted. The
more they talked, the more apparent it became that her craving
for Percodan was not a free, informed, adult choice.

Having acknowledged the feelings and experiences that had
led to this craving, he offered her oxazepam, a less potent drug,
an anxiety-reducing agent, that would help her bear the pain
without having quite the same addictive potential as Percodan.
This drug, he thought, was less likely to affect her capacity to
make choices as she learned to live with those things in her life
that caused her pain or began to take steps to change them.
"We're both taking a chance that this drug won't work very

well," he admitted, "but in the long run Percodan won't work either, and you and your husband and baby will be playing a risky game if you go on using it."

When it came to drugs, though, Barbara Reilly was not nearly so ready to gamble with S. as Dolores Clayton had been. "Why don't you just give me the Percodan," she demanded. There followed a tense exchange during which Barbara became visibly angry. "Who wouldn't be angry?" said S. "There's lots to be angry about." He wanted her to feel safe in expressing her anger, so that she could live with it instead of letting it dictate her decision. Living with anger, however, was not the same as making it or the situation that caused it go away.

In the end she agreed to a trial of oxazepam, though she wasn't very happy about it. She had not gotten what she wanted. S. asked her to make another appointment. "To get the most out of it," he added, "it would be good to have your husband come in with you. I'd like to see how his illness may be affecting yours, whether your load can be lightened in caring for him, and whether he can start helping you care for the baby." He hoped that she would keep the appointment.

In extending his trust to Barbara Reilly, S. spoke to what was best in her, the responsible wife and mother rather than the demanding child. People drift into blind trust or mistrust when they do not feel strong enough to trust themselves to make choices. By learning to make rational choices through principled gambling with a doctor, Barbara Reilly might learn to trust her own capacity for decision-making along with someone else's. As her trust and strength grew, she could see herself more as a person making choices under conditions of uncertainty. She could also begin to see those choices as having effects on others as well as herself.

As S. was learning in his practice, people look for certainty because it is easier to deal with than uncertainty, especially when one is alone. Uncertainty takes more effort, more mental and emotional energy. There is, therefore, only so much uncertainty that one person alone can stand. As a patient and doctor (or husband and wife, or parent and child) acknowledge uncertainty together and trust each other to recognize and deal with it, they become more certain of each other's support. This leaves them more energy to deal with their uncertainty about themselves. As they learn to trust others as well as be more comfortable with themselves, they can be more open to facing, rather than denying, what uncertainty there is out in the world and making it more manageable by turning some of it into probability. Uncertainty is decreased when it can be expressed in probable expectations, expectations that can be critically trusted: about oneself, about others, about reality.

Reestablishing Trust

Admitting his uncertainty was a gamble for S. But it was a gamble that he generally preferred to take. He might as well let people know that things might turn sour, since this was bound to happen sometimes whether he said so or not.

He was particularly sensitive to the issue of trust in the case of home birth. Because there were almost no other doctors in the area who attended home births, he did not have clearly agreed-upon professional norms to fall back on if his actions were questioned. Here, where he had less control over uncertainty than usual, he knew that he needed some help in putting the Probabilistic Paradigm into practice. He needed to be able to rely on the family's desire to assume responsibility, not only by participating in the delivery but by consciously taking on the risks. But he had his blind spots, as when his fear of reprisal from a disappointed family (which could have more serious consequences for him in an area where he did not have the support of his peers) led him to trust the family less. His wariness, in turn, led them to trust *him* less. Beneath the idyllic surface a home birth was a place where trust could be strained to the limit. On the other hand, the home birth situation provided a certain measure of safety for S. He could generally count on the kind of families who chose home birth to take up the slack in maintaining or repairing a trusting relationship when his courage and critical thinking failed him.

Margaret and Bill Benson were among the many couples who came to S. for a home birth without having known him previously. Unlike most families, however, the Bensons were disappointed by the way their birth went.

As with most of the families whose births he attended, the Bensons preferred that Margaret not have an episiotomy (an incision that widens the opening of the birth canal). This gamble, which the three of them had discussed in advance, had a high probability of success, since S. and the laboring mother could almost always prevent significant tearing of the perineum by various "natural" techniques. In Margaret's case, however, he neglected to perform one of these techniques—that of keeping his hand on the perineum while the baby's head was coming out so as to allow the perineum to stretch in a controlled manner. A severe laceration occurred, with S.'s lapse being a probable contributing factor. To compound his blunder, S. tried for an hour to sew up the tear at home, only to have to give up and admit Margaret (with her baby) to the hospital for treatment by an obstetrician-gynecologist. "Some home birth," thought Margaret.

Several weeks later Margaret came in to tell S. how disappointed and angry she and her husband were. After telling everyone how "great" her birth had been, she realized that it hadn't been so great. The pictures the family had taken of the birth showed clearly that S. had not kept his hand on the perineum. Naturally the Bensons blamed S. for their not having had a good birth experience.

S. accepted complete responsibility for his error. Margaret pointed out that the laceration might have occurred regardless of what S. had done (lacerations sometimes occur even after episiotomy). Still, S. made clear, his oversight probably had been a cause. He told her that he felt that he had let her down and thanked her for initiating the discussion of a subject that both of them found difficult to talk about.

Margaret mentioned that the family had noticed S. kneeling in an uncomfortable position during the delivery, but had not thought it their place to say anything about it. S. assured her that, were he ever to be her doctor again, he would want her to trust his willingness to listen and be corrected. As it turned out, it was not only the family that had noticed something amiss. Paula, the birth attendant, had seen S.'s error but had not called attention to it at the time for fear of causing the Bensons to lose faith in him. She hadn't trusted either S. or the family enough to let them see her take issue with S. "What happened might have been avoided," Margaret concluded, "if we had all trusted one another enough to risk taking the initiative."

S. told Margaret that he and Paula had agreed to keep an eye on each other in the future and correct each other when necessary. Nothing could change the outcome in Margaret's case, but she would at least know that other women might benefit from her experience. In stressing the need for a full and free interchange among the family, the birth attendant, and himself, S. was talking about a kind of trust that transcended hierarchical distinctions. It was not a matter of doctor versus nurse, doctor versus family. All had a stake in trust.

S. wondered whether Margaret would have liked him to have taken the initiative in exploring this problem with her, instead of leaving it to her to contact him about it. He took a chance and asked her. "Yes, I would have appreciated it," she replied. His failure to contact her had been an unconsciously chosen losing gamble, just as Paula and the Bensons had lost by not speaking up in time to correct S.'s error during the delivery. Building trust requires taking risks, and on this occasion S. and Margaret regained trust by speaking frankly with each other.

The photographs the Bensons took of the delivery would have been damning evidence in a malpractice suit. The Bensons, however, had built up enough trust during their brief prenatal relationship with S. to bring their grievance to him rather than take it to court. "We took this gamble together," Margaret explained. "You can trust us to know the difference between a mistake and bad faith." As she left, she shook hands with S. and said, "I hope we'll see each other again." The Bensons, who were already members of a prepaid health plan, were not to be among the families who adopted S. as their family doctor after going through a birth with him. But they were ready to consider him for their next home delivery.

From this encounter Margaret felt reinforced in her conviction that you could tell someone (even a doctor) that you were angry at him without having either one of you drop dead from the explosion. To confront someone with your anger, you had to trust that person and know that he trusted you. Her belief was strengthened that there is a middle ground between blind trust and vindictive retaliation. When you have come to trust someone over a period of nine months, it doesn't make sense to throw it all away because of one careless moment. Better to check out whether the person you thought was so good could really be so bad. You might confirm your initial trust or your subsequent disillusionment—or, again, something in between.

Betting on Oneself

What S. learned from this and other encounters was that trust breeds trust. What he did or did not do was only one cause of his patients trusting or not trusting him. He realized as well that his own observations and expectations of his patients' untrustworthiness influenced them to live up—or down—to his expectations. He also realized that, if he wanted to be trusted, he could not blindly trust himself. At times he would need to ask his patients or coworkers for help, as in checking that he manually supported the perineum during a delivery. When he felt himself to be under time pressure while making hospital rounds, he would ask the nurses accompanying him to watch him carefully and inform him of any omissions in his clinical procedure. In doing so, he was making a side bet that created an added immediate reward (approval or lack of criticism) for doing what was consistent with a larger, long-range goal (attending to his patients' well-being). Asking family members, birth attendants, or nurses to monitor his performance at crucial moments was a side bet that S. often made when he felt himself slipping into gambling in his own rather than his patients' interest.

In gambling on whether he needed help and whether he needed to make a side bet on his being trustworthy, S. was able to go beyond the mechanistic impulse to look to the patient or the situation for *the* clue, *the* piece of evidence that would decide the issue. Just as he made probabilistic estimates of the trustworthiness of his patients and coworkers, so he decided on a probabilistic basis whether he could trust himself. He would look at the context, including the patient, his own past experience with that particular type of problem, and how he himself felt at that moment. The "experiment" now took into account not only the patient, but the doctor as well. It included the feelings the patient evoked in him and whatever he could apprehend of the feelings he evoked in the patient. Whether he could handle a particular problem was a gamble, a gamble that he shared with patients so that he and they could approach it as carefully as they did other gambles.

What he learned from people such as the Bensons was to regard both himself and his patients as causes. Along with them he was taking a step away from the primitive thinking that saw causation as occurring either entirely inside or entirely outside himself. If everything were to be caused by the actions of others, then he would be powerless, and he would not be able to trust those who had power over him. If he himself were the cause of everything, then he would not need to trust anyone else, and he would soon become untrustworthy. ("Absolute power corrupts absolutely.") The primitive feelings of doctors tended toward the latter extreme—that of megalomania. But what about the primitive feelings of patients? These often took the form of frustration at the patient's lack of control over uncertainty. The very mistakes a doctor made (however unfortunate the consequences) served to demonstrate the doctor's power to influence events. What, then, was left for the patient to do but to demonstrate control in an equally negative way by the nose-thumbing gesture of noncompliance? If the doctor could be a cause of an unsuccessful outcome, so could the patient. So ran the perverse logic of primitive emotion.

It did not take long for S. to agree with the Bensons that the structure of the doctor-patient relationship was itself not conducive to trust. A relationship where the doctor, as "experimenter," held all the cards left the patient nothing to do but to trust blindly in "doctor knows best." When this trust was shattered either by errors on the doctor's part or by an element of chance that no amount of skill or goodwill could eliminate, blind trust turned to blind resentment. It was essential, then, for S. to involve patients in facing uncertainty by gambling with him. But it was equally essential for the patients' well-being. By becoming S.'s gambling partner (an active partner, not a silent partner who invested the resources of life and health without taking part in gambling decisions), a patient could learn where S.'s blind spots were and thus could *critically* trust this well-intentioned partner.

Even more important, by making choices, patients could test their own authority and power in an uncertain world. Like S. himself, they would now have the burden and the privilege of learning to trust themselves—the privilege outweighing the burden, since only a person who has some control over events needs to be trusted to use that power responsibly. Thus when misfortune occurred, doctor and patient both would know themselves to be strong enough to accept a fair share of the responsibility of the sadness and the fear. Both would know themselves to be a cause (so that they would not feel powerless), but not the only cause (so that they would not feel completely to blame). In a probabilistic world they would be able to share the sadness and the fear with that set of other causes called nature. Through the experience of gambling, on the other hand, they would feel that they had enough power and enough skill (the skill of gambling) to bear the burden of some of the responsibility and the sadness themselves.

There is a big difference between sadness and helplessness. It is easier to feel sad when one believes that there is a chance to do something about the sadness. When one has had some success in gambling in the past, the odds are that one will not be without hope or without resources in the future.

Living with Anxiety— and with Regret

S. learned that patients grew stronger through making choices, however much courage they needed at first to do so. He wanted the same thing to happen to him. He, too, did not always feel secure in the presence of uncertainty. He, too, was learning to make better choices.

He had gone through a considerable evolution, for example, in the way he treated those patients who chronically presented a variety of aches and pains that had no apparent organic cause and for which the likely diagnosis was "anxiety." He would explain to these patients, as he had to Dolores Clayton and Barbara Reilly, that feelings are manifested in bodily stresses and that it usually did not make sense to treat the mind and body separately. But what was the next step?

There was a time when he simply recommended family counseling as more honest and more effective than drug therapy. "That's the way you deal with these things," he would say. Then he would worry about whether the patient would come back, let alone bring the family in. As often as not the patient didn't come back, and S. was left to blame the patient or himself. Denying uncertainty in his presentation to patients, he was left with the anxiety of "Will they or won't they?" which he dismissed by looking for a certain determining cause—a flaw in their character, a diagnostic label such as "borderline personality"—when they "didn't."

Later S. became less mechanistic both about assigning responsibility for failure and about the values involved in making treatment decisions. While he still believed that the odds usually favored family counseling, he had come to realize that the world was such that some people could not change their lives. For these patients, sad as it was, drugs were better than nothing at all. Since no treatment was certain to work, S. presented patients with a series of options which he counted off on his fingers. One, do nothing and go on living with the symptoms. Two, get a second opinion about possible organic causes.

Three, take an antidepressant drug or a tranquilizer. Four, talk things over with S. or with someone else, with or without the participation of family members.

When S. left the choice in the hands of the patient or family, he felt "clean." No longer was he biased in favor of one choice or another. Whatever the patient wanted to do was fine—including not coming back at all. For a while S. thought of himself as "the transformed doctor." He certainly was less anxious, and he thought that he truly was practicing probabilistically.

After a while, though, he became dissatisfied with this approach as well. Previously patients didn't come back because he was too directive; now they didn't come back because he didn't seem to care. If he was too involved before, he was too detached now. He had made himself less anxious by turning away from uncertainty altogether, perhaps to avoid the anxiety he would feel if he faced it directly. The patients also could not get sufficiently involved in their own treatment, as a result of the packaged, take-it-or-leave-it way in which he presented the options. When it was a matter of choosing among "one, two, three, or four," patients were just choosing which option to consume instead of producing their own options.

So S. gradually learned to accept each case as having some unique possibilities. He now tried to help people see how they could create choices for themselves, choices to which his principles as well as theirs would speak. Without overlooking the fact that situations constrained people's choices, he helped people see their part of the responsibility for arranging those situations. All the while he helped them bear the responsibility by assuming responsibility himself in his interactions with them.

He recognized that if there could be said to be a "germ" that caused anxiety, this germ was uncertainty. He was willing to work with patients so that he and they could build up an immunity through measured inoculations of uncertainty in an active decision-making process. He, the doctor, was inescapably a part of that process. He took into account that anxiety was contagious, that anxious doctors made for anxious patients as well as vice versa. Of course, too little anxiety could be as bad as too much; he and the patient had to be careful to avoid quarantining themselves from uncertainty altogether.

How many transformations would he have to go through, S. wondered, how many layers of mechanistic skin would he have to shed before he could finally feel that he was doing it "right"? By now, though, having made some choices for himself, he felt strong enough to live with regret over the mistakes he had made, to know that he would someday live with regret over the mistakes he was still to make, and to trust himself enough to go on. His patients were growing to expect no less.

11

COMPLIANCE
VERSUS CARING

S. found that probabilistic medicine often was easier to think about than to practice. It was hard enough to practice in a world where there was little critical trust; it was doubly hard in the world of medicine, a world full of pain and fear.

When people came to S., they often were in pain. Even when they were not, they might well fear that they would suffer pain, either right there at the doctor's hands or in the coming months and years. Sometimes it was first the pain and then the fear, S. reflected, as in the case of an elderly woman with breast cancer. At other times it was first the fear and then the pain, as in the case of a man who had had a heart attack. Whenever this man would think about what intimate terms he was on with death, the pain in his chest would soon follow. Most often the two came together and were so intertwined that only when they became memory would they finally separate. Where there was sickness, there was always a heart broken with the pain of sadness for one's lost health (and sometimes youth). There was also the fear that it could mean facing death alone, or (where death was not yet an issue) that life would never again be the same.

Many of the people who came to S., therefore, were in no mood for probabilistic thinking. They wanted the consolations

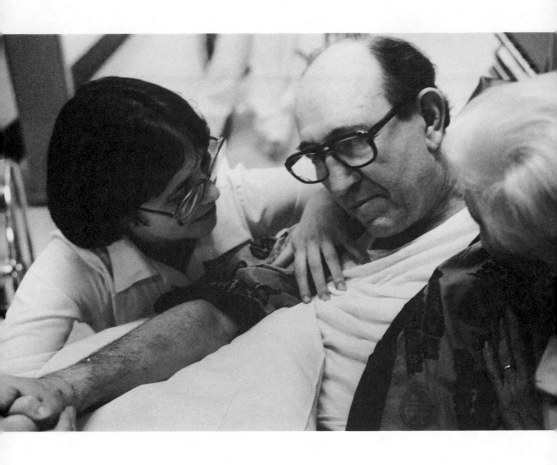

of certainty, the security of being told what to do. They wanted to be taken care of, and S. wanted to take care of them. When the pain and the fear got to be too great (as they could with any patient), it was understandable that S. would slip into the traditional doctor role and that his patients would slip into the traditional patient role. He would take care of them by telling them what to do, and they would comply with his edicts. Then there was little probabilistic reasoning, little of the spirit of doctor and patient gambling together. But S. consoled himself that at least the pain and fear could be held at arm's length.

S. would have gone on in this belief had it not been that his patients did not always comply. For example, they did not always take their medications as they had agreed to do. When he would ask them, "How can I take care of you if you don't listen to what I say?" he would feel anger and sadness. It was when he realized that the anger and sadness he felt were partly his and partly his patients' (for they, too, were angry and sad) that he stopped asking the question rhetorically as a reproach to his patients and began asking it seriously. How *could* he take care of patients who didn't comply? It was a question that he and they needed to answer together.

As they explored this question, S. learned that patients looked at the compliance issue from a perspective very different from his own. Taking medications often complicated people's lives. There was no saying how the medication would work—that it would work at all, or that it wouldn't make them sick—until they tried it. He couldn't tell them, as the advertisers did, "Try it; you'll like it." What he could do was to invite them to call him about any problems they had with the medication. But he could understand that they might throw up their hands if it didn't work right away. They might even blame him.

Remembering Mrs. Pinelli and her hypertension, S. realized that many patients weren't interested primarily in building a relationship with him. They came to him often as a last resort after finding that their pain didn't simply go away or respond to home remedies and over-the-counter drugs. They were looking for immediate relief, not a long-range commitment to deal with a problem. Little in their experience gave them reason to hope for anything more.

Compliance was a new term in the medical lexicon. *Caring* was an old one. Doctors had long spoken about caring for patients; only recently had patients' compliance with doctors been spoken of in the same breath. Reflecting on the current medical preoccupation with compliance, S. wondered whether caring could be separated from compliance in the doctor's office—or, for that matter, in the family. He wondered whether people knew how to care without exacting compliance in return. After all, they were living in a world where caring between husband and wife, brother and sister, parent and child—or anyone, for that matter—was often seen as part of an exchange.

In the course of his practice S. began to learn that he could take care of patients without insisting that they comply by treating his wishes as cookbook recipes. He no longer felt that he was engaged in an exchange or an implicit contract whereby a patient "owed" him compliance in return for care. Once he was able to untangle the question of caring from that of compliance, he could look afresh at the question that concerned him most: how one could care for people in pain and fear through the practice of probabilistic medicine.

What his patients helped him see was that he could best care for them when he neither demanded compliance nor adopted an indifferent, "anything goes" attitude. People sensed when he didn't care. To be involved with his patients, S. needed to stand by his own values while respecting theirs, and to support them in doing what he and they thought was right. Sometimes the outcome would not be what he desired, as often from the patient's choice as from what are called "natural" causes, and about some of these times there was nothing left to do but to be sad.

The "Hateful Patient"

An experience that taught S. to separate caring from compliance involved a patient who became so distasteful to him that his usual eagerness to care turned to a plea of "Oh, God, why won't she find herself another doctor?" It was only when his plea was answered and she found herself another doctor that he realized it hadn't been all her doing. She had become, in the words of a *New England Journal of Medicine* article (Groves, 1978), a "hateful patient." This had happened in the context of her relationship with S., a relationship that had been the sort of zero-sum game one would find in the mechanistic family. It had taken this doctor-patient relationship to make the woman, Mrs. Nagel, a hateful patient.

Mrs. Nagel was a woman of seventy whose cultivated speech and fund of medical knowledge seemed out of place in the cluttered studio apartment that S. would come to know as her home. Mrs. Nagel had hyperparathyroidism, a difficult to diagnose condition. Since hyperparathyroidism mimics the symptoms of other common conditions such as the flu, every instance of fatigue or loss of appetite became an opportunity for Mrs. Nagel to pit the family doctor's opinion against that of a specialist.

During her first few visits with S., Mrs. Nagel rambled on with complaints about other doctors until he finally felt he had to tell her to stop. She left his office in a huff, accusing him of not paying attention to her. He brooded about his "failure." Mechanistically, he considered himself to be the sole cause of her departure. Now it was "his" fault; before long it would be "hers."

Several months later she called him again and asked him to make a home visit. When he arrived, she began by apologizing for dismissing him so abruptly, but then proceeded to ramble just as before. Finally S. risked confronting her. "You know," he said, "if you keep talking about other things, I'm eventually going to tell you to get back to the subject at hand, and you'll just get so angry that you'll cut things off again, right? Well, then, I'll be glad to be your doctor if you'd like me to, but for us to get on with finding out what's wrong, you'll need to stop talking when I ask you to."

It worked. She complied with his wish. S. had shown Mrs. Nagel a picture of herself that she would acknowledge was accurate. In risking an uncertain reaction from her, in challenging his own mechanistic assumption that she would take off angrily, all because of him, he felt that he was also undermining *her* assumption that she could control *his* reactions (as she did everyone else's) by making him so angry that he would do something he would come to regret, and she would get to be the victim again. What he might also have done was to offer her the responsibility of asking him to stop talking when she saw fit. He might have said, "If you think I'm being unreasonable, tell me so." Although Mrs. Nagel was not responsible enough to handle much power in her relationship with S., this bit of equality might have given her some insight into what it was like to have a doctor's responsibilities. It might also have shown S. what it felt like to be on the other end of the judgments he made about the way patients took up his time. This reciprocity might have been the basis for empathy and trust between them.

S. was enthusiastic about his "breakthrough" with Mrs. Nagel, but in a probabilistic world the course of a relationship is not determined by the first encounter. S. had given little power to Mrs. Nagel within their relationship, but in a sense he had given her complete power. If he made all the rules, she could break them all, which she did by calling him several times a week with the same complaints. She let him know in the teasing manner of an unfaithful lover that she was seeing other doctors on the sly. S. felt that as her family doctor he would be able to sort out her maze of symptoms only if he were given access to the findings of the other physicians. Whatever his intentions, she interpreted his concern as a demand that she trust him blindly. She delighted in playing doctors off against one another, showing each of them how unimportant he was to her.

Such treatment wore S. down until he jumped at the provocation. He told her that he could not be her doctor if she called him all the time with insubstantial complaints and didn't tell him when she saw other doctors. He saw in her concealment of information a lack of trust in him, but in making an issue of this when there wasn't enough trust between them to begin with, he was unconsciously playing the jealous lover to her unfaithful one. His blowup gave her a pretext for walking away from him again.

The next week he called her—a first for him—and told her he had had "second thoughts." "Look," he said, "however you want to use me is fine. You're free to call me as often as you want and talk to me about anything you like. Tell me about the other doctors; don't tell me about the other doctors. You have your idea of what a family doctor is, and I have mine. For one thing, I need to be paid for my time. Medicaid doesn't pay for phone calls. If you won't come in and see me so that I can bill Medicaid, I'll bill you for the time we spend on the phone. There, my cards are on the table. I'll send you a letter which summarizes this conversation. If you want to sign it and return it to me, we can use it as a contract specifying the terms under which I'll take care of you." Mrs. Nagel thought this was a fine idea.

No sooner had he sent the contract than it was signed and returned by Mrs. Nagel. And no sooner did he allow himself an expression of relief than Mrs. Nagel called. She had found a loophole in the contract and was about to make use of it. "I need a home visit right now," she demanded. "I won't tell you over the phone why I think I need it. It costs too much to talk to you on the phone. I would much rather just follow the contract."

S. felt outwitted. She was complying with the letter, but not the spirit, of the "contract." The way he had written it, however, it was pretty clear that to follow it to the letter he would have to comply with her wishes. Now that the shoe was on the other foot, would he comply? He went to see her.

Again he had risen to the occasion; again it didn't last. A day after he had seen her at home, she called again with the same request. He responded that he would not go to her home again so soon for the same problems, but that she could see him in the office if she liked.

She became furious with him. "I pay you good money, so you've got to come and see me. Read that contract of yours; it specifies our deal. You're not holding up your part of the bargain. I am doing what the contract says I should, and you're not." Chagrined, S. nonetheless stuck to his resolve and asked her to renegotiate the contract. She refused, and he never heard from her again. He knew that she would continue to find other doctors. For his part he felt so drained that he would not call her back.

The burden of this encounter hung over him. A few months later he tried to examine whether anything he might have done could have made a difference. He did not want to fall back into the mechanistic pattern of blaming either himself or Mrs. Nagel, as if either were the sole cause. He no longer thought of Mrs. Nagel as intrinsically a hateful patient. As he got more deeply into probabilistic practice, however, it occurred to him that he would have had much to gain and little to lose in his last encounter with Mrs. Nagel by telling her explicitly (as he was telling her implicitly) that he didn't trust her: "Right now I don't trust you to be able to decide when you need a home visit and when you don't." He had since learned that even when you don't trust a person, you can still convey a degree of trust by saying so. Some people respond to being taken seriously in this way by taking on more responsibility for their choices; Mrs. Nagel might or might not have been one of them. Her life was predicated on the conviction that she didn't need to be responsible, since no one acted responsibly toward her. In the end S. failed to shake that belief. But one could hardly blame him if he, too, came out of that encounter feeling that life was a bit unfair.

As he continued to examine the case, he began to understand some of the reasons for Mrs. Nagel's anger and how he had contributed to it by his insistence on compliance as a condition for caring. Here was a lonely, elderly woman, scared to death of being made dependent by her progressively more debilitating and painful disease. No wonder she made so many calls and so many requests. Since she did not trust anyone, let alone herself, her solution to her pain and fear was to find as many doctors as possible so that she would not be completely dependent on any one of them. She felt that she could not trust anyone to stick by her in the midst of her intense pain and fear. She expected that she would lose Dr. S., and, sure enough, through her constant testing of S. she was not disappointed. Once again she would find herself all alone in the world.

As she saw the world, every relationship was a zero-sum game with one party or the other being to blame and thus somehow deserving the pain and the fear. She would "comply" with S.'s wishes so that she could later point the finger at him. She was eager to accept the contract, for it gave justification for her anger at Dr. S. when, as she had expected, he would not comply—to the letter—with the exchange it specified. In this way she could blame him for failing to protect her from pain and fear, and maybe even for having caused them in the first place. Blaming him let her forget for a moment how sad and precarious her situation was. It let her proceed with the illusion that, in an eccentric version of the *experimentum crucis,* removing S. as one would remove a splinter would produce the desired outcome of removing the pain and fear.

For his part it occurred to S. that his insistence on compliance might not have been entirely motivated by his wish to take care of her. An example was his initial demand that she tell him whenever she was seen by another doctor. By letting her know that he didn't feel able to care for her otherwise, was he making a self-fulfilling prophecy? By quickly jumping to spell out for her the consequences of her failure to comply, was he telling her that he was expecting, maybe even wanting her to fail to comply? In her "failure to comply," was she complying with the hidden message, implicit in the compliance model, that patients such as she are expected not to comply? He saw that her consulting other physicians had served some unacknowledged desires of his own. It meant that some of her demands for care as well as some of her anger would be directed at the other doctors instead of at him. It had also given him justification for the anger that he felt toward her. Thus he was able to win the power struggle and to rid himself not only of the anger engendered by this patient, but of the patient herself. Mrs. Nagel was being "compliant" with his hidden wishes when she was being "noncompliant" with his stated wishes.

Reflecting on his encounter with Mrs. Nagel, S. wondered whether by basing his caring relationships with patients on compliance he was treating grown people like small children. Was it any wonder, then, that some patients would respond like children and even attribute to him the magical powers of the mechanistic scientist, who by changing this or that variable could make their pain and fear disappear? When such expectations were disappointed, as sometimes they must be, anger would follow. By now, even when S. *could* make the pain and fear disappear, patients would be using the most primitive version of the Mechanistic Paradigm, whereby he was the only cause. They would need only the slightest provocation to consider him not only the sole cause of cure for their pain and fear, but of the pain and fear themselves. When treated as children, patients would fall back on a mechanistic notion of causality and would think of S. as they long ago thought of their mothers and fathers.

S. realized that, though he was using the criteria of the Probabilistic Paradigm, he was following them like cookbook rules rather than internalizing them as an interdependent system. Thus he could be drawn into Mrs. Nagel's zero-sum compliance game, an exchange relationship where he would make concessions to her as the price of getting his way. The two of them so arranged it that theirs was a competitive relationship, with the loser being "stuck" with the sadness that, together, they could not find a way to share. By being angry with each other, they attributed the sadness to the "fact" that the other was "making me sad," and thus named the other person as somehow the cause of the sadness.

Although both of them were thinking mechanistically, S., as a "scientist" in the Mechanistic Paradigm (not to mention his being healthy and having family and friends) ultimately had the upper hand. His initial reaction had been to steer clear of patients such as Mrs. Nagel. They took up too much of his time and energy and, he felt, took away from the care he could be giving other patients. He could feel sufficiently justified in his anger to label Mrs. Nagel "hateful," as if that were a classification to be applied to an individual rather than a result of interactions between people. On reflection, however, S. saw that he had swung over from the narcissism of total self-reproach to the paranoia of seeing this patient as the sole cause of her hatefulness. This enabled him to hold Mrs. Nagel's anger and sadness at arm's length, just as she had sought to hold her pain and fear at arm's length by being angry at him.

S.'s reconsideration of his interactions with Mrs. Nagel allowed him to accept his share of the responsibility for what had happened. He recognized that as long as he was operating on the compliance model, he could arrange matters so that with almost any patient the need to struggle against rather than work with him could come to the surface. He could get away from Mrs. Nagel, but not from himself.

S. resolved to become more conscious in forming relationships with patients that were based on shared rather than competing needs. Sharing between doctor and patient could not, of course, be total. It was the patient's life, the patient's health, that were on the line. Still, a caring person could share pain and fear that he could not directly feel. Instead of squaring off in a game that pitted the needs of one against the needs of the other, doctor and patient could gamble together to meet needs that were shared as well as needs that were not shared. With this hope S. stopped struggling to achieve compliance and tried to offer caring without strings attached.

Complying with Oneself

S. remembered Mrs. Nagel when he met Henry Kane, a twenty-year-old epileptic whose seizures were not well controlled. The kind of seizures that Henry Kane had could not be completely prevented under the best of circumstances, but matters were made worse by the fact that for periods of time he refused to take medicine. Henry had little experience in self-reliance; his family seemed accustomed to his being dependent and perhaps unwittingly encouraged it. While Henry was in the hospital after having fallen and cut his scalp during a seizure, he and S. arranged that he would be discharged to a halfway house, where his medications could be further adjusted and he could gain some distance from his family entanglements. Without telling anyone, Henry went straight home instead of to the halfway house. He also did not pick up his prescription and failed to keep an appointment with S. for a follow-up visit as was previously agreed upon.

At first S. stood in awe of the powerful forces that kept Henry as he was. How chaotic, how distrustful Henry's world must be. S. didn't see how he could continue to be his doctor. Then, remembering Mrs. Nagel, he called Henry. They set up an appointment. When the time came, Henry was there.

S. addressed Henry in a way that he had never quite brought himself to use with Mrs. Nagel. He was about to say, "Henry ..." when he caught himself. Though he often called patients by their first names, it seemed to have the wrong implications in the case of this grown man whose family still treated him as a child. "Mr. Kane," S. said, "it is very hard for me to believe anything you say after you behave as you do over and over again. I sense that your life is full of mistrust, and it hurts me that I, too, cannot trust you. I'll still be your doctor if you want to be my patient, so long as you know that right now I don't trust you."

Going by Henry's unresponsive face, S. couldn't tell if his words had even registered. But although he had lost his initial gamble of trusting Mr. Kane, he would still gamble on trusting him with the knowledge of his suspicions. After his experience with Mrs. Nagel he knew better than to assume that one brave gesture would create a higher level of trust. But perhaps it was a beginning.

What S. was doing was a far cry from what the drug companies implied he should be doing, i.e., manipulating the patient to achieve compliance. In their advertisements, such as the one entitled, "Patient Compliance: The Missing Link in Successful Control," the drug companies were marketing the second criterion of the Mechanistic Paradigm. They were claiming that, even if many causes were present, manipulating one cause, one variable (the "missing link"), would change the outcome decisively. The object to be manipulated was the patient. In the drug companies' mechanistic science patients were put into the role of compliant subjects who did everything they were told to do.

In Henry Kane's case, however, this was the role he already

had in his family, where he was, in effect, told to be sick. No wonder he couldn't do what S. told him to do. He couldn't comply with S. in being well because he was already complying with his family in being sick. If S. had tried to make Henry Kane comply, he would have put him into an untenable situation, as well as entering into a zero-sum game with the family over who was going to tell Henry what to do.

In his family Henry Kane had learned that he would be cared for only if he complied with his role as the cause of the family's troubles. When someone else got a cold, it was clear to everyone that Henry, "the sick one" who had always been prone to colds, had been the cause. When one or another family member met with a setback in the outside world, all would agree that the need to "take care of Henry" was the cause of it all. The more pain and fear was laid on Henry, the more he assumed the sick role, the more his brothers and sisters wanted to get away from him. And yet they were bound to take care of him by the same unspoken contract with which he was complying in being sick.

As Henry became more helpless, his brothers and sisters were all the more determined to show that they were different from him. But in the back of their minds lurked the fear that they, being of the same flesh and blood and the same genes as he, might not be so different after all. So they went to great lengths to show how different they really were. The way they showed it, however, was by taking care of Henry's every need while he was "sick," but having nothing to do with him while he was "well." Although their wish was to be as far away from him as possible, their behavior ensured that the ties of dependency that bound Henry to the family, and the family to Henry, would be far stronger than the genetic ties they feared.

S.'s task, then, was not to show Henry Kane how to comply; he could do that all too well. Mr. Kane was now in a weak, dependent position, and S. could not honestly treat him as he would most patients. But there were ways of caring for a person that did not involve manipulating him into compliance. Clearly Mr. Kane was not now able to internalize the principles of the Probabilistic Paradigm and practice them independently. Perhaps, though, he could begin by identifying with S. as someone who could do these things. In S., Henry Kane would have a model of a conscious gambler. If he liked what he saw in S.'s way of thinking, feeling, and acting, he might make it in some measure his own.

It would do no good to try to make Mr. Kane comply with anyone else's ideas about what he should do. What mattered was what he thought was right for himself. The real issue for S. was to see if Mr. Kane wanted to make a choice—to choose to be an independent, self-respecting human being—and then help him get beyond his fears and uncertainties so that he could live out that choice, i.e.: comply with his chosen self.

Henry Kane needed to learn in the most basic ways how to take care of himself—to get around the city, to achieve some financial independence, to manage his epilepsy without having it manage him, and even to articulate some of his thoughts and feelings. He was afraid to learn these things, since he feared that he would lose his family's support if he did. For the same reason he was afraid to stop having frequent epileptic seizures, which were a comforting sign of his dependency on the family. And yet he also was scared to death of the seizures and found them unpleasant and humiliating. This was the place where S. decided to try to break into the closed system of Mr. Kane's dependency. "Shall we take a chance on working together?" he asked him, hoping that at some level Mr. Kane would want to gamble on himself.

"Nothing ventured, nothing gained, I guess," replied Mr. Kane.

"What makes it so hard to take the medication?" S. asked.

"Well, what usually happens is that there is no way I can remember to take it three times a day. I need someone to remind me, but my family gets tired of it after a while. And once I stop taking it and have a seizure, it's a pain to start again."

The first gamble S. proposed was to switch to a medication that Mr. Kane would have to take only once rather than three times a day. "I'll bet that if we do that," said S., "you won't forget to take the medication so much. And the less you forget, the fewer seizures you'll have."

"Let's give it a try," said Mr. Kane. Instead of a "game" where he took his medication as the price of keeping S. in his corner, patient and doctor were now on the same side.

Even though their talks were still one-sided (for Henry Kane didn't yet trust himself enough to say what he thought and felt), S. carefully brought him around to a different attitude toward his illness and treatment. Since it was as yet impossible to stop the seizures completely, there was no reason for Mr. Kane to think that he had "failed," lost the gamble, if he happened to have a seizure. He and S. were going for a reduction of the probability, not an all-or-none result. Nor did Mr. Kane have to think, if he forgot one dose of his medication, that the bet was lost and he might just as well forget his medication altogether. True, he increased the probability of a seizure every time he forgot to take the medicine—and that was what they were try-ing to avoid—but he would raise the odds much more by forget-ting repeatedly than by forgetting once. So there was still every reason not to forget the next time. There was a thin line be-tween "it's okay to forget it" and "it's not okay to forget it," just as there was with patients who were gambling on themselves when they tried to stop smoking or overeating.

As in those cases, S. helped Mr. Kane understand that the consequences of a single lapse, in terms of the habits he was trying to learn, went beyond the physical consequences alone, which often were negligible. In the language of gambling, S. was setting up a side bet whereby Henry Kane could enhance his own self-respect every time he took the medication. As Mr. Kane put it, "You know, it's funny—the more I bother about myself, the more I think I'm worth bothering about."

On the other hand, S. thought it important that both of them understand that the consequences of forgetting a dose were not so dire as to mean that Mr. Kane would lose the whole of his self-esteem. "Who doesn't forget sometimes?" S. would say on those occasions when Mr. Kane would come in and tell him that he had forgotten a dose here and there. Though Mr. Kane would continue to forget once in a while, he did so less and less fre-quently. Moreover, when he did forget, he would resume the medication with the next dose instead of stopping completely and refusing to take it.

Controlling Henry Kane's seizures was an important first step in his treatment not only because he would be able to get around more confidently by himself if he were not subject to such frequent attacks, but also because his fear of being "out of control" during a seizure stood for his sense of not being in control of his life and in his family relationships. S. helped him achieve some control over the frequency of his seizures by familiarizing him with some of the known causes of epileptic attacks. Failing to take the medication was a cause. Drinking, which Mr. Kane had been doing with the tacit encouragement of his family, was a cause. Emotional agitation was a cause, and a person who kept his feelings pent up as Henry Kane did was often agitated.

As their relationship evolved, S. and Henry Kane were able to set up a regular visit schedule so that he could continue to count on seeing S. even without there being a crisis. He needed to see that, in contrast to his family situation, getting well did not mean that he would lose his ties to S. He could still count on S.'s care even after he stopped being completely dependent on S.'s presence. In time—and it would take time—Henry Kane would no longer have a stake in being sick. Now that he was beginning to identify with S. and internalize the principles S. followed, he could begin to deal with the uncertainty that he would always face, while knowing that others would work with him even if he was able to help himself. S., at least, would do so; perhaps those who lived with him would too.

In the months that followed, Henry Kane became more articulate. With S.'s encouragement he took an adult-education course in emergency medicine, a subject he chose out of his increasing awareness of and responsibility for his illness. Since the purpose of the course was to teach people to respond to just that sort of occurrence, it gave Mr. Kane a natural format for practicing the steps he and S. had worked out for him to take when he felt a fit coming on. First he would lie down. Then he would tell the people around him what was going to happen. "Don't worry," he would say. "It'll be okay as long as I can breathe. Keep the airway clear if it gets blocked. It'll just take five minutes, and then I'll be dazed for a while." This procedure had worked quite well at home with his family.

It happened that Mr. Kane did have a seizure in class. As he described it later to S., "It came out okay, and the people did the right things, but they were really scared, and afterward a lot of them didn't seem to want to look at me or talk to me all evening. And this was the kind of thing they're all supposed to be there for!" People have different ways of distancing themselves from what they fear, and just at that moment Henry Kane's family's way of smothering him with sympathetic attention was looking a little better to him. It did not surprise S. that Mr. Kane suffered a setback as his family drew him back into its protective folds. But while he had been changing, his family had been changing too. As the others in the family saw Henry take the gamble of stepping out of his sick role, and survive, they found the courage to do the same. S. was now able to begin working with the family as well as the patient to try to understand what had happened. Slowly the rigid roles that had characterized this family became more flexible, and the family began to break out of its mechanistic mold.

Over the next few years, as the family members learned to share the risks of gambling rather than load all the fear and pain of an uncertain world onto Henry's illness, their capacity to bear fear and pain grew. At the same time, the amount of fear and pain Henry's illness caused them became less as they began to understand the illness probabilistically. They were learning that epilepsy is an illness with many causes, some of which they as well as Henry could control. For example, as Henry learned to express his feelings, the frequency of his seizures decreased. His brothers and sisters learned to see that having one possible cause of epilepsy (some of the same genes) in common with Henry no longer meant being predestined to the same fate.

When they no longer had to differentiate themselves from Henry on the basis of who was caring for whom and who was complying with whom, the other members of his family could tolerate far more initiative on his part. They could be with Henry as a family, sharing experience and risk, rather than manipulating a passive, compliant, sick subject in order to hide from the uncertainty they could not tolerate.

Acknowledging Strengths
and Admitting Differences

The difficulties that S. encountered in caring for Henry Kane and his family and for Mrs. Nagel were exceptional. Even so, he learned something about caring from each of these cases. Caring sometimes meant supporting people in their efforts to comply with their own choices, as S. had done with Henry Kane. Sometimes it even meant supporting people when their choices did not comply with his own wishes, as he would like to have done with Mrs. Nagel. Having learned these lessons, S. could apply them when caring for less troubled families such as the Fowlers and the Neills.

When the Fowlers brought in their two-month-old, whose birth at home S. had attended, for a well baby checkup, they reported that the baby was fussing for several hours each evening despite all their ministrations. S. assured the couple that this behavior was normal. He explained it as a kind of developmental stage through which infants pass. "After all, he's still largely a reflex person," said S., pointing to the baby's easily elicited startle response. "There isn't that much he can do, and crying is one of those things. As soon as he begins to relate more discriminately to the world around him, you can count on this kind of crying coming to an end.

"Remember, we don't know what the experience he is having is like. We can't even assume that it's unpleasant. We just can't get inside his head. But you feel responsible to make him feel better, anyone would. And what you find out is that you can't do everything about it. Then you feel helpless, and maybe the baby does too."

S. knew how insecure many new parents felt. He believed that they were doing well, only they were the last to know it. His faith wasn't blind. Sure, there were things he encouraged them to do differently, but he did so in the spirit of refining an already amazing piece of craftsmanship, the family. All too often people simply are unacknowledged for being themselves. They are always being put down. Even the efforts of experts to assist can have the effect of undermining self-confidence. So he made a point of letting people know what a good job *they* were doing, and of offering them understanding and support. He also wanted to show them that he cared for them even though they were doing well. There did not have to be something wrong for him to care. He believed that the parents' feeling good about themselves was as important to a child's well-being as any of the traditional things he did, such as giving polio vaccine.

The more pain and fear there was, the harder it was for people to gamble with a doctor. S. began to realize that some of the pain and fear entered into his practice not from the patient's home, as with Henry Kane, but from the very fact of a person's becoming a patient.

It isn't easy to be a patient. People feel bad and find it difficult to express themselves (it is often hard even to describe a pain). They may feel stupid for being inarticulate, for having delayed seeking attention, or for having come for a trivial purpose. They may be ashamed to disrobe, particularly when they do not know the doctor. S. thought it essential to acknowledge this discomfort and to put people at ease so that they could provide better information and collaborate in their treatment.

When S. encountered patients who readily, even insistently collaborated in their treatment, he admired their courage in choosing to do so in spite of all the barriers. However, they often presented a different kind of challenge. There were some who insisted that the compliance shoe be on the other foot, that the doctor give them what they wanted, such as this or that tranquilizer, or they would take their business elsewhere. They presented S. with a difficult dilemma. He did not want to impose his values, yet he did not think that "anything goes" was a responsible position to take. So, depending on the patient and the request, he would try to work out some agreement. When an agreement simply could not be reached, he had to say, "Would you like me to refer you to another doctor for this?" More often he could continue to care for a patient or family while agreeing to disagree with a particular choice that they made.

It happened that way with the Neills, a professional couple in their late twenties. Elizabeth Neill had had three abortions in the past four years. The last of these had been performed by

S. Afterward he invited the couple to discuss contraceptive methods with him. As they spoke, it became apparent that the couple had previously spent a good deal of time examining the subject. "We've had this same discussion before with other doctors," said Elizabeth, "and the best we could come up with was the rhythm method. We've done everything. We keep track of the temperature, and we even use the mucus test." The couple's reasons for deciding against an IUD and the pill were based on an evaluation of the side effects of both. They rejected a diaphragm or condoms on the grounds that these would detract from the sensuality of their sex life. And they were both clear that they did not want to have children just yet.

After getting to know the couple better in the course of several visits, S. could not help but wonder whether their choice was not being constrained by an excessively rigid definition of sensuality made necessary by the otherwise fragile bonds between husband and wife. But the couple did not see that as a problem that they wanted to deal with just then. S. let them know that he disagreed with their choice, but that he could live with the disagreement and continue to offer them support and care. He and the Neills agreed to disagree for the time being.

Caring in the Midst of Pain and Fear

S. had come far in internalizing the Probabilistic Paradigm and applying it to caring for the frightened or pained patient. One such situation was blood drawing. It was especially difficult for S. when he encountered a person with a morbid fear of needles and of blood taking: Some people would faint right in the office. At first S. tried to tell these patients that this fear was not in their best interest. For example, to pregnant patients he pointed out that their inability to give blood not only interfered with prenatal care, but could become a significant hazard should a sample of blood or an intravenous treatment be needed in an emergency. He soon realized, however, that such statements, left by themselves, smacked too much of "compliance" and too little of "care."

Again his patients became his teachers. There was eighteen-year-old Ginny Meher, tears in her eyes, ready to walk out of his office: "No one is going to draw any blood from me. You're not going to stick me with a needle." Ginny had always been "scared to death" of needles, and now it was just too much. She had come to S. because her menstrual period, which had always been "like clockwork," was now, two weeks after its due date, yet to appear. She was worried when she walked into S.'s office. She was afraid that she might be pregnant and had no one, not her mother or her boyfriend, with whom to share that fear. Ginny's father was long dead, and she felt that her mother, a "very religious woman," would be "shocked." Tommy, her boyfriend, was away in the service, and this was something that she did not want to tell in a letter or over the telephone.

The urine test for pregnancy gave an ambiguous result. The results of S.'s pelvic exam were less ambiguous. He told her, "There is a good chance that you are in the very early stages of pregnancy." The thoughts that just then rushed through Ginny's mind were accompanied by a numbing, a deadening of her body, and by tears which came to her eyes but did not roll down her cheeks. After she had talked with S. for a while about the choices she faced, the thoughts were now of a different sort, but the feeling of deadness through her body and the tears poised on the edge of her eyelids still remained. It was when S. mentioned that blood would need to be drawn to confirm that she was pregnant that her outburst came.

She was surprised by her anger at him. "I am sorry, Doctor. I know that you want to help me, but I just can't stand needles." By now S. had realized that despite his best efforts to be helpful (and in part because of them), the fear and sadness that Ginny was feeling would have to be shared between them.

She had entered the office scared, thinking that she would hear "the worst": that she was pregnant. She was feeling sad ("robbed," she would later say) that something which under other circumstances would be joyful would now only be an occasion for pain. S. took great care to make the pelvic exam as comfortable as possible. He explained what he was going to do and how it was likely to feel at each step, referring to the illustrations and diagrams that lined the walls. He was so successful that during the exam she felt far calmer and safer than she did when she stepped through the door. She felt somehow reassured; she felt that as long as he took care of her, he would be able to keep the fear, pain, and sadness at arm's length.

So when Dr. S. reentered his office after the pelvic examination and told her that he thought she was pregnant, she was outraged. Although she fought hard not to show it, she felt somehow betrayed. The fear and sadness returned, and the gratitude she had felt toward S. during the pelvic exam, when she saw him as the cause of her calmness and confidence, turned into resentment. She couldn't help but see him now as the cause of her pain. This person who could ease her pain the way her mother had long ago when as a child she would bang her knee, this person who could ease her fear and make her feel safe the way her father had when he walked with her through a tough neighborhood, aroused in her both sadness and anger when the pain and fear came back. He had brought her the "bad news," and now she was more scared and panicked than before at the prospect that she would soon have to make a choice under conditions of uncertainty—to go through with the pregnancy or abort. She felt somehow "robbed" of her youth by the prospect of making that choice. It was one that did not make any sense in terms of the ambitions and ideals she had had while growing up.

"I know I am a coward, and I am ashamed of that, but I'm upset enough today," she told S. He felt that if she walked out of his office right then and there, feeling deeply ashamed, with the question of whether or not she was pregnant still a bit up in the air, she would not feel strong enough to make the critical choice that needed to be made. He decided to gamble rather than just watch her walk out. He did not tell her that she had to comply with his wishes and just *had* to have the blood drawn. He didn't doubt that she would have gone along with the blood drawing if he had phrased his request as an edict. But that would have resulted in her leaving his office completely dependent on him and as ill-equipped to deal with the uncertainty she would soon face as if she had left without the blood test, feeling independent but ashamed.

S. took a different approach, saying, "I wish I could tell you that this blood drawing is going to be painless, but it won't be. God knows, you're in enough pain already, but you've been in tough spots before." For the first time since she had entered his office, a smile crossed Ginny's face. "I guess you've had to deal with patients who've had a far tougher lot than mine," she said, "but they couldn't have been as scared as I am right now." He shook his head. "You're not the only one. Just now there's more than one scared person in this room." "You, scared?" Her voice had in it now both sadness and a certain relief.

They talked a while longer. At first it was in general terms about how much courage it took to allow oneself to be scared, to feel the pain, to face uncertainty. Ginny soon was sharing with S. her experiences with needles and doctors as far back as she could remember, and the thoughts and feelings she would have whenever she had to have blood drawn. Finally she said, "Okay, which arm?" "Your choice," he answered. She stuck out her left arm, explaining, "I am going to need my right one to write a letter to my boyfriend tonight."

S. went ahead and drew the blood, telling Ginny exactly what he was doing at each step: "Now I am rubbing your skin with the alcohol swab." "Now I am putting on the tourniquet." At each step she watched what he was doing and told him what she was thinking and feeling. She felt as if she was drawing the blood herself. At the end, when she felt faint, she heard him say, "If you feel like fainting, it's okay. It's safe—both you and I will be here to take care of you."

PART IV

FAMILY DECISIONS

12

DEATH
IN THE HOME

By now it was a familiar story. "Do you make house calls, Doctor?" asked the woman on the phone. He guessed that she was middle-aged. "My mother is riddled with cancer—breast cancer. The surgeons at the General Hospital said that there was nothing more they could do and that we should find her a local medical doctor. Now my mother is very, very weak and in pain. She doesn't get out of bed anymore, and she has a sore on her back. Since she had a stroke a few weeks ago, she has trouble talking and swallowing. She wants to stay at home, and we want that too. When could you come over, Doctor, and tell us what you think we should do?"

"Does she know that she's dying?"

"Yes, she's known it for a while now."

After S. had seen his last patient of the day, he checked the map, picked up his black doctor's bag, and headed into a neighboring town about ten minutes away from his office. "Nothing more to do," he thought. "Here I go again." He now felt the anxiety of being exposed to death and that of entering into a family's intimate life during a crisis. And it was always different in the home. The family would need support in whatever course they chose, support which he could give.

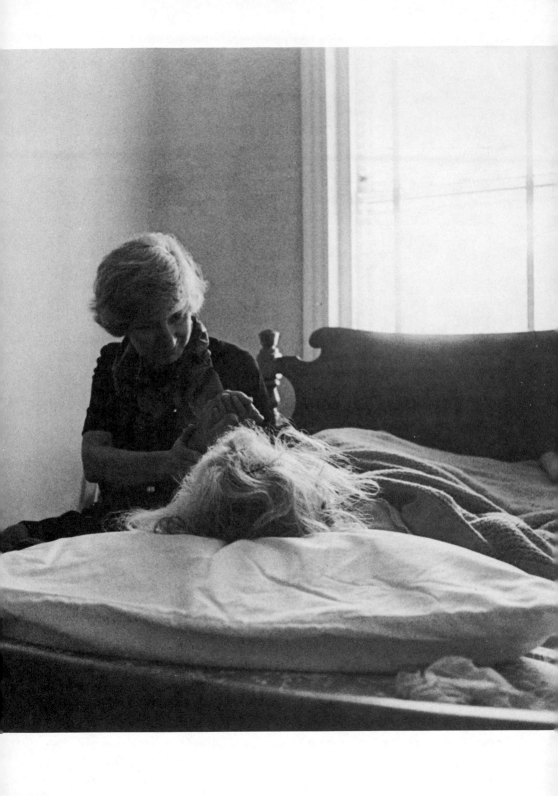

Eighty-year-old Mabel Gormley lived on the second floor of a two-family house on a quiet side street. Her daughter and son-in-law, Jessie and Norman Cavanaugh, lived on the first floor. It was not a fancy house or a fancy neighborhood, but the Cavanaughs, like their neighbors, were proud of the way they kept up the home in which they had been living for many years.

Another daughter, Jenny O'Farrell, lived nearby with her husband and two unmarried daughters. Both the Cavanaughs and the O'Farrells also had married children who lived in the neighborhood where they had grown up. This family did not fit the stereotype of the mobile nuclear family in contemporary American society.

Dr. S. introduced himself and was ushered in to see the old woman, who was lying in bed in her own bedroom. As he examined her, he saw how weak she was. There wasn't much skin on those bones. She couldn't sit up, and her chest didn't move much when she breathed. She was very deaf and very scared and very tired. What he said to her had to be relayed to her by her daughter, who leaned over the bed as she spoke. Mrs. Gormley was afraid, her daughter told S., that he would say that she had to go to the hospital. It was hard to tell, but while he was examining her she took his hand and squeezed it. After discussing the situation with the family in Mrs. Gormley's presence, he said, "Well, you asked me to tell you what I think you should do, but I'd say you have a choice to make."

Jessie Cavanaugh leaned over the bed again. "Mama, it's okay," she said. "The doctor says it's okay. You can stay." A look of relief appeared on Mabel Gormley's face.

S. went into the living room to speak with the family. He felt that although it might make him comfortable to speak to his patient in an extended fashion, it might not do her much good. So he tried to get a better idea of how she felt by finding out how her family felt. From his impressions of this family he decided that their statements probably did reflect her wishes. But he would be open to changing his mind.

Various questions concerned him. When Mrs. Cavanaugh had asked him on the phone to "tell us what you think we should do," was she asking whether they could responsibly care for their mother at home and how they might best go about doing so? Or was she asking him to be the one to tell the old woman that she had to go to the hospital? Was she becoming too much trouble for them? Did they feel themselves unable to undertake day-and-night nursing care? It would be very understandable if they felt that way. But if such were their decision, he did not want the responsibility "dumped" on him, as he had experienced with other families. He wanted to help this family shoulder the decision themselves.

Perhaps, though, he was being too wary. He didn't really have that feeling about Mrs. Gormley's family, anyway. Undoubtedly they had mixed feelings about what they were doing, and he thought it best that they be aware that they did.

"What made you decide that you wanted to keep your mother at home?" he asked.

"It's not our decision," replied Mrs. Cavanaugh, gesturing toward the bedroom where the patient lay. "It's my mother's decision entirely. She wants it that way. Give her the credit, Doctor. She's not the kind of person who'd let them keep her drugged in a nursing home."

The credit and the blame, thought S. "It's your decision too— all of you," he said. "After all, you'll be the ones who will be doing the work."

Mrs. Cavanaugh, who by now was doing most of the talking for the family, reminded S. that "it's my mother we're concerned about. The last thing we would want is for her to suffer because we decided to keep her at home."

"In some ways she may suffer less here than in the hospital," he reassured them. "You can do a lot to keep her comfortable, and she will feel better being among the people and things she has cared about all her life."

"And how about all the suffering she'd go through in a nursing home?" Mrs. O'Farrell broke in. "A few years ago, when she broke her hip, they put her in a nursing home for therapy after the operation. I went to visit her the first day, and it was as if she didn't know me. Whether she was heavily medicated, or whether she was scared out of her wits at seeing all those other people, I don't know. But I couldn't even make out what she was saying. Her speech was thick. This wasn't my mother. As soon as I saw her I knew she wasn't in her right mind."

S. commented, "The staff may not have been aware of how much she had changed. They may have assumed she was always that way. You could tell the difference because you knew what she was really like."

"I just couldn't take it," continued Mrs. O'Farrell. "I went right home and told my sister, 'We have to get her out of there.'" As she spoke, she glanced toward her twenty-two-year-old daughter, Audrey. "That night I told my husband and all my children, 'If I ever get to be that way, don't ever put me in that nursing home.'"

"It sounds like *you* have some very definite feelings about putting your mother in a nursing home again," said S.

"That same night my husband and I brought her home in an ambulance," Mrs. Cavanaugh related. "In just the few minutes I spent in that nursing home, I saw all kinds of drugs being mashed into ice cream for the patients. I turned to my husband and said, 'Those poor people. Whoever gets that concoction won't see the light of day for a year.'"

Her sister added, "In just one day she was stuffed so full of drugs that it took her until the next morning to regain control of herself. In a day or two, when the drugs had worn off, she was herself again."

"She felt at home," S. said gently.

"We think it was the drugs," reiterated Mrs. Cavanaugh.

S. doubted that it was only the drugs. "So you've all had experience with the way they treat old people in some nursing homes, and *one* of the things they do is to substitute drugs for people, for love." He was concerned that if they blamed drugs for everything, they wouldn't be able to choose freely to give their mother pain medication when she really needed it. Blaming everything on drugs was like relying totally on drugs. They needed to see *people* as a cause. "Who made the decision to put her in the nursing home?" he asked.

Jessie Cavanaugh was the first to answer. "It wasn't the doctor. It was the social worker who said she had to be in a nursing home. The social worker thought she was helping by doing that. The doctor didn't agree with her, but we didn't even know that. We thought, 'That's what the social worker says, that's what the doctor says, so that's what we have to do.' We didn't think we had a choice."

"You don't have a choice if you don't have anyone to take care of you," her sister went on. "But when there are people like us who want to help, the doctor should listen to them."

"The family makes these choices possible," S. explained. "I have had patients like your mother whose families were unable to care for them at home, or who didn't have families at all. In those cases the only choice I could live with was to put them in the hospital." As he spoke, he reflected sadly on the story of the doctor and the social worker. Everybody passes the buck, and nobody makes the decision. Either it's *"I'm* the doctor, and *I'll* decide," or "Don't look at *me."* Things just "happen," and nobody takes responsibility. Responsibility isn't a matter of ownership; it's a matter of sharing. He wanted to share responsibility with this family.

Just then Norman Cavanaugh spoke for the first time. "Jessie's father died in a hospital. He was thrown in a room with five other men; apparently they were all considered 'goners.' The nurses did what they could, but they all knew they were waiting to die, one after another. Is that any way for a guy to leave this world, with a bunch of guys in a room and nobody caring about them?"

"In this nursing home they have six or seven nurses taking care of one hundred people," said Mrs. O'Farrell. "They hardly have time to feed or bathe them, let along show them some concern. Most of these poor people die of a broken heart. They don't have anybody coming to see them and kiss them and hug them."

"As if those things didn't matter," said S.

"You can't buy love. Look at what people pay to go into hospitals and nursing homes, just to be drugged to sleep. Whether they give all those drugs to ease the pain or to keep them quiet I don't know."

"Sometimes it's hard to tell the two apart. Think what a better position you're in as a family. You have six or seven people to help care for one person."

Since S. couldn't get to know Mrs. Gormley by speaking with her, he asked the family what she was like. Since her radiation treatments at the General Hospital Mrs. Gormley had been going downhill fast. At first she just sat in her chair, afraid to get up. She said it was because of her fear of breaking a bone, but her wish to stay still seemed just as much a way for her to dig in her heels. Then she took to her bed. According to her daughters she was a shy person who wanted to be with people she knew best. Her biggest fear was that of being taken away from her loved ones.

S. wondered to what extent the fear of death is entangled with the fear of separation from the familiar. People are afraid of childbirth because they don't see it, don't know anything about it. It is the same with death. When people saw death and lived with death from their earliest years, perhaps it was not so overwhelmingly frightening, especially if they could see that the dead did not lose all contact with the living, that they were remembered. Death is an unknown. It is made even more fearsome and mysterious when it is put out of the way in sterile institutional settings, when the dying person is left alone in a strange place with all connection to the familiar stripped away beneath the hospital "johnny."

"My mother has a lot of courage," said Jenny O'Farrell, "but she also has a lot of fears. She's never wanted to take vacations or go out with groups of people. She's more comfortable staying at home."

"It takes a strong person to die away from home, but it also takes a strong person to die away from the hospital," S. commented. He was glad to see Mrs. O'Farrell take such a balanced view of her mother. Yes, her mother was a wonderful person, but she wasn't perfect. Dying at home was an expression of courage and also an expression of fear. It was a way for the dying person to say "no" to death. With that perspective the family would be better able to get through the tasks that lay ahead.

They had wanted to know whether they were "doing the right thing." He told them that he thought they were. He was willing to support them at home if they were willing to put in the necessary nursing care. There were no double-blind controlled studies to demonstrate that one choice was clearly better than the other. He doubted that there ever would be such studies. How could you isolate and measure all the variables contributing to the effects of treating patients with different medical needs and family situations at home versus in the hospital? Even if there were some data, he and the family would still have to make subjective estimates of what the probabilities meant in their situation, and of what their values were. They would have to gamble.

Either way, home or hospital, was a gamble. Most doctors thought only of the home as a gamble. In so doing they were simply showing a preference for the gamble with the more certain outcome. In the hospital you knew more or less what was going to happen. But the hospital, too, had its risks. As Dr. S. told Mrs. Gormley's family, either choice had its advantages and disadvantages. There was no sure thing. They had a choice between two gambles—going to the hospital or staying at home. (A third gamble, not yet available in their community, would have been a hospice, an institution that allowed the terminally ill to be cared for in homelike surroundings.)

S. made clear that he was not wedded to the choice of staying at home. The important thing was for the family to make the choice and to reevaluate the choice critically on a continuing basis. To do this they had to feel free to change their minds. "It won't always be easy," he told them. "There may be times when you'll want to change your minds. You should talk about these concerns when they come up. You don't have to keep your mother at home. The hospital is always there as a backup. My experience has been, however, that most families are able to get over the hurdles they face. Not all, but most. And it's okay with me if you change your minds."

It was not that he didn't have feelings of his own about the issue. His feelings were becoming clear enough to the family. At first he felt a bit ashamed of not being a bit more "disinterested" in the family's choice. He realized, however, that his role was perhaps to balance other social pressures. It wasn't easy to keep a dying relative at home these days with almost everyone doing the opposite.

"There are some things you'll need to do. For one thing it will be very helpful to rent a hospital bed from a medical-supply house. A hospital bed is higher, which makes it easier when you're turning or changing her. It goes up and down, and it has side rails to keep her from falling out. You can raise her head for feeding and adjust the angle for her comfort." He wondered, though, if the hospital bed was also a touch of "home" for a physician who found himself on strange turf. He had fantasies of yelling out for his order book and dressing the family up in white uniforms. He would have to be careful to avoid being carried away with these fantasies.

"Then you'll have to get to work on the pressure sore at the base of her spine. It comes from lying in bed too long in one position. Pick up a soft cushion filled with lamb's wool—that will take the pressure off that spot. Turn her from side to side every hour and apply ointment to the sore. This may cause her pain, but in the long run you'll be saving her pain. That's about all you'll need to know for the time being. I'll arrange for a visiting nurse to be with you during the day, and I'll come back in a few days to see what else you can do to keep your mother comfortable. We'll talk then about the things you may have to deal with in the later stages. Meanwhile, call whenever you need to, day or night."

Yes, S. thought as he was leaving, these were strong people. Sure, they were concerned about whether this was "the right thing to do." Who wouldn't be? In these times it was an unusual thing to do. How easy it was for him to fall into the professional trap of assuming that he was indispensable. Yes, they needed him, but not so much as he might like to think. They knew a great deal already. They only needed to be assured of how much they knew and how much they could do.

They did need some reassurance, of course. They weren't used to making such large decisions for themselves. In a way, they weren't used to thinking critically. Take Audrey, who had a dead-end job as a secretary in the very hospital where her grandmother had been given radiation treatments and sleeping pills. She had been taught to spell and define medical terms, but not to use them creatively. She was being paid to do her job, not to exercise the capacity for thought that her family had given her.

Her mother and aunt remembered more about what it was for a family to make its own choices. They had learned it from *their* mother, who—even more than they—had lived by her own labor. Her reward was that she would die at home, surrounded and comforted by her family rather than by machines and attendants. Of course, she had suffered in her life, but she had been able to teach her children something about critical thinking. They were showing the benefits of her teaching when they took her out of a nursing home and chose not to put her in a nursing home again.

In recent years this family had not had so many opportunities to make decisions that affected their lives. They were glad to have this opportunity, even if exercising it felt a bit like exercising long-unused muscles. They saw themselves in the mirror Dr. S. had held up for them: uncertain, afraid, yet strong underneath it all. They did have mixed feelings about doing all that work. But now that the choice was presented to them, they saw why it was important for them to do it. Perhaps they didn't want to think of themselves as abandoning their mother. But it was much more that they simply would not abandon her. What they felt was not guilt or shame so much as love. They just had to get used to the very new—and very old—idea that love didn't have to mean putting someone in a hospital.

Dealing with death aroused complex and contradictory emotions in S. It forced him to acknowledge his vulnerability as a doctor and as a human being. For one thing he could not help but share the pain, anger, and fear of the dying person and the family. The routine of the hospital, the orders and details, were no longer available to preoccupy him and deflect these emotions. Nor was the glamour of the intensive-care unit, the occasional life saved "just last week in the same bed," available to console him. For a doctor trained to treat and to cure, it was very difficult just to wait and let die.

Then, too, in the mortality of the dying person he treated, S. could not help but glimpse his own mortality. There were times when he looked away from that mirror, when what he saw there brought more pain and fear than could easily be borne. There were other times when he looked directly at it, when he sought out the opportunity to have a hint of what death was like. He tried to remember each death for the sake of the dying patient and for his own sake. There were times when he could see another side to death, when he could see it as the last gift of the dying person to the living. He was grateful, for that hint could enable him as well as the family gathered at the bedside to confront more consciously their own deaths to come. His thoughts turned to an essay of E. B. White's. He would return that night to underline a passage:

> I do not experience grief when I am down there, nor do I pay tribute to the dead. I feel a sort of overall sadness that has nothing to do with the grave or its occupant. Often I feel extremely well in that rough cemetery, and sometimes flush a partridge. But I feel sadness at All Last Things, too, which is probably a purely selfish, or turned in, emotion— sorrow not at my dog's death but at my own, which hasn't even occurred yet but which saddens me just to think about in such pleasant surroundings (White, 1977, p.89).

He had mixed feelings as well about his own undeniably important role in supporting the family of the dying person. There was a tinge of guilt, maybe even shame, at the voyeuristic, intrusive, busybody aspect of his going into people's homes when they were most vulnerable, most exposed. Did his calm, helpful demeanor mask a self-centered thirst for experience? Was that what he did it for? Did he just enjoy the kudos bestowed upon him? Did he do it so that he could glory in having lived with his own mixed feelings while trying to help the family make the best of the situation? Well, he thought, better to do the right thing for the wrong reasons than not to do it at all. He was hoping that it *was* the right thing, that it *did* help families. That was a better gamble, he decided, than to see himself as totally corrupted, a mere victim of these times, and let nature (no, not nature but "the system") take its course.

When S. returned a few days later, Mabel Gormley was resting as comfortably as her condition permitted in the hospital bed that her family had obtained. The family and the visiting

nurses had begun the nursing-care routines that he had out-
lined. Mrs. Gormley looked better, and everyone was pleased.

"Tell me, Doctor," Mr. Cavanaugh asked, "is there any hope?
If we do all the things you tell us, is there a chance that she
might rally?"

"No," replied the doctor. "She may have her good days and
bad days, but at this late stage there's nothing you or I can do
to stop the spread of the cancer, any more than the doctors at
the General could. You are caring for her, not curing her. Your
job and mine is to help her die in comfort, dignity, and love."
S. was careful to see that the family would keep sight of the
truth. And that meant telling the truth in a kind way, so that the
family would understand it without being driven to crippling
fear or denial. When this family brought up the possibility of
a miraculous remission, he gave them a straight answer. He
would not use uncertainty as an excuse to justify vagueness
about the odds. Vagueness was a means by which doctors—
including S. himself at times—could keep control over their
patients' and their own feelings. S. did his best to give his patients reliable probability information, along with some idea of
the margins of precision, so that they themselves could exercise some control.

As far as the family was concerned, there was no reason to
put Mrs. Gormley in the hospital unless there was some hope
of recovery. As Mrs. Cavanaugh put it, "People think that if you
don't go to the world's best hospital and spend all the money you
have, you're not doing the right thing. That makes no sense."

S. agreed. "You would have paid anything to save her if you
could have. But that's not what's at stake now."

The family did, however, have one major concern about providing home care. "What if something happens?" they wanted
to know. "What if there is an emergency and we don't know
what to do?"

"Things *will* happen," S. answered. "She is going to get
worse. She will have more pain. You will have to do more and
more for her." He explained the progressive deterioration of a
dying patient by drawing an analogy with pregnancy and birth.
"When we're taking care of a pregnant woman we watch for
possible complications that may cause us, along with the

woman and her family, to reconsider our decisions about the birth—for example, whether we will have the birth at home. The odds are very low, however, that any particular complication will occur, and there is a good chance that none of them will. With death we can be more certain—though not completely certain—that more and more complications will occur along the way: difficulty in eating, difficulty in breathing, loss of contact and communication. Perhaps *complications* is the wrong word, since these things are just part of dying. But whatever you call them, as time goes on, they raise the ante for taking care of someone who's dying at home. You recall my telling you that you could always change your minds."

"But, Doctor," Mrs. Cavanaugh objected, "you see these things all the time. For us they're all new."

"That's right. She is the only mother you have, and this is the only time she will die. I have to gamble a lot, and I win some and lose some. From that experience I get a pretty good idea of the odds. That's what I'm trying to share with you. I wish I had a crystal ball, but the best a doctor can do is to speak of probabilities rather than certainties." Still, he couldn't expect them to be as capable of detachment as he was, nor would he be capable of detachment if the dying person were a member of his own family. For she was their mother, and he knew how much more he had cared about his mother than any doctor had.

"Let's look at some of the choices you are likely to face in the coming days and weeks. By anticipating them, you may be able to make better, more conscious decisions. What if your mother develops pneumonia, as old people often do when they're ill? Will you want to treat it or not? Pneumonia used to be called 'the old man's best friend.' Now, though, we have drugs and machines that can bring people through it. It may not be easy to withhold those treatments from your mother even if that's the kindest thing to do."

The word *machines* brought up the respirators that could keep Mrs. Gormley going for days or weeks. Being away from those reassuring backup resources was one of the things S. found scary about treating people at home. Yet how often he had anguished over the plight of some old people, for whom the miracles of modern medicine—the machines that could keep them alive—had become a form of unwitting torture. "Please let me die!" they would say to the nurses behind the doctor's back.

It turned out that Mrs. Gormley's family had a pretty clear idea of how they felt about life-prolonging technology. "If it gets to the point where her life depends on a machine," they explained, "then we know that she wouldn't want any part of it."

Despite the family's statements on the matter, they still needed Dr. S. to explain what the machines would and wouldn't do. He told them that Mrs. Gormley would almost surely die within a few weeks. If a respirator were to be used to keep her alive beyond that point, it would not reverse the course of her illness; nor would it keep her conscious and able to communicate with her family. It would just keep her breathing. "Even so," he said, "I know how hard it is for a family to say, 'No, that's enough.'" This acknowledgment of the inevitable mixed feelings surrounding such a decision made it easier for them to make an informed choice not to use a respirator. As Mr. Cavanaugh put it, "A few days, a few weeks—at least we have some idea. Instead of it all being new to us, we have some facts to go on." In other words, S. was turning pure uncertainty into probabilities.

Another highly charged issue for this family was that of pain medications. "When she needs it," S. explained, "use this acetaminophen and codeine mixture for pain."

"But how will we know when she needs it?"

"Sometimes you will find yourself giving her the pain medication because she tells you she needs it. At other times you will be left on your own. Those are the times that are tough. It won't be easy to tell whether you are giving her the medication for her comfort or for your own—because she can't stand the pain or because you can't stand to hear her moan. Moaning is sometimes a signal that the person can't stand the pain, and sometimes a way for her to bear the pain. If her moaning means that she wants the medication, and if you don't give it to her, you will feel as if you're causing her suffering. On the other hand, if you give her the medication automatically every time she moans, you will be making yourselves more comfortable, but you also might be taking away from her what self-control and pride she has left, which is making her death bearable to her and you. Each time this choice comes up, you will be gambling that you understand whether she would prefer to have relief from pain or consciousness and clarity of mind. The more she is drugged, the less she will be able to share her last days with you. You will also be putting your own preferences into the equation. It might be worthwhile to sit down with her now, while she can still speak to you, and ask her on which side she would want you to err when in doubt."

"We don't have to ask her," Jenny O'Farrell stated emphatically. "As sick as she's been, there have been nights when she's told us, 'I've already had two aspirins today; don't give me any more.' She even said it the night she fell on the floor and couldn't get up. I know my mother. I'm the same way. Even in the hospital I wouldn't take sleeping pills." Mrs. O'Farrell could easily put herself in her mother's place. Someday she *would* be in her mother's place, and her daughter would be in hers. Audrey was getting some clear instructions.

"That's where a nurse in the hospital might have just given her an injection," said S. "But you listened to her because you are her daughter. This is one of the most helpful things you're doing for her—just listening and accepting and trying to understand her feelings, even the most painful ones, without falsely reassuring her. Since you do know your mother, you can trust your own feelings about her in a way that a nurse can't. Not only can you afford to spend more time with your mother than the nurse can, but you've had years already to get to know her. Since you know how she has lived, you can help her die the same way.

"You will have to find the answers to the problems that come up in your knowledge of yourselves as a family. All I can do is tell you about the situations I have seen families face. You will have to keep an open mind and choose what to do each time. And sometimes you will have to change your minds, and live with having made a mistake, and live with regret."

In a home visit there was always the feeling of being a guest on someone else's turf. In the office, even when one consciously tried, it was hard to shake the ingrained inequality of the doctor's and patient's roles. In the office it was so easy to see the patient, stripped of his or her life context, merely as a carrier of disease. So easy, then, to focus on the disease—to see treatment in terms of a magic bullet, of pills. Being in a patient's home left no doubt that the patient's autonomy, his or her capacity for deciding how much or little of modern medicine to take, was real, real in a family context, where the patient was connected to family members by long-forgotten yet still strong ties of nature and nurture.

This "case" had been going on long before S. ever got involved in it, as the patient had been sick a long time. But then the family had been living together and developing their own unique ways of getting along with each other and coping with the world for a long time also. Doctors had been involved with the illness only intermittently; the family had been involved continuously, minute by minute. Their decision to call S. had come near the end of a long chain of events. Though it would be a "cop-out," he thought, to say that his actions were of no consequence, it would be a fantasy to believe that he controlled the entire flow of events and decisions.

For S. questions like these made his participation in a birth or death at home more than a good human-interest story. It was a challenge not only to the heart, but to the mind as well. S. saw himself right on the frontier of scientific medicine, with all of the excitement and risk that he could ever hope to have.

He thought back to his first visit to the Cavanaugh home, when the family had shown some surprise that he so readily supported their choice. "Look at the facts," he had begun to tell them, then stopped himself. Another cop-out, he thought. As if all a doctor had to do was find the facts. Well-prepared house officers on rounds rattled off "the facts" on patients' charts as if any observer would see the same facts and then proceed to act on them. That wasn't the way it was, either on the hospital floors or out here in "real life." Those house officers changed the facts they looked at, and so did S. He was a cause of the decision to care for Mrs. Gormley at home, as were her children and grandchildren. If the family had been less willing and able to take care of her, the decision probably would have been different. If S. had not encouraged them to think that they and he would be "doing the right thing," the decision might well have been different. People, not facts, had made this decision.

S. also rejected the mechanistic interpretation that cancer was *the* cause of Mrs. Gormley's condition. While in the hospital she had been treated as though her problem was solely one of cancer. Once the hospital had done all it could about the cancer, it had "nothing more to do." For S. there was much more to Mabel Gormley than her cancer. She was a person with a history, a value system, and needs: needs for food, shelter, clothing, disposal of body wastes, relief from discomfort, and love. It was no accident that she wanted to be at home. She had always been at home. Home was where her supports were. It was where she had worked to support others: first as a mother who loved, taught, made food, and did so many other things that often are not recognized and appreciated. Then, as a grandmother, she did these things, somehow the same things and yet somehow so different.

This patient's condition was not determined unicausally by her cancer. It was the result of the interaction of a number of causes which would come and go as they had come and gone in her life, all depending on the context; for example, the pollutants in the air she breathed, the carcinogens in the food she ate, the feelings of anguish she had here and there felt while continually exposed to various stresses that could be felt even in her family's home. To respond to the special needs that cancer presented did not mean that all the other causes operating on and off in her life had to be ignored.

In medical school S. had learned to find the one correct solution, as one found the "facts," by experimenting. One could do an experiment, for example (or look up statistics obtained from such experiments), to see whether the home or the hospital provided a better environment for a person in Mrs. Gormley's condition. Actually, there had been and could be no such experiment, in part because Mrs. Gormley's condition could not be reduced to a set of controllable variables, and in part because the very act of experimenting would change what was being experimented upon. Now, practicing in real life under conditions of uncertainty, S. experimented by making a series of choices (gambles) and seeing what further choices they led to, all the while bearing in mind that all his actions, including his observations, were influencing the always tentative results of his experiments. Having made the initial decision to treat Mrs. Gormley at home, he and the family (as fellow experimenters) could see how she was doing and whether they were able to continue that form of treatment. Their choices, along with the illness and other causative factors, created new sets of circumstances requiring new choices.

Finally S. rejected the exaltation of objective data in favor of close attention to both objective and subjective (feeling) data. He took into account how the patient and family felt about where she wanted to die just as much as he did the report from the pathologist at that large hospital from which Mrs. Gormley had found her way back home.

S. was beginning to understand not only the kinds of gambles that the home and hospital represented for Mrs. Gormley, but also why many people did not see them both as the gambles they were. People thought you couldn't lose by going to the hospital, but only by staying at home. At home you could either win or lose. In the hospital, while you could lose as far as life and death were concerned, you somehow felt that you wouldn't lose because at the very least you would be doing the "right thing."

S. well understood that feeling. He knew what it was like to have someone close die in the hospital. He had been there many times. For the family it was always the same story: the visiting hours; the quick word with the private doctor; more frequent words with the nurses and house physicians; the trips back and forth. It all seemed so regular, like clockwork. The only hint of doubt, of the gamble, would come when you were home again, waiting for the call in the night that you knew would come but never knew when. Whereas when the person you loved was at home, dying where he or she had lived, you lived with the doubts and the risks day and night. Instead of settling comfortably into the thought that you had "done everything you could," you had much more left to do.

In reality, though, the hospital was as much a gamble as the home, as S. had learned in the case of K., the young child for whom he had unsuccessfully tried to make a "home" within the hospital. With K. the house officers had lost their "hospital" gamble. Whether S. would have won or lost his "home" gamble he did not know. But he had won enough such gambles since then to choose a similar gamble when he supported Mrs. Gormley in her desire to stay at home to die. Most doctors, like the ones who treated K., would have done otherwise. When he had begun taking care of patients at home, S. had felt uncomfortable about choosing a gamble that many of his colleagues would have regarded as unusual. But now it seemed like the least he could do.

Later that week S. received a phone call from one of the visiting nurses, who reported that Mrs. Gormley complained of considerable pain when she was moved. Because of this the family was not putting her on her bedpan, and she was urinating in bed, which in turn aggravated the bedsore. The nurse asked S. whether she should put a catheter into the patient's bladder, thus solving all these technical problems at one stroke.

S. did not order catheterization just yet. Instead he asked the nurse to work out a solution with the family. They might try to locate more precisely where Mrs. Gormley was feeling pain when she was turned. They might be more firm in reminding her that having to be moved was part of what it meant to stay at home. At the same time, they might explore any feelings they had that they were being cruel in causing their mother pain. Another approach was to increase the pain medication at the times when she needed to be moved. Then again, they could just have the catheter put in, at some risk of infection. But would it be such a bad thing for the old woman to die of an infection when she was about to die of cancer? In any case, S. wanted the choice to be made by the patient and her family rather than by the doctor and the nurse.

Again it was Mrs. Cavanaugh who articulated the family's decision: "No tubes if there's no chance of cure." She reminded her mother—and herself—why it was necessary to undertake the disagreeable task of moving her. After a while she sensed that her mother, even while continuing to object to being moved, still seemed more comfortable after being moved. She felt good at having been able to overcome her own reluctance to cause pain in the interest of sparing her mother what she felt was an unnecessary violation of her natural functions.

As soon as she got up each morning, Mrs. Cavanaugh would go to her mother's room, turn her, and clean the bedsore. After letting her dry off for an hour she changed her clothes. At eight thirty, when a home health aide arrived, Mrs. Cavanaugh went to work. She spent her lunch hour at home assisting the aide, then returned home for good at five when the aide went off duty. At that point it was up to the family. Mrs. Cavanaugh did what she could to get her mother to eat, but if she didn't, well, S. had told them that that might happen. Then the others trooped in for the evening. Mrs. O'Farrell (who, like Mr. and Mrs. Cavanaugh, had a full-time job) was there almost every night. Audrey and some of the other grandchildren came often, while others stayed away, saying it was "spooky." They, along with the ones who did come, were afraid.

The night was left to the Cavanaughs. Mrs. Gormley usually slept well, but if she was restless, her daughter would stay with her. Sometimes Mrs. Cavanaugh would wake up and hear her mother talking incessantly. If she sensed that she was not going to quiet down and become comfortable after a reasonable time, she would give her the pain medication. Mrs. Cavanaugh could go by her instincts about whether her mother needed the medication. It would be harder for a nurse to do that. She could adjust the medication to her mother's needs rather than the need to keep the ward quiet or get things done on schedule or keep harried personnel available for other tasks. As a result Mrs. Gormley needed little medication on the whole. Sometimes she didn't need any from one night to the next. It seemed that just being at home was half the medication.

Her last days contained many conscious moments. Although no one ever knew how much she was aware of as she passed back and forth from wakefulness to sleep to somewhere in between, her eyes always opened to the sight of the bureau, the mirror, the pictures on the wall—the things that had accompanied her through healthier and happier times. Her senses opened to sights, smells, and sounds of many years' familiarity. And into her fragile consciousness came her daughter Jessie, her daughter Jenny, her sons-in-law and grandchildren and even great-grandchildren, kissing her good night and good morning, kissing her hello and good-bye. They all had felt that they could do nothing for her, and yet they did a lot.

While Mrs. Cavanaugh did most of the physical chores, the others in their own ways worked too. It takes energy to move your mother onto a bedpan, and it takes energy to feel sad that she is dying and to extend to her some last kindnesses. People lose time from their own jobs when they take care of sick and dying relatives. This family gave up their leisure time to do something that was emotionally draining, that took as much energy as any job. The Cavanaughs and O'Farrells each, in effect, held down two full-time jobs.

No one would want to be reimbursed for loving someone. But the family could at least have been paid for doing the work of nurses, work for which taxpayers and insurance subscribers otherwise would have been billed. The economic system is not, however, set up to reward such work. People are encouraged to buy a gadget or a pill to help them do something they could just as well have done for themselves. Our economic system takes people's skills, processes them, and sells them back at a premium—just like food.

This family had to rediscover their capacity to do a traditional job. Their neighbors told them that they must be very brave to do what they were doing. Doctors, hospitals, even friends were saying that they couldn't or shouldn't be doing it. They themselves couldn't be sure. No wonder they needed a little encouragement from Dr. S! But they had something else besides his help; they were able to draw on memories of what it had been like to see someone die a generation or two before. Just forty or fifty years ago it had been a normal, routine thing to die or be born at home. Back then they didn't even take the body right out of the house as they did now (as if it would contaminate people), but held the wake at home too. Jessie Cavanaugh remembered how as a child of seven or eight she had seen her grandmother laid out on her bed. Maybe she hadn't fully understood, but she hadn't been scared out of her mind. So now when a friend told her, "If it was my mother, I just couldn't deal with it," she said, "You will when you have to." She began to have the feeling that she and her family weren't just doing it for themselves, but for others as well.

In the beginning what was particularly difficult for everyone was the strange feelings that came up when they were preparing to bathe the old woman, change her clothes, or clean up the mess that she could no longer keep from making. There is no getting around it; urine and feces smell bad. When a baby does it, somehow it's a sweet smell. Incontinence in an old person, on the other hand, turns a lifelong relationship on its head. Now the children and grandchildren were nursing someone who had given them life, taught them strength and competence. From this person they had learned how to live and work. Could they stand to see her fade away? Would they be able to see this once idealized person as flesh and blood and yet also as spirit still; reduced to childlike messing and yet still something more; powerless and yet still powerful? Would reality crowd out memory, or would memory crowd out reality? These unpleasant, scary things are what the sanitized medical apparatus (an unholy alliance of vested interests and people's own fears) shields people from. If the Cavanaughs and O'Farrells were heroes to take on a heavy burden of unpaid work, even more were they heroes to face these fearful things that taught them more than they had known about what a human being is. S. could see his task as supporting such extraordinary, yet everyday heroism.

Norman Cavanaugh had never imagined that he would get so uncomfortably close to his mother-in-law. "How can I do this?" he would think before entering her room. But then he said to himself, "Somebody's got to do it. I'll do it, that's all." Each day things got a little easier. It was amazing, he reflected, what people could do when they had to.

His wife was deeply troubled about violating her mother's privacy. She knew her mother as a modest, shy person "from a different era" who "wouldn't even tell us about the birds and the bees." Now she had to touch her mother in places where she never had before. She had to separate the physical functions of those parts of the body from the myths and fantasies that surrounded them. In touching her mother, she discovered something of what it must have meant to have her mother touch her in the same places a long, long time ago. In her mother's dying she had a glimpse, darkened and transformed, of her own beginnings.

The family also faced their fear of death. At first Jenny O'-Farrell could not get used to the idea that her mother was dying, that she was going to lose her and never see her again. All of the child's fears of being left unfed and unprotected were re-awakened. Yet day by day, as Jenny watched her mother suffer, the fear somehow dissipated. It came to seem right, or at least necessary, that her mother should leave her at this time.

Audrey, who in previous months and previous illnesses had tried to talk her grandmother out of being afraid to die, now just sat by her bedside and talked. It scared her to see her grandmother become less and less able to tell who she was, or who anybody was. So Audrey talked, not so much for her grandmother, who couldn't understand what she was saying, but for herself, because it made her feel better to pretend that her grandmother did understand. And as her grandmother got worse, she felt herself—felt everyone—getting better.

Audrey surprised herself. They all surprised themselves. Mabel Gormley's children and grandchildren "couldn't do anything for her"; but if all they could do was change her diapers, they still were doing something for her. And she still was doing something for them, even as she had long ago when she changed their diapers. She was giving them the courage to find out about themselves. It is said that a sudden death is more merciful than a "lingering" death. But Mrs. Gormley was not lingering. No longer physically or mentally active, she was actively a part of an exchange of strong feelings. As her own strength ebbed away, she was helping to produce strength in her family.

A sudden death may in some respects be more merciful for the person dying. Had she been offered the choice, perhaps Mrs. Gormley would have chosen a quicker death, like the one her son-in-law's mother had. The elder Mrs. Cavanaugh had been ill, but had not been considered near death when she suddenly collapsed one day while she was sitting in the living room talking with the family. The youngest granddaughter, a girl in her teens who only with great reluctance could bring herself to visit Mrs. Gormley as she lay dying, had been very close to her other grandmother. It was as if there hadn't been time to say good-bye.

The first snow of the season was falling on the night when, a few weeks after his first two visits, S. received an urgent call from the family. The patient was agitated, "out of her head," and her daughters felt that things were getting out of control. S. always found it disagreeable to leave his warm apartment once he was settled in for the night. When possible he made his house calls on the way home from the office. He especially dreaded being awakened during the night when he felt least confident about going out into the world to apply his incomplete knowledge. At two in the morning he had to make decisions without aid. Sometimes, though, it could not be helped.

As he drove through the night to the Cavanaugh home, he reminded himself that as a doctor he couldn't just leave the family with a parting word of advice and think his job was done. He remembered when he had prepared this family for the way a dying person might refuse to eat after a certain point. Family members needed to be told that this refusal was part of dying and not a sign of their own inadequacy. But there is no getting away from the frustration that people feel in being unable to do anything in the face of a refusal of food—in the face, that is, of death. S. saw it as part of his job (even if it wasn't taught in medical school or paid for by Blue Shield) simply to *be* with them to help them deal with that frustration. When he first spoke with Mrs. Gormley's family, S. knew that they would call him again and that he would come, even if his knowledge was not always what they needed.

Mrs. Gormley now looked very, very old. "It's okay," S. said to the worried family. "She is on her way out. I don't know exactly when, but it looks like we're getting near the end. This is the way people often are at that stage. Who can say what she's feeling now? It would be nice to be closer to her, but we can't be. She must be very frightened of dying. Who wouldn't be? The delirium is a normal response to that. You can look at it as a way of withdrawing, of blocking out the fright. It's nature's way of keeping people comfortable. Just accept it. Don't fight it. You're doing fine."

At this time he brought out into the open an anxiety that many of them (especially the younger ones) must be feeling. "One of you will discover her in bed dead—cold, blue, lifeless. How will you feel about that? Who would want to be the first to find her?" Along with the near-certainty of Mrs. Gormley's death was the large, looming uncertainty of who would have the responsibility of finding her dead. It was like a wheel of fortune, a game of chance with no skill attached to the gamble. In speaking about this with the family as a whole, S. sought to reduce their anxiety in advance, as well as to encourage a common sense of responsibility by making it clear that this was a gamble that they all shared. Whoever found her dead would not be at fault.

Two days later Mrs. Cavanaugh went to her mother's room and found her blue and breathing very slowly. She was crossing the threshold of death. She was clear-browed and calm, like someone looking forward to the long, long rest that she had earned by all her suffering. To her daughter she looked beautiful. Mrs. Cavanaugh, who had long resisted the idea of her mother dying, felt at ease now. This was the way her mother had wanted it. Somehow this was so much easier to accept than to have had a call from the hospital telling her that her mother had died.

The family members assembled around the old woman's bed. No one of them alone would bear the responsibility of finding her dead; they were assuming that responsibility collectively, as a family. The gathering was like one of the deathbed scenes on which the literature of past generations turned, but are rarely found in our own. Although Mrs. Gormley had no opportunity for final instructions and explicit farewells, each person in turn was able to step up to the bed and kiss her good-bye. Soon her breathing stopped.

After she died, the family called S.'s office as he had instructed them to do. Since S. was not on call that night, it was one of his partners who went out to the home. This was another way in which home care required cooperation. The same doc-

tor couldn't be on call every night—not if he wanted to have a
family of his own.

The doctor pronounced Mrs. Gormley dead, filled out the
death certificate, and stayed with the family until the undertaker came to take the body. "How many doctors would do that
nowadays?" said Mrs. Cavanaugh to her husband and sister.
His presence gave the family a lift, a bit of encouragement
when they needed it.

A few days later S. spoke with the family by telephone. They
all agreed that Mrs. Gormley had "died well." As Mrs. Cavanaugh phrased it, "The whole thing was like a puzzle that fell
into place as she was dying." Still, S. added, she *had* died. They
would all have to live with that.

For S. the last piece in the puzzle was never quite in place.
Even though the patient was dead, the family was still alive. A
doctor who was not concerned with the family would have
considered the job done when the death certificate was signed.
S., whose reaction to Mrs. Cavanaugh's first call had been to
wonder whether her family really even needed him, had to
remind himself that his job was not done. Although Mrs. Gormley was dead, she continued to live in the thoughts and feelings
of her family and continued to influence their lives.

So S. would stay in touch with the family (who by now expected no less). After all, not only Mrs. Gormley, but the whole
family had been his "patients." He had tempered the savage
fantasies that the young children (and their elders) brought to
great-grandma's death with the sad, but far gentler reality. He
had figured out a lot of little ways for everyone, himself included, to say good-bye. Everything he said and did in that
house had an effect (he hoped therapeutic) on the family; but
when he submitted his bill to Medicare, he would not be able
to name the family as the patient.

S. was touched when, a year later, on the anniversary of Mrs.
Gormley's death, he was invited back to the Cavanaugh home
to review the experience with the family. Norman Cavanaugh
spoke for the whole family when he said, "For me this has been
a new part of life that I'm learning about. As I get older I'm
trying to adjust to death myself. It seems it's not as terrible as

I thought it was. It's just another thing that we go through. We're born, we live, and we die." For his wife this new acceptance of death, an acceptance that came from having "seen" it, was only a small consolation for the seeming unfairness of her mother's having had to suffer as she did. Jessie Cavanaugh, it seemed, still had mixed feelings. "Who wouldn't?" said S.

Audrey certainly did. "It was the most important experience of my life," she exclaimed. "Not that I'd want to go through it again with my own mother. This was hard enough to accept as it was."

"It will take a lot of courage," Dr. S. cautioned her, "but you'd be surprised how much courage you have, just as your mother was surprised this time." Later, in the course of a discussion of medical treatment in institutions, Audrey said, "When I watched my mother take care of my grandmother, I pictured myself doing the same for my mother in thirty or forty years. You'd never put *her* in any nursing home!"

Along with everyone else, S. shared his reactions to the experience. "It was very special for me as well. In order to come here I had to open myself up to all my own fears about dying. I also learned something from it as a doctor. You handled things beautifully. What we all learned I can share with other families."

The family expressed concern that it was so hard to find a family doctor. They had a family doctor from years back, but he was too old now to make house calls. "It's a sad situation when you can't get a doctor to come to your house," said Mrs. Cavanaugh. "You can't get an old, sick person to the office, so the only alternative is to put her in the hospital."

S. managed a wry smile. "So doctors, who should be keeping people out of hospitals, sometimes are a cause of people being put *into* hospitals."

"And once they're in," Mrs. O'Farrell volunteered, "it isn't the doctor who takes care of them, but the nurses and aides. So what's the difference if a person stays home? You can have nurses at home too."

S. was made uncomfortable by all the praise that was being directed at him for his extraordinary involvement with this family. He enjoyed basking in their appreciation, of course, but at the same time he felt angry and sad. What a commentary on modern medicine and modern society that the experience of making decisions and exerting control even in the midst of death should be so novel for people. "Why does this have to be something special?" he asked. "This should be the way it always is."

"Absolutely," said Mr. Cavanaugh. "Why should this be such a 'brave' thing to do? It's perfectly normal. I think everybody ought to face something like this. It would be a good experience for anyone."

"Nobody encourages people to do this," S. interjected. "Doctors don't encourage it because they're scared too. They're afraid other doctors will criticize them for doing something risky. Doctors are a little afraid of something they aren't used to doing, just as families are."

He spoke to them again about uncertainty, about which Norman Cavanaugh commented, "The only certain things are death and taxes, and we've made the best deal we could with both." S. reviewed with them the principles that had guided them and the gambles they had chosen together—how they had turned out, and how else (being gambles, after all) they might have turned out. He mentioned also some gambles that they had not chosen—*could* not have chosen, things being as they were. They were not wealthy people who could arrange their schedules to suit their convenience and hire servants to do the "dirty work." They did not live in a community (who did?) where they could choose to have their neighbors come and help care for an elderly person. These things, in all probability, they could not change. But it was good to be reminded every once in a while that the world did not have to be as it was.

There came a moment when deep emotional currents could be felt beneath the surface of the discussion. When they spoke of the decision not to prolong Mrs. Gormley's life by artificial means, Mrs. Cavanaugh was quick to give S. all the credit. "I'll tell you who made that decision, folks," she stated, pointing a finger at the physician. But S. reminded her of their discussions. He wanted it to be remembered as a decision for which they all bore some responsibility.

Other things were said that day that were very satisfying for

S. to hear. When he asked the family how they felt about not being reimbursed by Blue Cross for nursing services, someone said, "That's okay. We got something out of it." Someone else added, "When we remember our mother, we will remember the way she went out of the world and the things we did to help her."

But there were mixed feelings too—probably more than they could easily admit to a doctor. Mrs. O'Farrell gave an inkling of these with this enigmatic utterance: "Sometimes it's harder when you're close to someone. There's more to cope with when you're close."

S. glanced at Audrey and thought of the concluding paragraph of Kafka's *Metamorphosis,* which describes a family that has been released by death:

> Then they all three left the apartment together, which was more than they had done for months, and went by tram into the open country outside the town. The tram, in which they were the only passengers, was filled with warm sunshine. Leaning comfortably back in their seats they canvassed their prospects for the future, and it appeared on closer inspection that these were not at all bad, for the jobs they had got, which so far they had never really discussed with each other, were all three admirable and likely to lead to better things later on. The greatest immediate improvement in their condition would of course arise from moving to another house; they wanted to take a smaller and cheaper but also better situated and more easily run apartment than the one they had, which Gregor (the dead son) had selected. While they were thus conversing, it struck both Mr. and Mrs. Samsa, almost at the same moment, as they became aware of their daughter's increasing vivacity, that in spite of all the sorrow of recent times, which had made her cheeks pale, she had bloomed into a pretty girl with a good figure. They grew quieter and half unconsciously exchanged glances of complete agreement, having come to the conclusion that it would soon be time to find a good husband for her. And it was like a confirmation of their new dreams and excellent intentions that at the end

of their journey their daughter sprang to her feet first and
stretched her young body. (Kafka, 1948, p. 132).

Together with grief there is relief at no longer having the dying
person in the house to attend to. Energy that was drained by
dying can go back into living. The family can acknowledge this
(without being overwhelmed by the shame that such a feeling
can bring) when they have had the dying person in the house
and have known what it took to care for her.

13

BIRTH
IN THE HOME

One of the greatest satisfactions S. had as a family doctor came from being able to experience all stages of life, and with them an extraordinary range of human feelings. Within a single night, for example, he might witness a death and then a birth. Having just left a family stricken with sadness, he might ring another doorbell to find a family at a moment of hope and confidence.

One of the best times for families to learn to gamble consciously and take their destinies in hand was during the months of pregnancy and the intense hours of labor. The positive energy and hope that a family invested in a birth (a momentous event, yet one that the family could prepare for) made it an ideal time to learn a way of thinking that could be applied to other situations in medicine and in life. Birth combined the predictable with the unpredictable, skill with chance. It was a series of gambles over a nine-month period in which changes in strategy, anticipated and unanticipated, might occur at any time. Moreover, the sort of gambling a couple would engage in, especially if this was the birth of their first child, would be the basis upon which the couple could begin to define itself as a family, the husband and wife growing to become also a father

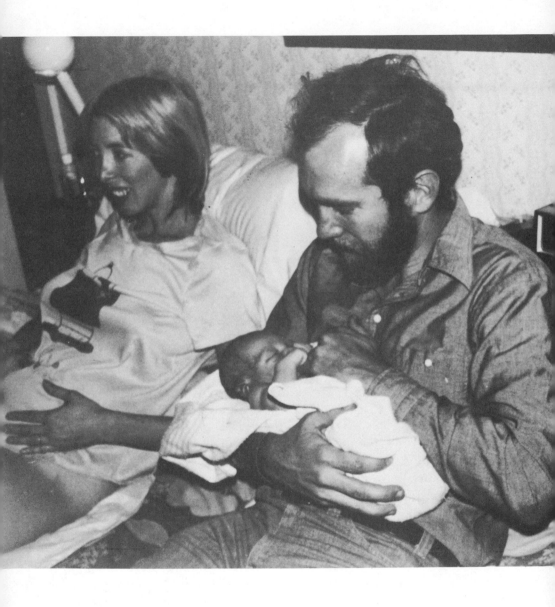

and mother. This was true for any birth, but it seemed most true for a home birth, in which the gamble had an extra dimension. Here none of the participants, least of all S., were likely to forget that they were gambling together.

Initial Visit

S. breezed into his "prenatal" office to meet a couple interested in using his practice for maternity care.

"Hello, I'm Dr. S. Welcome."

"I'm Roberta Johnson and this is my husband, Bob Williams."

"I understand you're pregnant."

"That's right," Roberta replied. "I'm three weeks late with my period, and the pregnancy test I just had here was positive."

"Were you planning a pregnancy at this time?"

Roberta and Bob exchanged glances. Finally Roberta said, "I guess it was a bit of a surprise. "We're getting used to the idea by now, though we've had our ups and downs about it."

Before S. had a chance to explore these feelings further, Roberta quickly added, "We came here because we'd like to talk to you about a home birth. We understand that your practice is one of the few that do home births."

"Yes, we're open to the idea of home birth. What makes you want to have one?"

"Several things. First of all I just don't like hospitals. I find them very unpleasant places. I've had some really bad experiences with sick relatives in hospitals. To be perfectly truthful with you, doctors are not my favorite people. Also, hospitals are for sick people, and I don't consider pregnancy to be a sickness. Sure, I know that things can go wrong and a hospital might be necessary, but I'd like to cross that bridge when I come to it. The other thing that scares me about hospitals is that they do things to you—like using a monitor, IV, and episiotomy. I think that when you're at home you can avoid those kinds of things. Also, you can have all your familiar things around. You can have your friends and family there. It's your own place—you know what I mean?"

"Are you familiar with the changes that hospitals have made in their maternity services to make them less 'hospitallike'?"

"The birthing rooms? I've heard about them, and I guess they're a step in the right direction, but still I'd like to try a home birth if it's possible. Even though this is our first child, I've done some talking and reading, and at this point I think that I want to be at home. We'd like to hear your views."

"Okay. A home birth is fine if your medical history, physical examination, and pregnancy course don't show significant risk of any problem that would be hard to handle at home. Also, you have to be willing to accept the risk that is there. You need to know that even though everything looks okay going into labor, you could die and your baby could die—that's the ultimate kind of risk that I mean. Now, let me soften that a little. Having a baby anywhere carries a risk of death—a small risk in these times, to be sure, but there nonetheless. The hospital has its kind of risk and the home its kind. I'm not saying the home is less safe than the hospital for the low-risk mother. There's no evidence I know of to support that claim. But you must understand that a situation could conceivably arise in the home where your having been in the hospital instead would have made the difference between life and death. It may be only one in a thousand or more, but if you're the one, it's a hundred percent for you."

"I know there is risk, but I don't think I'll be the one," Roberta interjected.

"It would be nice if the things we don't want to happen to us wouldn't happen to us, but we can't count on it. No matter how skillful I am or how well prepared you are—that is, assuming neither of us makes a human error—there is a tiny but real chance beyond our control that there will be a tragedy. You've got to face that just as I've got to. I put it to you straight because I'm not here selling home births or, for that matter, hospital births. I appreciate the benefits of home births—I've learned to appreciate them because they've been important to quite a few families I've worked with—but I'm not ideologically committed to them. We have wonderful home-like births in the hospital, too. My concern is that you have a good birth experience, wherever you have it." He paused, and they all shifted a little in their seats.

It was S.'s practice to bring up the subject of death early on with couples choosing home birth, but not with those choosing hospital birth, even though the risk of a tragedy, as far as he could tell, was no greater in the one setting than in the other. While the home might not be more likely to be a cause of death than the hospital, it was a different cause. Having a baby die at home would heighten a couple's sense of personal responsibility for the tragedy and could make it harder to live with. It was easier to be angry at the hospital than at oneself.

Bob broke the pause. "One of the reasons we've come to you is that we'd like to have maximum control over the pregnancy and delivery. We understand, correct me if I'm wrong, that you involve patients actively in decisions affecting them."

"That's quite correct—with, however, one 'but,' which is that sometimes in labor things can happen so quickly and so unexpectedly that there simply isn't time to talk. You've got to move and move quickly. That's where trust—in both directions—comes in. So during labor I'll have to take a more active role."

"I can understand that," Bob responded.

"Let me get back to home birth for a moment," said S. "The determination of risk is ongoing. We look at the choice of home versus hospital all the way along during the pregnancy—right into labor and beyond. If the odds change for the worse and technical maneuvers available only in the hospital can lower the overall risk, then we'll have to shift to the hospital. Just as we have to accept some risk in the hospital, so we have to accept some risk at home. The question is, when does the risk at home become unacceptable? We have a printed policy—you'll get a copy—which spells out what we think are unacceptable risks. For example, aside from risk factors such as age and complications of prior pregnancies (which wouldn't apply to you), an unacceptable risk could come from an illness such as diabetes or high blood pressure, or from a complication such as prematurity or lack of progress in labor. Our policy also states that you have to be within twenty minutes of one of our backup hospitals, and that you have to have certain supplies ready in your home for the birth. You'll need to take childbirth education classes as well, so that you'll know what you're doing by the time you go into labor. We won't deviate from our policy unless you come up with some good reasons why we should. And after you go into labor, I don't find it so easy to accept 'good' reasons."

"You make it sound so technical; it sounds like you have as many rules as the hospital," Roberta replied.

"It may sound that way at first, but what we're interested in is coming to an agreement, rather than your obeying a rule. Read the policy over and let me know any special conditions in your case that might justify our having a different understanding from what is spelled out here. The more we can anticipate what may be special about your labor, the more we can come to an agreement ahead of time about when to move to the hospital if that becomes necessary. That way I won't have to make the decision myself during labor." He paused. "Basically you have the freedom to have the kind of birth you want. It is your birth, after all."

Roberta's expression changed. "If anything happened to my baby, I'd never forgive myself."

"Never is a long time. Anyway, responsibility is a tricky thing. You are responsible for your choices, but things still happen which are beyond your control. Even when you *can* blame yourself, that doesn't mean you don't ever forgive yourself." For a moment they were all silent. "Well, this has been a hard discussion, but a necessary one; the odds are that you'll do fine with a home birth. By the way, I never did get around to asking you what kind of work you do."

"I'm an urban designer," Roberta replied.

"And I'm a computer programmer."

S. noted their occupations in the record. "Any questions?"

"We'll save them for the next visit." They looked at each other. "We're pretty well agreed that we want to come to this practice."

"Let's set up a visit soon so we can do a physical exam and go into your medical history. Let me walk out to the front desk with you and make sure you get all the literature, our policies and fees, and the phone number of the birth attendant, Paula. Be sure to get in touch with her. She'll be working with us right along."

Physical Examination

S.'s prenatal room was more like a classroom than a doctor's office. There were diagrams on the wall showing the anatomical structure of the female pelvis and changes in the uterus over the course of pregnancy. S. referred to them as he did the physical examination. On the ceiling over the brown wooden examination table was a humorous poster showing how to build a rainbow. Women found that it took the edge off a sometimes awkward situation and, rather than being distracting, allowed them to focus on what they and the doctor were doing. S.'s office was in many ways nonstandard. It reflected the suggestions of his women patients and colleagues. Stirrups were "optional," and there had never been any takers.

"I've always disliked this part of the examination," Roberta muttered as she placed her feet at the corners of the table and shimmied her buttocks down to the edge.

"What's it been like for you?" queried S.

"I don't know. I feel so exposed. I'm a little embarrassed, I guess."

"Who wouldn't be?" S. replied. "When I started doing pelvic examinations, I was embarrassed too. Let's talk a little about the exam before we begin. I need you to participate in this pelvic examination. It's not something I can do alone. Before we get to the rectal exam, I'll feel your uterus and ovaries. Now, these organs can't be touched directly. All an examiner can do is get a sense of what's between his or her hands, the one pressing up from below in the vagina, the other pushing down from above on the lower abdomen." S. brought his hands together by way of illustration. "By your relaxing, you allow the examining fingers to come closer together to feel what's in between."

Roberta nodded.

After checking the tone of Roberta's perineal muscles and commenting on the importance of toning exercises, S. visualized her cervix with a lighted speculum. With a mirror Roberta could see it too. She propped herself on one elbow and with her other hand brought the mirror down to her buttocks. "Well, what do you know," she said with a look of surprise on her face. "It's so small. How will the baby ever get out? Bob, come on over here and take a look."

After they had finished looking, S. withdrew the speculum. "Now let's check the measurements of the birth canal. I'll feel for the landmarks I pointed out to you on the wall charts. As I do, I'll tell you what I'm doing." Following this part of the exam, S. was able to say, "Feels like a roomy pelvis. Good."

Next S. positioned his hands for the bimanual examination. He could feel Roberta tense up.

"Now what I want you to do is to 'let go' of the tension in your muscles, and I'll let you know if I can tell the difference. Now let go. Good. Now, let go some more. Great. I can feel most of your uterus except on the right. Yes, that's the muscle to relax. Fine. Feels almost six to eight weeks size. Now your right ovary —good. And the left—good. Now the rectal exam." "Ugh." Roberta winced.

"All done." The bimanual and rectal exam had taken sixty seconds. S. withdrew his hands. "Why don't you get dressed; I'll be right back," S. said as he left the room. When S. returned, Roberta was dressed and seated. It was easier now for them to speak as equals.

"You were very helpful," S. said.

"So were you," she replied.

"How did you feel about the exam? Was it comfortable for you?"

"Okay, I guess. Better than usual. As I mentioned, it was a little embarrassing, though after I spoke up, I felt more at ease. Pelvic exams have always been uncomfortable for me since I first had them. I guess I still tense up, even now."

"You didn't say anything about pain today. Does that mean that there wasn't any?"

"Well, for the most part."

"You mean there were parts that were painful that you didn't tell me about?"

"Well, yes."

"What stopped you from speaking up?"

"Oh, I don't know. I guess it's awkward for me to tell a doctor what to do."

"I see. Look, if you don't tell me, how can I know? The easiest way for me to know what you're feeling is for you to tell me."

"I'll keep that in mind. Okay, tell me, did I relax enough for you to do a thorough exam?"

"Yes, it was a good exam. You should have no problem with a vaginal birth. Of course, you can't be sure till you're in labor, but for now everything looks okay. Speaking of labor, the pelvic exam reminds me of labor in this sense: as the baby moves down the birth canal and begins to stretch out the perineum, one of the ways to help ease the baby out is to let yourself open up, as you did during the pelvic exam. Also, when the head emerges or, as we say, 'crowns,' we let the perineum stretch out ever so gradually—to prevent tears and minimize the need for an episiotomy. We'll tell you to 'push,' or to 'pant' so you won't push. In other words, we'll let you know how your perineum is responding. Just like today when I let you know when you were relaxed, or weren't."

S. turned to Bob. "What do you think of all this?" he asked him.

"Sounds good to me. It was interesting to see Roberta's cervix and hear about toning up the pelvic muscles." He grinned. "Of course, I can't tell you how the exam felt. I've always thought that Roberta was some kind of sissy with her fear of going to the dentist or gynecologist. I guess her antsiness today is part of the same thing."

"You've not been exactly sympathetic?"

"No, not exactly," Bob replied. Roberta nodded her agreement.

S. noticed that Bob was still grinning. He guessed that Bob, too, had been embarrassed. A form of sympathy, he mused. "Well," he said, "it might be good to review with each other what went on here today. One thing among many that you can learn about during a pregnancy is how you respond to each other's feelings."

Roberta changed the subject. "We'll be seeing Paula, the birth attendant, today right after we're through. I've kept a three-day record of my diet, and I want to go over it with her."

"As far as general precautions are concerned," said S., "nutrition you've already taken care of. Smoking is a risk to the baby —smaller size and greater chance of respiratory infections after birth. Alcohol can harm the fetus. I'd stay away from alcohol and other drugs, including over-the-counter medicines, especially during the first trimester (the first three months of pregnancy). Also, be sure to use a seat belt when you're in a car. As your uterus grows bigger, use just the lap belt under your uterus and around your hips down low. Everyone else in the car should buckle up, too, because if you're in a crash nonrestrained passengers can fly into you. All of these things will help you exert some control over the outcome of the pregnancy. You can't completely prevent problems in pregnancy, but you can avoid some risks. Even though, together, these measures might make only a few percentage points' difference in rates of complication, each point counts."

After Bob and Roberta left, S. reflected on his parting words. Here was a place, he realized, where he advised families to gamble so as to avoid an extreme outcome. A pregnant woman who was used to smoking or drinking would be more or less uncomfortable if she stopped. S. thought it "right" for her to accept the high probability of such moderate discomfort in order to avoid even a low probability of serious harm to the baby. This was the same argument that other doctors gave for accepting the moderate discomfort of giving birth in the hospital instead of at home, and yet he did not agree with them. Some families placed a high value on the comfort and integrity of their home life; some families placed a high value on the pleasures of smoking and drinking. He was inclined to honor the one set of values, but not the other. At the same time, he would not attend home births in cases where he thought it unsafe to give birth at home, and yet he would attend births where the mother-to-be had disregarded his warnings against smoking or drinking heavily.

Although he was not entirely comfortable with these inconsistencies, he realized that different gambles were appropriate in different contexts. Besides, he was not about to pretend (to families or to himself) that he did not have values.

In asserting his values, however, he did not want people to conceal from him the way they lived or to avoid coming back to him out of a fear of "failing" and disappointing him. Though he worked out agreements with patients by which they would stop smoking or lose weight or take pills for hypertension, he wasn't about to stop being someone's doctor because he or she failed to live up to such an agreement. His commitment to the patient as a person went beyond his commitment to a way of treating a particular disease. Nonetheless, S. felt his open-mindedness strained to the limit when someone was careless with the life and health of an unborn child. That, to him, was an unprincipled gamble.

S. also sought to have the father share in the increased concern for safety and health that made itself felt during pregnancy. It was another way in which a family learned to share the gamble rather than gamble against each other. What might start as an agreement by the father to share the inconvenience of wearing seat belts or giving up smoking out of fairness to his wife might become a real commitment to better living habits on his part, which would benefit the entire family. These were the kinds of choices that changed individuals into family members.

A Principled Gamble

If a concern for his professional reputation was only a thought that crossed S.'s mind when he cared for a dying patient at home, it was an ever-present preoccupation when he attended a home birth. Here he was clearly flying in the face of accepted obstetrical practice. Talk about gambles, he might even be risking his livelihood. S. hadn't entered this professional lion's den without very careful thought and evaluation of the evidence. It was barely a generation since birth, seemingly once and for all, had moved from what was considered the unsafe setting of the home to the scientific security of the hospital. In the 1930's and 1940's there were good reasons for preferring the hospital. But conditions change, causal relationships change, the odds change. Now it was possible for the low-risk mother to have sanitary conditions, adequate monitoring of fetal health, and prompt initial care of emergencies outside the hospital. S. believed it to be a gamble worth taking, but he was willing to change his choice of gambles, just as he had done once before when he started doing home births. He had chosen that gamble on the basis of new information, and he would need further information to reevaluate it. So he was documenting each home birth and subjecting his overall experience with home birth to both internal and external critical review. Even as the home birth service that he and his partners provided was becoming better established, he did not let himself forget that it was still a pilot project. Although he did not think it likely that on the basis of the evidence they would decide to discontinue the project, he was not about to close his eyes or his mind.

He had carefully examined the evidence drawn from studies done in many countries on the safety of out-of-hospital births. The findings pointed to the same conclusion—either no differences or the home had better outcomes for low-risk patients. This was true in Holland with its fifty percent of births in the home compared with Sweden with its one hundred percent in hospital, in England before births shifted sharply from home to hospital in the 1960's, or in the United States in the 1970's where in one study more than one thousand births at home were compared with a matched comparison group in the hospital (Kitzinger and Davis, 1978). It was true in a 1979 report by the Maternity Center Association of New York City of its three-year experience working in an Upper East Side town house birthing center staffed by midwives (Faison *et al.,* 1979). Not only were the center's births safe, they were only one third as expensive as hospital births during a time when soaring health-care costs became an object of national concern. (Despite these data the center, which housed all of two birthing suites, was bitterly opposed by the obstetrical community in New York.) Although the existing studies left something to be desired, S. thought it a good bet that no strong link between site of birth and safety would be found.

To be sure, the standard of safety set in the best of today's hospitals was impressive. In university hospitals such as the ones S. worked in, the neonatal death rate for babies born after at least a thirty-seven-week gestation and without congenital abnormalities was calculated to be 4 per 1000 (Neutra *et al.,* 1978). Whether that figure could be equaled or improved in the home was hard to tell, especially when the data could not be viewed out of its social context. It was one thing to do home births in Holland where the entire health-care system (including the emergency transfer apparatus) was supportive; it was another thing to develop a service in an American city where the congested traffic could not always make way for ambulances, and where most obstetricians could barely restrain their hostility toward home delivery. For the comparison between home and hospital to be fair, resources comparable to those lavished on the hospital setting would have to be invested in perfecting the home birth support system, including transfer to hospital.

S. could envision, for example, a modern version of the famous flying squads of England, where mobile vans were equipped with the trained personnel and equipment necessary to give anesthesia and perform emergency surgery. Expensive? In itself, yes, but it would very likely cost less to provide mobile backup for home births than to have everyone give birth in the hospital. As long as society did not appreciate the potential savings, however, home birth would not be fully supported. S. was left having to be more tentative than he otherwise would have been in his advocacy of home birth for his place and time. His own work as a home birth practitioner—with its close attention to safety, its excellent outcome record, and the appreciation it brought from families—was the best advocacy he could offer.

It was not only his own work, he reflected. He would not have been able to attend home births at all had it not been for the open-mindedness of some established obstetricians who made their hospital services available to him even though they had reservations about home birth. And couples like Bob and Roberta, by choosing home birth at a time when it was not yet fully accepted, were taking a gamble on principle, one that would benefit other families in the future as well as themselves.

Families like Bob and Roberta typically took an interest in the social, economic, and political implications of the controversy over site of birth. As their relationship with S. progressed and they became more comfortable with one another, and as the uncertainty that surrounded their own upcoming birth gave way to a shared understanding of probabilities, they could discuss the broader picture. There were, for example, the implications for hospitals and obstetricians if out-of-hospital birth were to become a widespread movement. In one sense there were significant cost reductions to be realized. But at whose expense? So long as the profit motive lurked unacknowledged in the background, rational debate—let alone critical choice—would be difficult.

Electronic fetal monitoring was a case in point. Monitors produced a continuous tracing of uterine contractions and fetal heart rate, allowing for early detection of signs of distress in the fetus. In just a few years the use of monitors had become almost standard obstetrical practice. Although fetal monitors were being used almost as routinely as anesthetics or infant bottled formulas had been in the past (it was the "lunatic fringe" of the preceding generation of women who had begun the now well-established return to breast-feeding), they had not been demonstrated to make a significant difference in the care of the low-risk labor (Neutra *et al.,* 1978). (About high-risk labors there was little question.)

This evidence notwithstanding, an unacknowledged, profitable, and (in our society) almost inevitable alliance between well-motivated, dedicated academic obstetricians and manufacturers of fetal monitors had, it seemed to S., almost prejudiced the outcome of the debate before it could get off the ground. Many obstetricians claimed that there was no such thing as a low-risk labor and feared not to use monitors lest a malpractice suit for a misadventure be based on this omission. Of course, monitors were not available in homes, further casting doubt (for those who saw things that way) on the wisdom of out-of-hospital births.

S. and his partners were the first family doctors in the city to be interested in maternity care in recent years. At the same time, midwifery had again been legalized in the state (although not for home births). The family doctors and midwives, together with the families they served, were reclaiming an area of medicine that had long been exclusively controlled by obstetricians. In calling upon the obstetrician for consultation and support rather than for direct care of the low-risk pregnancy, the new practitioners were, to be sure, carving out for themselves a slice of the economic pie. But they and the families also were creating a new philosophy of birth, one which held that birth was not a medical problem, although medical problems could occur along the way. This critique of established practices had already helped bring about changes in hospital birth procedures, such as the use of birthing rooms.

The out-of-hospital birth movement was one expression of a revolt against professional dominance. By working with families like Bob and Roberta, S. was aligning himself with an important shift in public values. In so doing he was more than willing to give up some measure of control and play by mutually produced rules. Whose birth was it, anyway—the family's or the doctor's? S. had to catch himself whenever he lapsed into the jargon of his medical-school days when he, the doctor, "delivered" babies. To be accurate, he now said that he "attended" births. He was quite clear that mothers were the ones who delivered babies. The difference in words was not incidental. It reflected a different understanding of birth and a different way of arriving at decisions.

Some of the new experience S. was acquiring was painful, as much because of peer disapproval as because of his own failures and the accidents of nature. If things fell apart in the hospital, the doctor was largely cushioned against criticism by the safe institutional setting. But if a serious problem occurred at home, everyone would say, "I told you so." He remembered how awkward he had felt when he had to bring in Margaret

Benson (Chapter 10) for suturing an extensive perineal laceration (something that at times is unavoidable in home or hospital). He could read the disapproval on the faces of the doctors
and nurses he called upon to help him. So far he had had only
one death—a stillborn who had died during a very short labor
before he and the birth attendant had arrived. This death undoubtedly would have occurred even if the mother had planned
a hospital delivery. That may have been the "one in a thousand." Although stillbirths occur in hospitals too, in the home
he had to call in the medical examiner to investigate. It was not
only a sad but also an anxious moment. S. felt as if he were on
trial and feared that a complaint might be raised. But the examiner found that it had been an unavoidable death.

S. had to guard against the extremes of disabling fear and
complacency. He rehearsed emergency procedures while keeping the rarity of emergencies in perspective. Yet he knew that
he could not stand apart from his environment in the manner
of a detached scientist coolly manipulating experimental variables. Like it or not, he lived in a climate of opposition which
affected his emotions and in turn his actions. What others
thought of his choice of gambles affected his self-esteem; it
might also affect his ability to think clearly. He was concerned,
for example, that, to avoid disrupting a rich family experience
and exposing himself to criticism in the hospital, he might
deny to himself that there was a real need to transfer someone
for whom it was no longer safe to be at home. Because he was
aware of these potential "experimenter effects," he established
principles to guide the choices he had to make under pressure.
For example, he and the birth attendants agreed to observe
each other closely and voice disagreements openly. By trusting
each other enough to subject their uncertain perceptions to
each other's scrutiny, they sought to be worthy of the trust
families placed in them.

For S. the risk of failure and the excitement of achievement
that characterized medical practice were two sides of the same
coin. He enjoyed the emotions of birth, wherever it took place:
the pain, fear, laughter, joy, relaxation, closeness—the sense of
drama and triumph. Still, there was something special about a
home birth. Even though the home did not contain all the life-

saving technology of the modern hospital, there was nonetheless a kind of security there, along with a warmth that the hospital could not match. (The traditional image of distant flickering lights across a field from an isolated farmhouse on a cold winter night came to mind. Maybe that's how it felt as he arrived.) Perhaps the relaxed atmosphere—the friends and relatives (including children), the familiar surroundings and food, the quiet lights, the sense of celebration, played an important part in supporting the laboring mother. She didn't have to go anywhere; she just stayed put. Where was she more at home than in her own home? The trappings of the home were collectively a cause, one among many, in a successful outcome. They were not the only cause, though, as those who left things to chance in an unattended home birth appeared to think. These families, in S.'s view, were engaging in the same kind of unicausal thinking as those who regarded the hospital as the sole cause of a good outcome.

S.'s role as a doctor, too, was only one factor among many. He was a cause, but the kind of cause he was varied from one home to the next. Sometimes the most important thing he did was to contribute to the family's peace of mind. He sometimes transformed a tense scene into a confident one simply by reassuring a couple that all was well with baby and mother, even though it might not feel that way at the moment. The reality of it was often changed merely by his observing and being there, which enabled all concerned to feel that if the crunch came (and at rare times it would), he would be there to do what needed to, and could, be done.

Pregnancy and birth provided an exciting opportunity for S. and a family to work together probabilistically. Every case represented a unique and ever-changing combination of causal factors. No two labors were exactly alike, physically or emotionally, and no two families responded to the stresses and strains in exactly the same way. Every family had its own values, its own way of supporting the laboring woman through her pain, its own way of expressing and discharging tension. For some the home would be a source of anxiety, for others a source of comfort. When did a woman really need hospitalization? When did a labor become "prolonged"? At what point in the vast range of variation did the "normal" become "abnormal"? These questions called for highly sensitive, individualized judgments. They were questions of value and questions of probability. S. could estimate the probabilities only by drawing upon his and others' past experience in attending births, his experience with a particular family, and the family members' experience with one another.

Life would be a lot simpler if he could ignore the changing pattern of causation over the course of pregnancy and birth, ignore the effects of his procedures on what he observed, ignore the effects of the woman's and the family's feelings (not to mention his own) on the outcome. Wouldn't it be nice if he could have one answer for everybody! Given that he was concerned with value (avoiding serious complications), he originally had found it hard to be concerned as well with probability (how likely such complications were to occur). He was trained to be oriented toward extreme outcomes—the tragic death, the dramatic rescue. And indeed, the hospital was a good place to be if an extreme outcome was at all likely. On the other hand, it was good to be at home if all was expected to go well.

Whenever he became too preoccupied with avoiding maximum loss, he thought back to the well-meaning physicians who had scheduled exhaustive diagnostic tests day in and day out for the starving child K.—or for elderly patients, some with incurable illnesses, who needed rest more than anything. Beneath this dueling with the specter of maximum loss lay the fear of death. Though it was the patient's death that was in the forefront of a doctor's mind, lurking in the background was a concern with his own.

Just as he could not give everyone the same answer, so he could not tell anyone that the same answer was right from beginning to end, even over a nine-month pregnancy. For S. the beauty and the difficulty of childbirth lay in its being a developing, unfolding event. A woman's body was undergoing progressive physiological modifications. A child in the womb was growing, ever more noticeably, to the point where it came to dominate the feelings, thoughts, and actions of everyone in the family. To this new presence the family's life was continually adjusting itself. How could one be sure that the answer that seemed right at the beginning of this process would still seem right at the end?

Roberta and Bob came to Dr. S. in October. The due date for their baby was estimated to be June 15. In the eight months that intervened any number of complications could occur, along with the normal, but never quite predictable evolution of parental feelings in the mother- and father-to-be. The gamble would be constantly changing, right from the initial meeting, history-taking, and physical examination. S. would be on the lookout, as Roberta and Bob would be, for any changes that might tip the balance in favor of the hospital gamble as against the home gamble. There were some cases where the initial gamble was to choose a hospital birth, but that gamble was changed to a home birth as the pregnancy progressed. Still, he was much more on the lookout for events that would change a planned home birth to a hospital birth than vice versa. He hoped that, as experience with home birth grew, this would not have to be the case.

Nausea

The leaves had stopped falling when Roberta, ten weeks pregnant, came to Dr. S. in despair. "I'll tell you, this morning sickness has just about done me in. I spend about four hours each day absolutely miserable—retching and sick to my stomach. Paula said to take some pilot crackers while I'm still in bed in the morning and then to eat frequent small meals, but nothing helps. I have never felt so awful in my life. When will it end? It makes me wonder whether it's all worth it."

"Well, I'm sure you already know that nausea is a common, possibly even normal part of early pregnancy. It doesn't harm the baby; nor does your temporarily eating less affect the baby's growth. It's related to hormonal changes and rarely lasts more than three months, usually less. I know that three months or even one day is too much, feeling the way you feel. The point is that it does end. When the things you've tried don't work, some women choose medication. According to the best evidence we now have, the medicine we prescribe has not been found to be harmful to babies, and often provides relief. Nevertheless, lots of women stay away from it unless forced to the wall, because they fear harming the baby."

S. thought it extremely important to be attentive to what were called the "routine" or "common" problems of pregnancy. Engaging with Roberta on the common, everyday issues was a way of developing trust for the big issues that lay ahead. There was nothing routine about this nausea to Roberta, just as there was nothing routine about Mrs. Gormley's death to her family. S. had to guard against automatic responses. If he was really listening to Roberta, he would know it by feeling closer to her by the end of the interview. On the other hand, the fact that dealing with morning sickness *was* routine to him enabled him to give her some perspective on her suffering.

"It must be hard to be so uncomfortable physically when you've had mixed feelings about this pregnancy in the first place. Do you want to talk about those feelings?" he asked her.

"Yes," she replied. "They have been on my mind." Roberta then confided to S. her worries about holding onto her job after the baby's birth, her concerns about the changes in her relationship with Bob, and her fears about the pain and discomfort of childbirth.

"Just now you're really feeling the costs of having a child. I don't blame you for wondering whether it's all worth it. Your nausea has brought these normal worries to the surface. I wouldn't blame you if you changed your mind altogether. But you should ask yourself whether morning sickness is a good reason for changing your mind. I mean, to take an extreme example, you could get rid of the pain from a tooth extraction by killing yourself. Or—and this is something you'll be facing soon—you could yell for pain medication (which we don't give at home) at the first twinge of discomfort in labor. If you can get through this morning sickness, you'll be better prepared to face that crisis when it comes. You want to be careful not to

relinquish your power to make important long-range decisions
with and for your family (including this unborn child) by trying to make those decisions when you're in pain."

"You mean it won't be peaches and cream from here on in?"
she replied with a sad smile. "I guess I will be giving up some
things to have this child."

As often happened in S.'s experience as a family doctor, a
medical symptom had revealed a deeper problem, in this case
an unresolved issue in the family. Why did it have to take a
symptom—physical discomfort—to get people to talk about
something so natural, so understandable, so *permissible* (if
permission were his to give) as mixed feelings about an event
that would irrevocably alter their lives? He marveled that so
many couples had to be with a doctor to air their mixed feelings, even to each other.

Being a family had gotten so complicated. It used to be that
people just had children automatically, whatever anxiety they
felt about it—and wasn't there always some anxiety? Now there
was often doubt as well. These days it was accepted that a man
and woman might question whether they wanted to have a
child, but often they weren't equipped by experience to ask
each other that question and answer it together. Often they
acted not as a family but as competing individuals, with the
child as a new competitor that the mother had to "cut in" to the
game by depleting her own reserves. Some birth techniques
seemed to emphasize the baby's comfort at the expense of the
mother's, while some feminists contended that the mother's
well-being was of primary concern.

How could a family get beyond such an either-or situation,
a zero-sum game where one player lost when another won,
and the doctor (or lawyer) was always there to take his cut? S.
remembered the "cones in the bottle" game, where if the
players competed with one another, no one ended up ahead;
instead, the cones all got stuck at the neck of the bottle. He
resolved to stress the principles of cooperation and fairness as
issues for families. The sharing of risk was a principle which
needed to be observed within a family if the family was to
gamble wisely.

The Rubicon Crossed

For eight weeks during the winter Bob and Roberta attended childbirth education classes, where they supported and were supported by couples at different stages of pregnancy. At the same time they continued their regular prenatal visits to Dr. S.'s office. S. kept an eye out for anything that might indicate possible complications, such as protein in the urine or high blood pressure or blood sugar. He also was attentive to the couple's changing attitudes. He knew from experience that a couple that came in one week expressing doubts and fears about a home delivery might come in the next week saying, "This home birth idea is the greatest thing!" S. cautioned them against such denial of doubt. "Keep an open mind," he would tell them. He wanted them always to remember that they were a little afraid, so that they might not ever be too afraid.

Similarly, they needed to be aware of their responsibility without being awed by it. More than one agitated parent-to-be had alternated between wanting to lock the doctor out of the house and passing the whole thing off with false assurance: "Don't worry, honey. Dr. S. will take care of it all." Whenever S. heard the words (or the sentiment), "You take care of it, Doc," he was quick to disclaim such sweeping responsibility and power. Both he and the family needed to be aware that the responsibility was shared.

These mixed and shifting feelings often were tied up with doubts about the pregnancy and about the couple's future as a family. When Roberta and Bob came in for a prenatal visit on the Ides of March, which marked the end of the sixth month of pregnancy, it appeared as if all doubts had been resolved. Roberta looked relaxed, pleased, and perfectly healthy.

"How do you feel?" S. asked her.

"Great. It's funny now to think about the time I was almost ready to give up on this pregnancy."

"Well, I guess by now you've crossed the Rubicon," said S. He wanted to give the couple a chance to articulate whatever mixed feelings might remain.

Roberta laughed. "Oh, yes. We haven't been thinking along

those lines for a while now. At this point I guess we're as clear as we'll ever be that we want this child. Pregnancy, childbirth, and beginning a family have brought to the surface all kinds of feelings for me. All of a sudden I'm going from being my mother's daughter to being a mother myself. I've learned a great deal about myself and my own family too. Not all the things are pretty. But I am learning to live with these mixed feelings."

Bob smiled. "And I'm learning to live with Roberta living with mixed feelings. Until this pregnancy I always expected her to be Ms. Joy and Comfort. But when we found out that she was pregnant, other feelings came up for her, feelings of anger and sadness. She trusted me to bear with her while she expressed those feelings. That gave me courage to express some of my own. All this has been tough, but it has drawn us closer."

The Hospital Visited

Roberta waddled and Bob walked into the room. By now she was thirty-two weeks along. S. reviewed her record. Her blood pressure and weight gain were normal and there was no protein or sugar in her urine. The measured size of the uterus was "right on target."

"Well, your exam looks good; how was your visit to the hospital?"

Bob replied, "The birthing room was quite nice, much nicer than I had expected."

"But it's still a hospital; there's no getting away from it," added Roberta.

"When you need the hospital," said S., "there's nothing like it. In fact, I wouldn't be willing to attend births at home (since there are alternatives available) without a well-equipped hospital twenty minutes away to back me up. The hospital obstetricians bend over backwards to involve me and the family in decisions requiring our participation, like whether or not to do a cesarean section. There is far less of this 'play by the rules or else' than at some other hospitals I could tell you about. Given the fact that the hospital staff—both nurses and doctors—are strangers to the families we work with, I am impressed with how accommodating they are."

"I'm glad to hear that," Bob replied. "I think you're right. It is comforting to know they're there. It almost feels as though we're getting something for nothing. After all, we won't actually be paying the hospital to serve as a backup unless something goes wrong and we wind up there. So we get our peace of mind for free."

"On the other hand, by choosing a home birth, you are cutting the costs of care, yet have no incentive to do so."

"You mean, for example, our insurance won't pay for the birth attendant."

"Right, even though you will be saving your insurance company and its subscribers well over a thousand dollars."

"It's a crazy system, isn't it?" Roberta reflected.

"Unless you're in it for the money," quipped S.

To which Bob reacted, "I guess gambles that are best for profit are not always best for people."

"Anyway," said Roberta, "we're willing to consider the hospital if things go wrong. You know, if the odds change. It's easier to think about the uncertainty now that we're sure that we want the baby after all."

S. smiled. "I'm feeling increasingly comfortable working with you. See you in two weeks."

Coming to an Agreement

Through the spring, as new green leaves replaced those that had fallen during the difficult early months of Roberta's pregnancy, the prenatal visits focused increasingly on the delivery. Whereas S. usually preferred to wait until patients brought up difficult topics, the time was now growing short. Since one of the tasks that remained was to prepare the couple further for getting through labor without anesthesia or pain medication, at the thirty-four-week visit S. said, "You know labor is going to be painful."

Roberta responded, "Yes, we've gone over that in our childbirth classes. I've talked with a number of women about labor pains, and it's the kind of thing that's hard to imagine until you're actually having it. I know that I can use the breathing that we've learned, the massage, and all that."

"It would be nice if study would make it painless," S. sighed.

"But suppose I need something too. Do you bring pain medicine with you, just in case?"

"No, we don't use pain medicine at home. I know you've been over this in your classes, but let's go over it again. First of all, many of the reasons drugs would be necessary would also require care in the hospital anyway. But more important is the fact that drugs, even when they are carefully and critically used, as they are now in most hospitals, can depress the vital functions in you and your baby. So, even though the additional risk is slight, we don't feel it is a risk that we want to take at home. In the hospital it may be a different gamble, since the kinds of problems that drugs can create can generally be handled by the equipment and expertise available there."

"You mean that if I want to keep my options open I have to go to the hospital?"

"Yes. It's like with many other choices: take one turn on the road, and you can't take the other. You will have some choices at home that you wouldn't have in the hospital, but pain medication isn't one of them."

"But can't we just play it by ear and see how bad the pain is going to be?"

"Well, you know how I feel about keeping an open mind. But there are times when you have to commit yourself to a gamble ahead of time and stick to it on principle. I think that you have to decide about analgesics *before* labor. I say that because it's almost too hard a decision to make while you're *in* labor. Many women, particularly in first labors, reach a point where they feel that they can't make it. They've practiced all their skills— breathing, massage, knowing what's happening to their bodies

—all that. And they reach a point where they feel like they're falling apart. 'Do something! I can't go on!' " S. said, raising his voice and flailing his arms, eliciting a smile from the couple. "And then we say, 'You're okay and the baby is okay.' It's hard to reconcile the way you feel—which might be awful—with reassuring words like these. Now, if you ask a woman who feels like that whether or not she wants pain medication, what do you think the answer will be?"

"I can imagine what it will be."

"Right. It's almost not fair to expect someone whose feelings are so intense to think rationally."

"In other words, we ought to decide ahead of time, when we can still think clearly," said Bob.

"There are several things to consider," S. continued. "First, when you feel that things are at their worst, when you're 'falling apart,' you're usually in transition—the time when the cervix is dilating most rapidly. In other words, you're almost to the top of the mountain. If you can hold out a bit longer, then you'll be in a position to push, which many women feel gives them a new kind of control over their pain. Second, what you're talking about is several hours of pain out of a lifetime. I've not yet known a woman who in retrospect would have wanted to have the pain medicine she didn't get. Third, this is an opportunity to learn about pain and sort out what part of it comes from fear. There are few other situations in which pain is normal—that is, doesn't mean that there is something wrong—and comes and goes so that you can observe it and yourself. Here's your chance to experience it for what it is."

"Sounds like she'll have more control over it than I will," Bob said animatedly. "I don't know if I'll be able to stand it."

"That's a good point. I'm glad you brought it up. The people around a laboring woman often have difficulty tolerating her pain. They have the urge to do something; they feel responsible. Also, the woman might yell and scream and accuse those around her of not caring, of sitting on their hands. Husbands we've known have had the impulse to throw us out of the house and move right to the hospital. It's hard to be with someone who's so uncomfortable and not do something. It's hard to say no to a request for pain medicine unless you're honoring a prior agreement to do so. It's almost asking too much of anyone to be with someone who is in pain, and yet not feel responsible for it. If you don't do something for her this time, you might wonder whether you can ever look her in the face again. Under these circumstances just being with someone isn't easy, and it's not the same as doing nothing."

"Like when I'm in a funk, it's hard for Bob to take. He tries to humor me—he'll do anything but just leave me alone." She turned to Bob. "And when I tell you to leave me alone, you get upset. Sometimes you go and take a walk, but that's not what I meant."

"Well, I must own up to it," replied Bob, "that I can get pretty upset with Roberta when she's in one of her moods—like around her periods."

"Well," continued S., "here's your chance to talk through what a person can do that's most helpful to another in distress. We've got to remember, Roberta, that the pain will be yours, all yours, not ours. But that doesn't mean we are turning our backs on you. We're going to support you in your decision to handle the pain without medicine. Our job is to keep cool if and when you feel you're falling apart."

"But what if the pain gets to be too much?"

"I'll be keeping an open mind and listening closely to the messages I get from both of you. Even though we're now committed to no pain medication and home birth, you'll need to trust that I know you well enough by now to recognize when the pain gets to be too much. Also, all this discussion presumes a normal labor. If there is a problem with the labor, then we'll be dealing with a different set of issues."

"Well," she said, "you have certainly seen me in some pain already, like during the pelvic exam and when I had the morning sickness. Bob can be of some help to you too."

"I'm counting on that," said S. "And remember, I'm committed to being your doctor all the way, whether the birth is at home or in the hospital."

"That makes me feel much more comfortable about going ahead with a home birth without pain medication," said Bob.

"I guess that up till now being in pain and being alone always meant the same thing to me," Roberta remarked.

Bob looked at her. "You've never said that to me."
"I guess I've never quite said it to myself."

A Crisis of Confidence

It was an unusual request over the phone to "talk things over in the next day or two." Roberta's office was on S.'s route between hospitals, and she and Bob agreed to meet him there. S. was glad to be able to see them at her workplace.

"I'm glad that you could see us on such short notice," began Roberta, now thirty-six weeks pregnant, "and that you could come to my office." She paused and then continued, "It's hard for us to say this, but now that we're coming down to the wire with this birth, we're having some second thoughts about you as our birth attendant. Let me say that basically we like you a lot and think you're a good doctor. But a few things have happened which alone might not mean anything, but taken together have shaken our confidence in you somewhat.

"First, there was the time when I sprained my ankle early in the pregnancy and you told your assistant to wrap the wrong foot. Second, when we did that screening test for blood pressure complications during labor and it was abnormal, you didn't react to the report; your nurse practitioner overheard your assistant in the hall and told me to increase protein and fluids and to rest on my left side for an hour twice a day. Finally, when you noticed the yeast infection in my vagina two weeks ago, you disregarded it; yet when I mentioned it yesterday to you you started me on medication. I guess what we're worried about is that you'll overlook something during the labor. We felt we had to discuss these concerns with you now."

S. swallowed hard. "Do you feel the same way, Bob?"

"Who doesn't make mistakes? I'm not as concerned about each item as is Roberta, but the fact that she's concerned is what concerns me too."

S. then spoke to each of the points, admitting error in part and also legitimate differences of approach. "In some cases I change my own mind as to what's the best gamble. But I can understand your doubts. What can I say? I'm the one who keeps stressing the importance of trust. I certainly have more trust in you for sharing these doubts about me. I'm unhappy about the mistakes. I also erred in not working out the options with you about that yeast infection. That is our agreement when the treatment for a problem is uncertain, and I broke the agreement. I wouldn't blame you one bit for asking me to bow out."

Roberta shook her head. "Well, I'm glad we can agree that you've broken the agreement. As I said before, we really want you to be there, but we wanted to reassure ourselves that we have a common understanding."

"I feel better too," said Bob. "At least we know that if differences arise, we can see them for what they are."

"And I appreciate your talking with me about this," S. replied. "I'd like to attend your birth. I'm looking forward to it."

"Good, we're looking forward to it too. Come, let me give you a tour of the office."

For S. to say that he looked forward to the birth was an understatement. He still found it hard to acknowledge to his patients the degree to which they inspired and educated him. As long as he could hear them, they would help him become the kind of doctor he wanted to be. On the other hand, recognizing that he was a cause wasn't always easy on his ego. Moreover, he had to guard against the pitfall of becoming "just one of the family" and slackening his professional alertness. Notwithstanding the egalitarian doctor-patient relationship he fostered, with its active family participation and negotiation, there were still decisions that he alone would have to make. That was what people expected him to do—especially when it came down to labor. If a move to the hospital was called for, he could not allow himself to be swayed by the family's disappointment or by his own. If the family was ready to run to the hospital for pain medication when in fact labor was progressing normally, then, too, he would have to speak with authority, though in such a way as not to compromise the family's participation in the decision.

On the Alert

At the thirty-seven-week office visit Roberta's urine showed a moderate amount of sugar. S. then drew a blood sample for sugar (glucose) determination. The report came to his desk first thing the next morning. The blood glucose was mildly elevated.

That was the thing about "normal" pregnancy. You never knew for sure whether or when it would turn into something else. The presence of sugar in the urine late in pregnancy was very common and most often normal. Usually it resulted from a temporary and harmless change in the capacity of the kidneys to recover filtered glucose. But it could also signify diabetes, an impaired capacity to process sugar in the body. A glucose tolerance test could help make the distinction.

S. was on the alert for diabetes because, without producing any symptoms at all, it could increase the chances of a stillbirth as well as result in an extra large baby that would have trouble passing through the birth canal. Furthermore, a baby born of a diabetic mother was prone to complications at birth such as breathing problems and low blood sugar, sometimes accompanied by seizures. The diagnosis of gestational diabetes was one that S. much preferred to make—when he had to make it at all—before rather than at birth. He well remembered one nine-pound-plus baby, one of his first home births, who stopped breathing and turned blue for seconds at a time. S., who had already left the scene, had to return to the home. The baby's breathing was shallow. S. packed everyone into his station wagon and drove to the hospital. It was scary. The baby did well while tests done on the mother showed a diabetic pattern.

This was not a good way to discover minimal diabetes, and S. never forgot the lesson. In fact, there was a danger that he might be overshooting in the other direction: finding the borderline cases of diabetes where there were no good data on outcome and treating them like high-risk pregnancies. It was understandable that he was sometimes overcautious, since he practiced in a milieu where many of his peers believed that there was no such thing as a low-risk pregnancy.

"Hello, Bob," S. said on the phone. "This is Dr. S. calling. I want to let you know about the report on Roberta's blood sugar. It was on the high side—not much—and I'd like to recheck it."

"Funny that you should call. We were just about to call you. Roberta's waters broke about ten minutes ago."

"Really!"

"We've already called Paula. Here's Roberta now. I'll put her on."

"Hi. It's hard to tell how much came out, maybe a cup of clear stuff. I was in bed, and I just felt it coming out, so I sat up. It soaked the floor. It's still coming out."

"Are you having any contractions?"

"No, not yet."

"Well, sounds like you're about to go into labor. You're just at thirty-seven weeks, which is our cutoff point for home birth in terms of prematurity. Paula will call me after she sees you. If you go into labor, we'll make a decision about home or hospital."

"Okay. Hey, what was that you were telling Bob about my blood sugar?"

"It was a little elevated, and we'll have to deal with that. But we may not have time to deal with it in the way we would like. Right now we'll have to see whether you're indeed going into labor."

The Birth

S. slowly put down the phone. It was still May, and Roberta's due date was June 15. "Uh, oh," he said to himself. "Could be trouble." He caught himself. "Well, a gamble different than expected, anyway." Whether Roberta had diabetes was still an open question. Moreover, premature babies were at greater risk of complications at birth. It was a risk he was reluctant to take. And if Roberta didn't go into labor following the breaking of her bag of waters there would be another problem: the danger of infection. Once the protective membranes had broken, bacteria from the vagina could enter the uterine cavity, infecting it and the baby. Infection could break out with lightning speed, and the monitoring techniques to detect its earliest signs —temperature rise, elevation of the white blood cell count, and the appearance of pus cells in the leaking fluid—were good but not that good.

So there was some danger in waiting. Traditionally, if Roberta's cervix was "ripe" for labor, labor would be induced, but that would mean no home birth. "Watching and waiting" also had its advocates, though. But it was one thing to watch and wait in the hospital and another, in the eyes of those opposed to home birth, to do so at home. In the home, too, a traditional obstetrical view was that the couple couldn't be trusted to take the temperatures and to refrain from activities like sexual intercourse and tub baths which might flush bacteria up the birth canal.

If you had a woman in the hospital, you could at least control what she was doing. You could place her in an *experimentum crucis* where you didn't need to trust her and her husband to follow the rules themselves. Many of these "rules" had arisen in impersonal clinic settings where trust was minimal. They might make sense as a response to this lack of trust. Once established, however, the rules took on a life of their own.

So here he was, here they were, faced with another decision with a number of elements: borderline maturity, borderline blood sugar, and ruptured membranes without (as yet) signs of labor. He caught himself momentarily wishing he had a pocket computer with a programmed decision analysis. But what good would that ever do? There was no way he could place this unique patient into a preexisting statistical category, and even if he could, placing her there would still be a judgment, a gamble. Talk about gambling—twice in one morning new gambles had arisen.

When Paula called, she reported that mild contractions had begun. Paula had a "sense" that this baby was of good size and that the labor would proceed normally. She felt that the couple's wish to stay at home was reasonable even though there was a question of prematurity.

S. felt a load on his shoulders over the question raised by prematurity and possible diabetes. The answer he came up with was: "Share the dilemma with them. Let them know that there may be a slightly increased risk for the baby and that the hospital on a technical level might offer some advantages. Review with them, in these changed circumstances, some of the things that make the home gamble different from the hospital gamble: the greater variance of possible outcomes, the slightly greater chance of a very negative outcome, and so forth. Remind them that they had agreed to go to the hospital in circumstances like these, and that if we're going to change the principles by which we're gambling, we should do so consciously."

Thirty minutes later Paula called again. She had just checked Roberta and found her cervix to be dilated to four centimeters, a sign of labor. That issue, at least, seemed resolved. S. asked to speak with Roberta and Bob. He presented the choice and the risks to them, and they strongly indicated their preference to stay put even if it meant slightly modifying agreed-upon principles. "Well, as long as you've given it some thought," said S. "It's a decision we all have to take responsibility for."

Paula felt surer than ever about the home birth. S. respected her judgment. From experience she had learned what the probabilities were, and she had a good understanding of the situation. "Okay, Paula, call me when things heat up."

S. went back to seeing patients in his office with Liz, a medical student. There were a few progress reports through the day. By late afternoon a milestone was reached when the baby's body rotated from a "posterior" position (with the face pointing to Roberta's front) to an "anterior" one, optimal for labor. Paula, who had worried about the slow progress until that time, had found useful and reassuring Roberta's mother's observation that her three labors had been just that way—starting slowly from posterior and speeding up following rotation, which had occurred, as it now had in Roberta's case, relatively high in the birth canal. Maybe Roberta, too, would follow this "family" pattern. This was the kind of data that the probabilistic approach, sweeping wide in its search for relevant information, was more likely to take advantage of than the mechanistic. In its own way it was as useful as any statistically constructed labor curve.

About eight that evening, with the day's last patient waiting to be seen in the office, Paula called back: "She's at eight centimeters. You'd better come. Her contractions were so mild I didn't check her until now. I'm amazed that she's moved so fast."

"I'm on my way. Would you check with Roberta to see whether it's still all right to bring that medical student we talked about a few weeks ago, Liz, to watch the birth. She's welcome to come? Fine." S. put down the phone and poked his head into the office of one of his partners. "I've got to go. Come, let me introduce you to Mrs. B., whom I was just about to see. I'll tell her I've got a delivery."

S. grabbed the oxygen tank and home birth bag, a big black kit designed for veterinarians and chock full of equipment including emergency drugs, plasma, IV tubing, needles, syringes, specula, laryngoscope, and infant resuscitation breathing bag. He asked Liz to take Roberta's medical record and the "ultrasound" instrument from the OB examining room. The ultrasound was useful in recording the baby's heartbeat during the final contractions when the heart might no longer be in easy range of the stethoscope. They packed S.'s car and drove off.

Even though it was after rush hour, traffic was still heavy as he crossed the bridge connecting two parts of the city. Heavy spring rain had delayed many in getting home. He was getting frustrated as the traffic backed up. "Talk about uncertainty," he thought. "When you deliver in the home, you don't control the conditions under which you get there." He was getting angrier at the traffic until he remembered the time in the hospital when he couldn't find a free nurse to assist at a delivery because so much was going on at the same time, as well as all the times when obstetric nurses delivered babies because the doctor didn't get there on time. He realized that he was getting angry because he was comparing what was happening now with an ideal standard of hospital perfection—the perfectly oiled machine. The machine didn't always work perfectly either.

Fifteen minutes later they turned off the major artery. "Right at Williams' Market to the third house on the left," said the directions. Shabby three-decker wooden homes. Past two men working on a car at the corner under the streetlight. A truck trailer was parked on a side street. The neighborhood was just as Paula had described it after her preparatory home visit two weeks earlier.

They quickly unpacked the car. The birth kit and oxygen tank were heavy; the sidewalk slippery. Up the stairs to the porch. The door was unlocked. A young man greeted them and directed them to the bedroom in the rear. A quick glance told S. that things were not under control.

That was an understatement. Roberta was, simply stated, panicking. "Do anything—take me to the hospital, give me an anesthetic, anything—but end this pain." Bob was even more unnerved. He looked like he could barely contain his anxiety and anger.

It was time for firm action. S. quickly put on a sterile glove and persuaded Roberta to hold still long enough for him to check her cervix and the position of the baby. Paula simultaneously applied the ultrasound to Roberta's abdomen, and the reassuring hoofbeatlike sound of the baby's heart was broadcast through the room for all to hear.

"Roberta, you're fully dilated!" S. exclaimed. "You can begin pushing now. You're over the hump. No wonder you felt like you were losing control. You're fine and the baby's fine. Relax! I know it hurts, and you're okay—do you understand? Now let's all get to work to get this baby out. There is more work to do, you know. Now, Bob, you come around to her side. I want you to keep eye contact with each other during contractions."

If ever S. had to give an example of how he couldn't observe the "facts" without changing them, it was now. He was prepared to go even further if necessary. There were times when he had to remind a couple of the agreement they had made to have a home birth. They had wanted this kind of birth, and he had been willing to support them. He didn't think they should let the passion of the moment overturn a well-worked-out plan. If it came to that, he would remind them that if they wanted an anesthetic, they would have to move the whole show to the hospital. There were times when a firm hand was called for.

"First, let's position you better," he told Roberta. "Lying on your back isn't such a good idea. Let's prop you up with these pillows behind your back and get gravity working for you. You'll be in a better position to 'push' if this makes you comfortable, and the baby will get more blood from the placenta."

For the first time he could pay attention to the people present. There was Jim, who had come to the door; his wife Sarah; and Alice, Roberta's mother. A whining dog was locked up in an adjacent room.

"Now you don't have to push now, Roberta. Try and see if it helps you feel better. The baby will be born whether or not you push." He had to speed up his probably too lengthy instructions because another contraction was starting up and competing for Roberta's attention.

Half an hour later Roberta's face was flushed and moist. She was no longer available for verbal interchange, although between contractions she could nod her understanding of the observations and guidance of her coaches. S. noticed, almost in passing, that she was no longer breathing in any special pattern when she wasn't bearing down. Breathing techniques were a central part of natural childbirth instruction. The couples whose births S. attended (at home or in hospital) learned the techniques, but learned to use them selectively, as needed.

S. didn't insist upon any particular set of rules for breathing. Here, too, there was choice, just as there was in the matter of "pushing the baby out," which women traditionally were told to do. With S. they pushed only when they were comfortable doing so. Unless, of course, delivering the baby quickly was important. Then the mother would be told to push and to push hard. Speedy delivery was in order, for example, in the case of abnormal and noncorrectable slowing of the fetal heartbeat, signifying possible fetal distress. In general, though, what babies needed to be born was time and patience. Much of the interventionist mentality of obstetrical practices, especially in the past, it seemed to S., had to do with the pressures, economic and otherwise, to hurry things along.

By now Paula had stopped applying warm wet towels to Roberta's perineum. The lore of midwives was that this moist heat increased blood flow and stretchability of the tissues. She continued circular movements around the vulva, stretching the by now pursed-out lips with her gloved and oiled fingertips between the lip and the emerging head.

Sarah held a mirror near Roberta's buttocks so that she could see the baby's head emerge. "Here's your baby. Put your hand down here and feel the baby."

S. checked the baby's heart after each contraction. Paula predicted that several more contractions would do it. S. positioned himself on his knees next to Roberta in order to assist Paula with an extra pair of hands for the baby. With the contractions Paula told Roberta, "Pant, don't push," so as to decrease the expulsive force. Just after the last contraction eased, Paula asked Roberta to push "just a little; easy, easy." As Roberta bore down, the head slid through the stretched vulva. S. felt around the neck and reported that it was free of umbilical cord, which sometimes becomes twisted around the neck and needs to be disentangled or cut so that the baby can be born. He then suctioned the mouth with a nozzled rubber bulb.

At this point S. asked Roberta to bring her hands down to grasp the baby as it emerged. This freed his hands to support the perineum and ease it over the shoulder as the baby slid out. "It's a girl!" Roberta had delivered her own baby!

The baby cried lustily and pinked up. Roberta and Bob cried too. "Apgar eleven," said S., turning to Liz. The Apgar score, the standard rating scale of newborn function (named after anesthetist Virginia Apgar, who first proposed it), takes into account color, heart rate, quality of respiration, muscle tone, and responsiveness to stimuli. A perfect score, often seen in unmedicated births, is ten points. "Apgar eleven" is a way of saying "better than perfect."

S. wrapped the newcomer in a warm receiving blanket and asked Roberta to put her to breast. She sucked immediately, and her mother's uterus contracted in response. Within minutes the placenta, assisted by gentle tension on the cord by Paula, emerged. S. breathed a sigh of relief. One of his major concerns was the possibility of hemorrhage that revolved around delivery of the placenta. Paula inspected Roberta's vagina and reported that there were only a few "skid marks," i.e., small, superficial tears which required no stitches. No episiotomy had been done, and these small tears would heal on their own.

Amidst all the celebrating, though, S. had to keep an eye out for any signs of bleeding. In situations when the uterus was lax and there was bleeding, the husband would be asked to suck his wife's breasts (if the baby did not) to stimulate the reflex clamping down of the uterus. This was unnecessary for Roberta. Of course, there were always the drugs (Pitocin and Ergotrate) as a backup if these maneuvers, coupled with massage of the uterus, failed.

S. caught Roberta's eye. Her face was relaxed. She was beaming and overwhelmed. He felt he would never forget that expression.

While Paula was cleaning Roberta up and repositioning her, S. checked the baby and recorded his examination findings in the record. He gave the baby vitamin K and treated her eyes. Paula filled a rubber examining glove with ice cubes, tied it at the wrist, and applied it to Roberta's perineum to reduce swelling.

In the relaxed afterglow, while the new parents enjoyed the privacy of the bedroom with the baby, the other participants reviewed the birth over tea, a birthday cake with the newborn's name already iced on it, and Sarah's guitar music. "I'm glad you stood by the family's wish for a home birth," S. told Paula. He turned to Roberta's mother, with whom he had had only passing words in the heat of the delivery, and asked her how she had found the birth.

"Well, I was dead set against the home part of it. It's not easy to overcome what you've been led to believe is the right way. But let me tell you, I was so out of it when Roberta was born that I barely remember what happened. You've got to hand it to these young people and to people like yourselves for being so sensible about what you're doing. I think it's great. I'll never forget it. I wish my husband had lived to be here too."

"I have to thank you as well," S. replied. "You made an important contribution. Do you know that your telling Paula about your labors—turning from posterior to anterior—was the piece of information that tipped the balance in favor of staying at home instead of deciding that labor had stopped progressing?

And just your being here—what a source of support that was for all of us."

Just then Bob came in with a tray of wineglasses filled with champagne. "Well, we almost, it felt, came to blows," S. remarked to him. "And here we are. We can say that we lived through some pretty strong emotions. I'll never forget it. When I see you again to check the baby, I'll know that we sweated it out together and that we handled our emotions just long enough to get through—but emotions there were!"

They embraced. S. knew that he was doing all the talking. He also knew Bob well enough to know that he was speaking for both of them. It was the trust that Roberta, Paula, and the two men had developed that had enabled them to contain the frustration they felt with one another and to produce the result they had all worked for. S. and the family could build upon this trust in the future. For a family doctor birth was just one episode (though a uniquely important one) in working with a family.

All agreed that this had not just been the birth of a baby, but the birth of what in this family was a new idea—the idea that a family could consciously make decisions *as* a family. All of the questions they had faced together, all of the decisions they had made—whether to have the baby; the choice of a doctor; the planned home birth; what to do about the morning sickness, the elevated blood sugar, the borderline prematurity; the difficult yet unmedicated labor—had built toward something larger: a way of gambling consciously at the important moments in their lives. "You could have made the same sorts of decisions in a hospital or birth center," said S., "but since you wanted to do it at home, I'm glad that you were able to."

Just as each successful experience of gambling during the pregnancy (whether the gamble itself was won or lost) gave Bob and Roberta added confidence for approaching the next, so the overall experience would lead them to believe in themselves a bit more, even amid all the pressures (and these weren't going to go away) that could undermine any family's belief in itself. It wasn't blind confidence; they had lived through things that easily could have gone wrong, and they knew it. They would always have to face uncertainty, but with a growing capacity to turn it into probabilities. As they learned what they could accomplish, they would rightly set higher probability estimates for success in the things they attempted. And with a growing backlog of consciously held experience, successful and unsuccessful, they would not interpret each new success— or failure—as meaning that the world had only a friendly—or demonic—face to show them. Together, they were becoming rational instead of reactive human beings.

PART V

CONTEXTS

14

MEDICAL MILIEUX

While Dr. S. visited patients in their homes several times a week, few of these visits were to help someone die or be born. But the births and the deaths, with the special character they took on in the home, served to remind him of some important, yet often unasked questions about the visits with patients that constituted the major share of his daily experience. Where did they take place? Who was visiting whom? How did the site affect the nature and quality of care? Did people (himself included) make decisions differently in different sites? If the questions were not asked, the choices could not be made consciously.

S. saw patients in a number of different places: his office, their homes, hospitals, nursing homes, and just about anywhere in an emergency. He sought to learn and teach critical thinking in all of those sites. But to do so he had to learn and teach critical thinking *about* the sites. He and his patients had to think critically about the probable consequences of choosing one site rather than another. For he knew from experience that things do not remain the same when taken out of one context and put in another. Even something as concrete sounding as a symptom has little meaning outside the

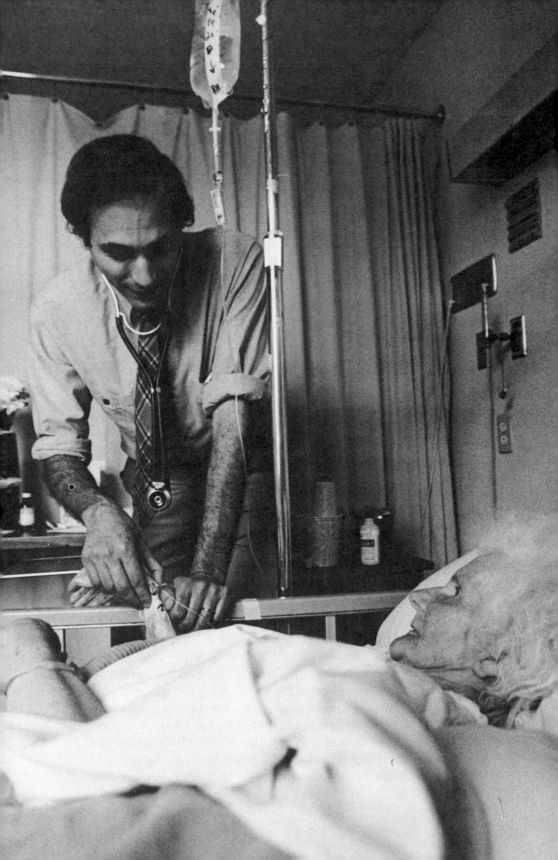

contexts in which it appears. S. sometimes "cured" patients who suffered chest pain (what doctors call *angina pectoris*) on exerting themselves in a stressful job situation when he told them to "take it easy" and move around less. S. removed the symptom by changing the context; in a different context it might reappear.

As with the disease, so with the treatment. Although it cannot be said that the site completely determines the type of care that is given, it does have an effect. It has the largest effect when people take it for granted, when they do not realize that they are making a choice. Going to the hospital or staying at home is a choice people make that in turn makes other choices more likely, though not inevitable. In the hospital people can become passive before the operation of technology; in the home people can become passive before the operation of nature. By being aware of the implications of their choices, families and their doctors (as S. well knew) can make better choices of site and better choices within whatever site they choose.

These days the hospital (or, in chronic cases, the nursing home) has become a habit—i.e., still a choice, but one made by default. At one time the sick were cared for in the home. Illness was something that happened—and was dealt with—within the family. In those days no medical technology could do any better than home treatment. Today many people who otherwise would have died are alive because of hospitals and hospital technology. Still, patients and their families need to consider in any given case whether they are entering a hospital or nursing home because it is the right choice in that situation or because they have drifted into it, swept along by the currents of habit formed under the Mechanistic Paradigm.

What is profitable for a few tends to become the habit of many. S. aimed to break the institutional habit and reopen the home-versus-hospital question as a conscious choice for families. They hardly needed to hear a case made for the hospital when so many social and economic pressures combined to push them in that direction. On the other hand, some families now were making a case for the home because they wanted to retain the power of choice through the course of the illness, rather than surrender it to institutional personnel.

There are some visits that one doesn't like to make, like the last social call on an old friend who is moving out of town. And there were some house calls that Dr. S. didn't like to make: the ones where he and the family faced the painful, at times agonizing decision of whether an ill person—especially an elderly person—should stay at home or go to the hospital. The patient, if he or she was alert enough to know, rarely equivocated: Stay at home! "Don't put me in a nursing home. Whatever else you do, don't do that!" On the other side was the view of an involved relative such as a son or a daughter (if the patient was fortunate enough to have one): "My father simply can't take care of her anymore; he's old and sick too. And we haven't any room at our house. Besides, we're working people; who would stay with her?"

S.'s role in all this was an equivocal one. A family that wanted to keep a sick relative at home would look to him for support. His involvement made home care a viable alternative. A family that didn't want to take care of the patient at home might find it easier to attribute the decision to him: "The doctor says you've got to go to the hospital." In such cases S. would say, "I don't want to be the bad guy to your mother, who is my patient, after all. The fact is that she could stay at home if you could take care of her there. Tell her that, though you love her, you can't do it anymore. If you had unlimited money and if there were more supports for families, then you could do it and would want to. But that's not the way it is."

The hospital, one anguished daughter had pointed out, was a place where her mother could get used to being cared for away from home; this would make it easier to place her in a nursing home. That was the idea—to make the transition in palatable stages: from home to hospital, then from hospital to nursing home. On such visits S. felt more like the sheriff evicting an old friend than a family doctor sending a patient to the hospital to get better. If the patient got better, she would probably go to a nursing home. If she got worse, she would go to her eternal resting place. Either way the hospital would be a way station.

That was how the hospital made things easier for the family. It also made things easier for the patient—and for S., the doctor.

He remembered a woman in her eighties whom he had treated at home for a blood and joint disorder. She spoke only Portuguese, and S. could communicate with her only through her niece. He had left the two women with written instructions and what he had thought was a clear mutual understanding about the medications the patient was to take, only to find on his next visit that nothing had been taken as he had ordered. The patient had run out of some medications without telling her niece; her niece had changed S.'s instructions without telling him; and the old woman had ended up taking some things he had told her *not* to take. S. was left puzzled and confused about what medications the woman had actually taken. No one—not the patient, not her niece, not S. himself—had assumed the responsibility of seeing that what they had all agreed to was carried out.

At that moment the controlled environment of the hospital looked very attractive to S. There he and the patient and family did not *have* to take responsibility. On the other hand, even if they wanted to take responsibility, they still could not. Insofar as taking responsibility itself was a cause of a successful outcome, there would be costs, for each act of taking responsibility increases one's capacity to take responsibility, and each failure to take responsibility diminishes that capacity. In fact, S. considered fostering that capacity to be one goal of treatment.

In the hospital responsibility was diffused among different "services." If the patient had a fracture of the hip, which was often the final straw, she would wind up on the orthopedic service. Chances are that the orthopedist wouldn't know her and would defer to a social worker, who wouldn't know her either. The family doctor, who had no clearly defined role on the orthopedic service, could easily hide in the fuzziness of responsibility made possible by specialization. In fact, it took a lot of conscious effort on S.'s part to remain involved at all— asserting himself on the ward, with the social worker, with the house physicians who welcomed excitement and challenge, but who weren't always as interested (nor were they expected to be) in the "routine" cases where the job was to make an ailing elderly person more comfortable and to extend her conscious life.

S. was aware that he brought a mind-set to the care of his patients that was different from the one that he had learned in the hospital and that was still current there. His mind-set, like that of the hospital physicians, could imprison as well as liberate. Each setting had its own bias. To remind himself of the strength of those biases and of the need for critical thinking in any setting, he would recall three cases: one that showed the hospital in all its glory and all its excess, one that revealed the mixed blessings of the home, and one in which critical judgment (together with an appreciation of the family context) enabled him to use hospital technology to advantage.

S. was asked to see Evelyn Dewey by her longtime friend and former neighbor, Florence Peterson, who had been given his name by the Visiting Nurse Association. He arrived late one winter afternoon at her first-story, one-bedroom flat after having gotten lost in a neighborhood unfamiliar to him. A quick look around the apartment told a lot: an obese, elderly, white-haired, pleasant (even charming) woman who looked less than her ninety-one years, sitting in a chair, huffing and puffing; red, oozing, swollen legs. Dishes and garbage in the sink; unmade bed; clumps of dust on the floor. How long had she been this way? She must have slipped gradually, over many months, into what at a glance looked like congestive heart failure.

"She hasn't seen a doctor in twenty years," said Florence, a woman of about sixty. He didn't need to be told that it had been a long time. Could this have been prevented? He doubted that congestive heart failure could have been prevented, but its effects could have been tempered. He was often called in late when the disease was advanced. It wasn't ignorance; frightened old people wished so hard for it not to be true that their better judgment was impaired. The slow, insidious process by which the heart slipped into failure made it easy to deny that it was happening at all.

At first Evelyn Dewey seemed to have her wits about her, but the longer S. stayed with her, the more her mental deficiencies —what doctors usually called "senile dementia"—became apparent. The questions by which he tested her reasoning and memory (such as "How much is 7 from 100?" and "Who is the president of the United States?") were always painful to ask, no matter how gentle he tried to make them. Her answers confirmed his impression that she was mildly intellectually impaired, but still could reason and feel.

He checked her over: blood pressure in the normal range; rapid pulse; clear lungs (a surprise—he had expected to hear the sounds of fluid in the lungs); swollen abdomen probably full of fluid so that the liver, which he had expected to find enlarged with backed-up blood, couldn't be felt; legs very swollen.

"Looks like it's your heart. It's not pumping as strongly as it needs to," he concluded as he returned his examining equipment to the black doctor's bag.

"I think it's my arthritis. That's why I can't walk. My heart's just beating fast from all the excitement. I'll be okay. Don't know why you're all making such a fuss," she said.

Florence thought otherwise. "Since Christmas, about six weeks ago, I've come in once or twice a week to do the shopping and pay the bills. But I can't take care of her, and there is no one else. I think she needs to go to hospital."

"I agree," replied S. "Some time in the hospital to get things under control, and you could be in shape to come home again."

"No, that's out of the question. I'm staying right here, period. I'm an old woman, and my family is all gone—except Florence here, who's like family to me. All I have left is here."

S. could sense that Evelyn valued living longer less than she did maintaining her pride and autonomy. He knew there was little point in arguing with her. Who was he, after all, to tell her what to do? "Okay, let's give it a try. If treating you at home works, great! If not, then you may have to go to hospital." He knew that by meeting her halfway and allowing her to participate in the decision, he, a stranger, would be building up trust which could be tapped for the more difficult decision that lay ahead. Later he made sure to explain to Florence that they were taking a gamble, so that she would share in the responsibility.

After drawing several tubes of Evelyn's blood for chemical analysis, S. gave her two prescriptions. "One is for digitalis, which is a heart tonic," he explained. "The other is for a fluid pill to help get rid of the excess water and salt your body has stored. I'll call the VNA nurse to see you tomorrow; she'll give you an electrocardiogram. I'll be back the day after." He left his phone number on a piece of paper in case she needed to call him before then.

He doubted that it would be all that simple. He questioned whether she could or would take the medications as directed. In this first visit he hadn't checked her medicine cabinet, which he often liked to do. Was she like so many other older people he had met who maintained a veritable "drugstore" of medications collected over the years, some of them out of date or no longer in use, trying a little bit of this and a little bit of that?

The next day the visiting nurse called S. back to say that she hadn't been able to get into the apartment with her portable EKG machine. Evelyn hadn't been able to get out of her chair, where she had sat since S. had left the night before. All that time she had held in her urine and hadn't been able to get to the pills that Florence had left for her. The nurse had had to call Florence, who hurried over from work with the key and helped her get Evelyn to the toilet.

While driving for a second time to her apartment, S. pictured Evelyn Dewey sitting immobile in her chair. How much like Mabel Gormley, he marveled, who in her dying days had sat as if glued to her chair, afraid to move for fear of disrupting the tenuous equilibrium that kept her frail body functioning. He wondered whether it was just a coincidence that Evelyn had declined so precipitously right after his visit. Was she frozen in her chair by her illness or from the fright of having been seen by a doctor, what with the looming threats of nursing home and death that his presence must have brought menacingly close? Had the gentle questions he had asked her not been as gentle as they might have been?

When S. arrived, he articulated as a conscious decision what everyone must have felt was a forgone conclusion. It was time to go to the hospital. Florence persuaded Evelyn to go by reminding her of the days when she had been a volunteer driver for the Red Cross. "Think back, Evvie. For twenty-five years you took people to the doctor or the hospital and back home again. Well, now it's your turn."

S. phoned ahead to the emergency room at City Hospital to

tell the house officers about Mrs. Dewey. He didn't know the doctor at the other end, and the exchange felt impersonal, although proper. "After you get a look at her, give me a call. I want to see her before we take the next step."

Evelyn and Florence left in an ambulance. Evelyn thought she would be back soon. S. told himself later that he ought to have discussed with her the probability of her ever returning home, which—not for "medical" reasons, but on other grounds —was not very good. This was to be her farewell to independent, private living. S. was being the sheriff again.

S. came down to the emergency room after the doctors there had called him back. They agreed with his diagnosis of heart failure. They, too, noted the absence of fluid in the patient's lungs or distension of the veins in her neck—findings that, if present, would have completed the picture of garden-variety heart failure.

"The team from the ward will be down soon. No need for you to wait. We'll take care of everything." It seemed so natural, so polite, for them to make this gesture. And so easy for him to leave. He had many other things to do, among them getting home to dinner on time for a change.

He caught himself. A real "family doctor" would not leave his patient here among strangers without personally making the transfer to the ward and letting the staff know that he was her doctor. He, like everyone involved in the case, was concerned with the patient's well-being. Yet he had let himself become preoccupied with getting home for dinner, just as the house officers and nurses, with their greater emotional distance from the patient, were attuned to their own convenience as well as to the pressing needs of other patients. That was the whole point of having a family doctor—someone who stood at varying distances from the case, so as to be able to see it from the patient's and family's "personal" viewpoint as well as the "professional" one of the trained physician. If S. didn't look out for his patients, who would? Yet it was not always such an easy thing to do.

In this case it was to be harder than he yet knew. He stayed with Evelyn in the emergency room, so that all the procedures done there were undertaken in consultation with him. In any event, the initial tests, such as the EKG and chest X ray, were not much of a strain on the patient. Their benefits were clear, and their costs were relatively low. But what would happen when Evelyn was on the ward and the prospect of further tests arose? S. would no longer be with her. He later realized that he ought to have instructed the ward personnel to inform him immediately of any significant changes in his patient's condition, even during the night. He might have told them, "She's an old woman; she's frightened; she's been sick a long time. Let's do only what we need to do and look for small changes over time." He might have said these things. . . .

In the emergency room Evelyn was given additional digitalis intravenously along with oxygen administered through nose prongs. The chest X ray showed a massively enlarged heart, an accumulation of fluid in the left chest cavity outside the lungs, and an increased amount of fluid in the lungs themselves.

The ward team, too, was struck by the massive swelling of Evelyn's legs and the absence of distension of her neck veins. The latter could be explained, consistent with the likely diagnosis of congestive heart failure, by her dehydrated state. This explanation would make further testing unnecessary. But the ward team thought of another possibility, especially in view of her labored breathing: pulmonary embolus. According to this hypothesis blood clots had formed in the veins of her legs. Some had broken loose and, having been carried by the venous system through the right side of the heart into the vessels of the lung, had lodged in the branches of these vessels. So, following their commitment to thoroughness, they phoned Dr. S. and urged him to authorize a lung scan, a procedure that involved injecting radioactive dye intravenously and then counting the radioactivity over the lung fields.

It seemed like a reasonable step to S. as well. It was hard to argue with the house staff when they were right there on top of the situation, while he was at the other end of a telephone line. He couldn't take a look at Evelyn and see how she was doing. And if he disagreed with the house officers' recommendation, they might ask him to come in and look for himself. Besides, S., too, was afraid of "missing something." In this instance it didn't take much for him to be drawn into the prevailing mentality. "Maybe they do know something that I don't," he put it to himself. And he was quick to acknowledge that they did know a lot about acute care, since they saw acute illnesses every day that he only ran across occasionally.

The lung scan was negative—no signs of embolus. Struck by the bulk of Evelyn's abdomen, the house doctor had also requested an ultrasound examination. This test bounced sound waves off her intraabdominal contents and gave a scan picture of her abdominal structure: it revealed a lot of fluid in the abdominal cavity, a finding consistent with heart failure. No new information.

Once in her room on the hospital floor Evelyn was thoroughly questioned and examined by an intern and again by a resident and a nurse. They all wrote detailed notes in her record listing her various problems and the plans to attack them. Among the problems were heart failure, heart murmur, confusion, and weakness of her left arm and leg, this last suggesting that she had had a stroke on the right side of her brain sometime in the past. That part of the brain is known as the "quiet side," since in most people it does not control such functions as speech or memory. Often no one, including the patient, notices a mild stroke when it occurs on this side.

Evelyn was finally settled in late that night in a room with three other seriously ill patients. Her vital signs—temperature, pulse, respiratory rate, and blood pressure—were taken every four hours, day and night. The nurses and aides were always running in and out; if it wasn't Evelyn's vital signs being taken, it was someone else's. The treatment begun at home and in the emergency room was continued. But an important component of that treatment—rest—was being neglected.

By the next day Evelyn, who had hardly slept now for several days (a fact which everyone had overlooked), was more confused. The treatment for heart failure continued, and plans were made to do the studies that would shed light on the list of identified problems, all of which represented stable, "underlying" causes rather than variable causes such as stress, fatigue, and disorientation.

The next morning Evelyn went to the X-ray department for plain films of her skull and a repeat chest X ray. While she was

there a phonocardiogram (sound analysis) and an echocardio-
gram (sound picture) of her heart were performed. She then
went to the nuclear-medicine department for a brain scan. The
brain scan gives a picture of the distribution in the brain of an
intravenously injected radioactive solution. Following this was
an electroencephalogram. S. missed her on his rounds because
she was getting these studies. Sadly, but predictably, none of
the studies added much to what was already known. They had
been motivated by the hope of an unexpected breakthrough
and the need to avoid future regret.

By evening Evelyn looked much worse: increasing shortness
of breath, confusion, irritability. In her lucid moments she
complained of pain in her back. The original intern being off
that night, the house officers on call, fearful that she would die,
asked and received S.'s permission by phone to do three things.
They wanted to tap her chest with a needle to draw off the fluid
in the pleural cavity which was compressing her lung, and
then to give her morphine, an old remedy for pulmonary
edema. Morphine was a two-edged sword. It could relieve the
sense of suffocation; it also depressed the drive to breathe. So
while it helped with one problem, it left another in its wake.
Hence the third request—if necessary, to pass a tube, which
would then be attached to a mechanical respirator, through her
mouth into her airway.

In addition to the symptoms observed by the house officers,
there were ominous changes in the electrocardiogram. These
signaled a malfunction in the rhythm of the heart, likely due
in large part to a toxic reaction to the digitalis, although so
many things were now happening that it was hard to quantify
the contribution of each. If not dealt with, this dysfunction
could lead to heart standstill or to ventricular fibrillation—a
rapid quivering action of the heart which renders it ineffectual
in pumping blood and unable to sustain life. This dysrhythmia
had to be treated, so the drug lidocaine was administered intravenously. It quieted down the heart, but also irritated Evelyn's brain, so that she became more confused. Because she
looked so bad, her vital signs were now ordered hourly—
whether or not she was sleeping at the time. She was also
moved to a small single room near the nurses' station so she

could be watched more closely. The room had no windows or plants. The contrast between her new "home" and her old apartment couldn't have been more striking. The change would have been disorienting even to a younger person with intact senses and mind, yet none of the tests that the house officers relied on could measure its impact. An *experimentum crucis* cannot measure the fluctuation of feelings, including those caused by the experiment.

While the hospital functioned efficiently and smoothly, S. couldn't help being struck by the succession of new faces, every eight hours, who tended to his patient. He barely knew them himself. How must it have been for someone in Evelyn's condition? When did visits become visitations?

Evelyn's deteriorating condition made it necessary to increase the frequency of blood sampling from her veins to monitor her changing chemistries. Since respiration was becoming an issue, blood had to be taken from the artery in her wrist to measure oxygen levels. Each puncture made Evelyn wince. Sometimes she had to be stuck several times to draw blood. Her bruised arms told the story.

By now Evelyn was moaning and restless. It appeared likely that she was having a reaction to the morphine. So she was given a morphine antagonist, which, while it could reverse the effects of morphine on her consciousness, could also depress the respiratory drive in its own right and therefore make mechanical respiration more likely.

That night S. spoke to Florence Peterson on the phone. She expressed confusion, anger, and concern. "She looks much worse. I can't for the life of me understand why a woman that age has to be subjected to all those tests. She's exhausted. Why can't they just leave her alone to rest?" Florence's words echoed S.'s concerns and spurred him to honor his own inclinations. Things had gotten out of hand.

The next morning S. found Evelyn wildly thrashing. She had knocked away the oxygen mask. She only half knew where she was.

Finally S. acted. Turning off the oxygen and the room lights, he told the technician who came to draw blood that he had changed his mind. He sat down next to the old woman and asked her where her back hurt. Then he rubbed her back, talking softly to her all the while. He told her what a good person she was and how much he enjoyed being her doctor. He told her that her heart was doing better (which it was) and that she just needed a chance to rest. Unlike some of the young nurses who, winking to each other at what seemed her childish complaints, tried to assure Evelyn that this or that wouldn't really hurt, he let her know he understood that she was suffering. Evelyn seemed to enjoy the back rub until finally she fell asleep.

S. had never done anything like this before. He, the doctor, was doing something that was normally left to nurses and aides, assuming they weren't too busy with vital signs and IV's. After all the technical work was done, he saw that a simple act was needed just to make the patient feel good. He took the responsibility of giving the back rub himself instead of delegating it to the staff. An hour of his time—the *doctor's* time—just being with a patient! The staff could take their cue from that.

While he was rubbing Evelyn's back, S. reflected on his feelings toward her, toward the house officers, toward himself. He realized that he had been ambivalent all along—on the one hand reluctant to tax Evelyn's meager strength, on the other hand afraid to "miss something." It really was a case of the left hand not knowing what the right was doing. Busy with other patients in other places, he had let fear and inertia gain the upper hand. Talking to Florence and actually seeing the state Evelyn was in had made him conscious of his mixed feelings. Had he still been ambivalent, he would have come down hard on the other side and thundered at the house officers for being callous and destructive. But it was hard to be angry at them when he recalled that he had gone along with their decisions. A system of thought and action that was bigger than all of them together had led people of goodwill—himself as well as the house officers—to do the wrong thing. Still, it wasn't enough to blame the system. The only way to counter its influence was to take responsibility. He would set the example.

Leaving Evelyn sleeping peacefully in her room, he ordered the digitalis temporarily stopped and reduced the frequency of vital signs to once every four hours. He gently reprimanded the house officers for their overzealousness, including himself prominently in the critique. He had been angry with these less experienced physicians, but he felt that he should deal with them as thoughtfully as he dealt with patients, and he knew that putting them on the defensive was not the way to help them learn. "We've done a good job so far with her heart failure," he explained. "She developed it over many months, and it will take a while to reverse it. Let's not rush things. She's an old woman who has been through a lot. She's tough. Look what she's survived. Now let's give her the day off. None of these neurological conditions you've been looking for are ones that we could or would treat anyway. There's a high cost to finding out about them, so why bother? Let's just let her have some ice chips, plenty of good nursing care, and visits from her friend Mrs. Peterson. Yes, she could die; whatever we do, we'll have to take that chance."

He was telling them frankly that this was a gamble, whatever course they chose. The gambling skill that the house officers best understood was that of avoiding the maximum loss (death). They would have to learn other skills in order to gamble well. House officers also had a limited time perspective, since they usually only saw patients during a brief crisis of acute illness. As Evelyn Dewey's family doctor S. was in a position to remind them that patients generally have a long life span before and after hospitalization.

It was only natural that the house officers exaggerated the importance of the tests and treatments they performed, as if these constituted an *experimentum crucis,* and were not fully aware of the duplication of procedures that often occurred. In the case of K., for example, to each month's new rotation of interns every fever K. ran called for a spinal tap. A family physician would have observed a succession of six spinal taps, each one further straining K.'s system without revealing anything new. Such a physician would have seen the cumulative effect of medical investigation on K.'s health, instead of assuming (as one who observed only one test could reasonably assume) that each test simply documented the child's condition without changing it. Yes, S. thought, it was tough to be just one person trying to temper the effects of a hospital machine that could continually throw fresh personnel into the breach. But being just one person had its advantages too. It gave one the perspective of continuity, which in turn made it possible to practice probabilistically.

After S. spoke to the house staff, an embarrassed intern apologized. "I had no idea she was ninety-one," she said. "She looked much younger, and I thought we had to go all out to pull her through." S. later wished that he had clarified the issue further, both to the intern and to himself. The intern was saying, in effect, "I didn't know you were just letting her die peacefully." The issue was not whether or not to try to save this patient. The issue was what course of action had the best chance of saving both her body and her soul. K. had been as young as Evelyn was old, and no one could say that the house officers had not "gone all out to pull him through."

S. had not then had the authority to turn off the hospital machine. Now he did. The machine was turned off.

In a way it seemed that the machine had come close to killing Evelyn. In a way it seemed that it had saved her life. For her condition improved, and after about ten days she was out of danger. The signs of heart failure were almost gone. Her weight had come down due to the loss of both retained water and accumulated fat. S. had observed that obesity was often a factor in the problems of the elderly. At her new weight Evelyn's heart, assisted by the digitalis and diuretics, had less work to do. He knew from experience that to have gotten her to lose weight preventively would have been next to impossible. In this respect, ironically, the trauma she had gone through had reinforced the beneficial effect of her medications.

S. made it a point to phone Florence daily during the critical period. It was the beginning of a working relationship that would result in her becoming a patient of his too. At first Florence felt embarrassed to have spoken up as she did. S. praised her for having done so. "You know her best. We value and need your opinion. People seem to think that doctors always know what to do. Well, as you see, we don't. We know how to use our machines, but don't always know whether to use them. We need help from the family. So keep on speaking up."

Florence made clear that what had sustained her in her advocacy was Evelyn's strong "will to go on." In the darkest moments she had cheered Evelyn on by telling her, "You're fighting for both of us."

S.'s relationship with Evelyn Dewey herself was a different matter. He regretted that he hadn't better prepared her for the hospital. In retrospect he knew just what he might have said: "I wish there were some way I could continue treating you at home. But none comes to mind. We gambled, and we lost. Now we'll have to gamble again by going to the hospital. I wish I could say that I'd be there all the time to look after you, but I can't. I'll be just one of many doctors there, and you'll be just one of many patients. We'll continue to gamble together, though we'll now be playing less and less according to rules of our own making. It will be easy for us to lose touch, to get lost in the shuffle of the machine, with its rules and its tempo, that is the hospital. Well-meaning people may perform test after test on you without explaining why. Sometimes you have to use your own good sense and say no to them, or at least ask questions when something they do doesn't make sense."

What could he say to her now, though? She might well have reason to doubt whether she still wanted to gamble with him as her doctor. He had to admit that he had made mistakes. Her judgment about what might happen to her in the hospital had been better than his. Now, however, given what he and she had learned together, he was in as good a position as anyone to help keep the hospital apparatus off her back.

S. felt a bit foolish rehearsing monologues for situations that had already happened or that would never happen. For now he would have no need to speak in serious terms with Evelyn Dewey. She was very easy to please these days, remembering as she did only what had happened the moment before (or, perhaps, a long, long time ago).

As Evelyn's physical condition improved, her mental deficit became more apparent. Her memory was much more impaired than at home, as were her attention and reasoning capacity. Heart failure, drugs, lack of sleep and nourishment, and the hospital environment all could have contributed to her disorientation. S. could not sort out the relative impact of each causal factor. But he knew from experience that to take a person with failing eyesight and reasoning out of her environment with its familiar cues—where she could see and understand things half from memory—would likely break down whatever it was in her that resisted final deterioration. In the hospital she would learn that she was going to be taken care of by others, like it or not. If she had any yearnings to make a meal for herself or put on her street clothes, she was judged to be "going crazy." If being denied these things made her cry, that, too, was "going crazy." What was there to do but go crazy?

Through her illness and hospitalization, Evelyn had suffered an irrevocable loss of independence. She had recovered physically; but, then again, all she ever did was get out of bed and sit in a chair by the window. Who could know whether her heart failure might reappear if she tried to do more? The very idea of "symptoms," he was reminded, was context dependent—the context here being one of very limited functioning. Asking whether Evelyn still had a heart problem was like asking whether a tree falling in an uninhabited forest made a sound.

In the months that followed, for a combination of medical, financial, and geographical reasons—and some plain old red tape—Evelyn Dewey was moved several times from one nursing home to another. She didn't seem to mind, though the moves were a strain on Florence, who had to make all the arrangements. At least Evelyn was able to get into a nursing home reasonably quickly, unlike many other elderly, chronically ill people for whom a nursing-home bed could not be found because it was not profitable for nursing homes to accept people on state assistance. The majority of these patients stayed in acute-care hospitals at enormous expense to the taxpayer, sometimes even forcing hospitals to turn away people who were in immediate need of acute medical care. At least Evelyn, as a widow without assets, was not in the position of elderly couples who were compelled to divorce so as to preserve what savings they had (or perhaps their home) and at the same time qualify for government aid for the ill partner. The irrationality and cost (in human and financial terms) of the system saddened S.

Ordinarily, as old people move around, they have to change doctors. S., however, remained with Evelyn throughout. At each new home he let the staff know that he was her doctor. In him and in Florence, he was telling them, their new charge had friends at court. S. was grateful for the opportunity to get to know Evvie (as he, like Florence, was now calling her), thereby "getting in on the tail end of a long life." The feelings he had for her, though, were mixed: "We've done it again. The miracles of modern medicine have saved another old person. But for what? What will her life be like now? A succession of nursing homes? What kind of life is that?"

In the heat of the struggle for life many an old patient had told him, "Let me die." How could he tell whether or not someone meant it? Though many survivors remained indifferent to the gift of renewed life, some were reinvigorated. What about the ninety-year-old woman who, after all but giving up on herself during a stormy six-week hospitalization, told S. during a home visit two months later that she was "on top of the world"?

S.'s first reaction was to doubt whether feelings and values could ever be interpreted as accurately as, say, lab tests. But a blood pressure reading taken under duress can be as misleading as a feeling insensitively registered. Both require care and attention; both require interpretation. A blood pressure out of context has as little meaning as a woman in labor screaming for pain medication or an elderly patient saying, "Doc, please let me die." Does that statement mean "Please take the pain away" or "I really want to die"? Does it express a stable preference or a momentary delirium? Given that people change their minds, is this patient changing her mind? A doctor who has known the patient in good times and bad, or who is consulting with members of the family, can often make a good judgment, just as a doctor with a good sense of pathophysiology can detect mechanical and procedural artifacts in lab results.

"Without a sense of context," S. reflected, "critical thinking is lost."

No wonder S. thought twice about hospitalization when he was called by the superintendent of a low-income housing project to see eighty-one-year-old Frank McMillan. What he found in the third-floor, walk-up apartment was a short, obese, disheveled, elderly man with massive swelling and redness of his legs from toes to hips. Serum oozed from sores on his inflamed shins. Mr. McMillan could not walk because of the pain in his legs, which he attributed to "joint trouble." Like Evelyn Dewey, he may have found the idea of arthritis a lot less scary than that of a heart condition. Unable to breathe when flat in bed, he had been sleeping upright in a chair for three weeks. One look told S. that Mr. McMillan was probably in advanced heart failure. One look was about all S. got, since he couldn't do an adequate examination without the patient's being able to lie down.

S.'s reflex reaction, even after all that had recently transpired, was to send this man immediately to the hospital. Mr. McMillan pleaded with S. to try to treat him at home. "It's Joe, my brother. He's mentally retarded," he said, gesturing toward a man standing in the doorway, who looked to be in his sixties. "There's no one to take care of him."

"Well," said S., "we agree that something has to be done. I think it's risky for you to stay at home. I can't get the information here in the house that I need in order to treat you effectively. I'd be taking a real chance myself to treat you without knowing more. You could get worse, you know. You could even get worse from any treatment I might prescribe, and I'd be to blame."

Those objections didn't impress Mr. McMillan, who again pleaded for care at home. "I'd just as soon die in my chair," he said.

S. thought back to Evelyn Dewey. "On the other hand," he said, "it's true there's a risk in going to the hospital too. And then there's your brother to consider."

For a moment S. seemed lost in thought. Mrs. Dewey's case was teaching him how the risks of staying home had to be balanced against the risks of going to the hospital. Elderly patients risked being harmed by procedures or drugs intended to help them—risks that became greater in the hospital setting. There the elderly were met with a great enthusiasm for diagnostic procedures which, while they might help in their care, could also drain their strength. They were exposed to microorganisms that often had become resistant to the usual antibiotics and therefore set up infections that were difficult to treat. In a strange environment they were vulnerable to disorientation and depression, especially at night. Their confusion itself then needed to be evaluated, resulting in more tests and procedures to determine its causes: whether a drug effect, a change in the salt concentration of the blood, and so forth—until the only explanation left was the change of environment itself.

S. continued, "You know, Mr. McMillan, it *is* a gamble either way. Thank you for reminding me. Seeing your swollen legs almost made me forget. Why, it's like betting the horses—that's what we're doing. I'll tell you what. I'll gamble with you at home for a week. I'll draw some blood, give you medicine to drain some of that fluid that's causing the swelling, and have the visiting nurse come tomorrow to take an EKG and begin to make other plans for your brother just in case you have to leave here. Is it a deal?"

When S. was satisfied that Mr. McMillan would do his best to get better at home, he shook hands with him and called it a deal. He then called someone from the Visiting Nurse Association and discussed with her how Mr. McMillan might be made more comfortable in his home.

S. could understand Mr. McMillan's feeling about his home. He himself felt comfortable there. Seeing patients in their homes made it easier for him to remember that he was (as the office and hospital settings sometimes led him to forget) a human being. Physicianship somehow had become hard to reconcile with humanity, as represented graphically by his own creature needs. When people offered him a cup of coffee, his professional upbringing cautioned him not to accept it. What an upbringing it had been! Years earlier, during his internship, while working in an intensive-care unit for newborn infants, he and other interns had been shamed into not eating and not going to the toilet, let alone sleeping, during their thirty-six-hour rotation stints. As if taking five minutes to attend to one's human needs was going to harm a baby. Everyone knew that it wouldn't, of course. But there was the tiniest hint of doubt, and in the world of the Mechanistic Paradigm that was enough.

In the home S. found it easier to be himself while also being a doctor. During the hours he spent at a home birth, for example, he ate, drank, used the toilet, took his shoes off, and sometimes even took a nap right there with his "patients." It was a relief for him to experience this kind of wholeness. All the same he had to concentrate on doing the things for which doctors are needed. He couldn't allow the informality to lull his judgment.

In the weeks that followed, Mr. McMillan (S. never felt comfortable calling him anything else) slowly improved. He did well enough to stay at home, thus saving Medicare $300 a day (the average daily cost of hospitalization for heart failure in that community in 1980) minus the modest reimbursements given to S. and the visiting nurse. Joe was able to go on living in the shelter of his brother's household, where he did the shopping and helped with the cleaning and dressing changes.

As S. gradually stepped up the medications, the swelling in Mr. McMillan's legs was reduced, and he felt better. He lost weight, though not as much weight as Mrs. Dewey had lost in a much shorter time. "How am I doing?" he kept asking Dr. S. He was delighted to hear that he was making satisfactory progress. "Let's keep going and keep an open mind on this," S. told him. "Call me if anything seems wrong to you."

The trouble was that S. never fully got him out of heart failure, as he had done with Evelyn Dewey. In the hospital Mr. McMillan would have been put on bed rest and oxygen, but at home, where he had more control, he refused to lie down on account of his breathing difficulty. Spared the acute crisis Evelyn had gone through, he remained more comfortable than she had been and for that very reason was less receptive to heroic measures. The home setting introduced its own bias—that of allowing the patient to live much as he always had. Influenced by that bias, S. did not wish to intensify the treatment very rapidly.

That autumn Mr. McMillan died in his sleep. He died peacefully in his home, in his chair, as had been his wish. It had not been his wish that his brother Joe be left alone to take care of himself. Contrary to his expectation, however, Joe at last report was still living in the apartment and was doing well on his own. Joe didn't want to have much to do with Dr. S., but from time to time S. asked the visiting nurse how he was coming along. He wished Frank McMillan could see his brother now.

*   *   *

People went to the hospital to be cured and stayed home to die. The hospital was set up primarily to save lives. Everything about the hospital made it possible for patients to believe that they were there to be cured, and that there was no other place where they could be cured. Outside the hospital it was difficult —psychologically as well as economically and culturally—to mobilize the resources needed to have the best chance of saving a life.

Evelyn Dewey and Frank McMillan were in some ways similar; neither of them wanted to die in a place where they wouldn't want to live. But Mr. McMillan unquestionably was more fatalistic about death than Mrs. Dewey. He expected to die, and there were some compromises he would not make to live. She "fought like hell" even in a situation that had its degrading aspects. It was likely that their expectations had affected not only their own internal resistance but the performance of the people who were caring for them. S. wondered if it would be stretching things too far to say that they both got what they were looking for.

Evelyn left the hospital with her life saved and her life at home ended. While it would be impossible to separate the effects of all the causal factors that operated on her in that setting, S. considered it probable that her heart had been strengthened by digitalis (which improved its contractions), diuretics (which drained her excess fluid), oxygen, and a salt-restricted diet. With the exception of an opportune weight loss, all of these factors would have been—in fact were—part of S.'s treatment plan on the basis of the physical examination, chest X ray, and EKG. Further testing failed to modify his original impression of Evelyn's condition. (He wished more doctors would follow the old medical-school adage, "If you hear hoof-beats, don't look for zebras.") In all likelihood the tests had created at least some of the abnormalities revealed by subsequent tests, and the remedies then applied had created further abnormalities to be remedied.

It is conceivable that the treatments that appeared to have worked for Evelyn could have been given her at home if proper support had been available there. But it was not available, as is often the case in our society. Evelyn was put in the hospital so that she could get the nursing care she couldn't get at home. One reason doctors put patients in the hospital is simply to have them rest and be taken care of. Often, though, it doesn't work out that way.

In the hospital it is easy for physicians (unless they stop and think about it) to perform unnecessary procedures simply because the means for doing so are readily available. In medicine as elsewhere, technology is used *because it is there.* Actually, diagnostic testing should be considered *less* necessary in the hospital than at home, because, with the patient under more or less constant observation and all necessary personnel and equipment at hand, the staff can respond much more quickly and effectively in the event of a complication. Less necessary —but still the machines are sitting there waiting to be used. And who would want to live with the regret of not having done an easily available test that had even the tiniest chance of providing lifesaving information?

In Evelyn's case S. had fallen into that way of thinking along with everyone else. In Mr. McMillan's case, too, he had reason to be self-critical. Perhaps he could have done more of the things for Mr. McMillan at home that apparently had been beneficial for Evelyn in the hospital. Why had he not increased the medications more rapidly? Why had he not worked harder to have Mr. McMillan agree to lie down for part of each day, with oxygen being administered during those hours to assist his breathing? Why had he not insisted that Mr. McMillan follow his diet and get more rest? Perhaps because with Mr. McMillan, in his own home, he hadn't had the power to insist —and hadn't had the time and the will to persuade the patient to act in his own best interest. Perhaps, too, it was because he himself had not been thinking critically.

There was no way to tell why one patient lived and the other died, or what judgments one might make about the way the one lived or the other died. They were two different people. Still, S. thought in retrospect that he had probably given too much treatment to the patient in the hospital and not enough to the patient at home. His decisions in each case had been influenced by reflex responses to the site, with all its customary associations. As a result, although both patients did a lot better than they might have elsewhere, it could be argued that neither received optimal care.

In the hospital S. had responded mainly to the acute aspects of the case; in the home he had responded mainly to the chronic. The home was not seen, by families or by doctors, as a comfortable setting for acute care. Like the hospital, it had its own tempo and its own rituals. In accepting both the hospital and the home on their own terms, had S. unwittingly accepted the assumption that scientific medicine could be practiced only in the hospital? Was there a way to practice scientific medicine at home without bringing the hospital into the home and making a family feel like strangers in their own house?

S. could envision alternatives, such as a kind of infirmary or halfway house that would offer hospitallike nursing care while being equipped to provide acute care when necessary. (Nursing homes often did not do this.) Given the choices available in the present, however, he would need to be aware—and to make others aware—of the large influence of site on medical decision-making. This awareness would help him make decisions that would be better both in context and in spite of the context. He now knew what a struggle it could be to maintain one's critical consciousness in a context that drew people in until they were simply overwhelmed.

This could happen both in the home and in the hospital. It was possible—and necessary—to think critically in either setting, and yet each setting contained special barriers to critical thinking. Nonetheless the two were not equivalent—not when all the forces of society and the dominant contemporary habits of thought and feeling drew people to the hospital and, once there, to mechanistic choices and procedures. S. would, of course, recommend home or hospital care to his patients in keeping with their wishes and with his own sense of what was medically appropriate. But to enable families to choose rationally between the home and the hospital, S. would often need to emphasize, as a balance against the force of the hospital habit, the values to be found in home care. To take a value-neutral position, when judgments are skewed by habit, is just to let habit run its course.

* * *

Critical thinking (and the welfare of his patients) also required that S. keep an open mind about medical technology and
use it to advantage when its use was called for. A case in which
he did so, while working in a hospital outpatient clinic, was
that of fifty-six-year-old Albert Riccola, whose daughter
brought him to the clinic for treatment of a severe headache
that had lasted for four days. S. was not the first doctor to see
Mr. Riccola on this occasion. One doctor had diagnosed mi-
graine and prescribed pills. Another, going by the patient's
unshaven appearance and history of heavy drinking, had concluded that his headache was caused by alcoholic withdrawal.
(He had in fact stopped drinking just when the headaches
began.) Still, his daughter was not satisfied. Speaking on her
father's behalf (since he spoke only Italian), she shared her
concern with S. "He isn't himself," she said. "He used to drink
every day, but he also used to shave every day."

S. wasn't satisfied, either. Noticing the visual contrast between the unkempt father and the well-groomed daughter, he
questioned why this man would suddenly depart from his habitual way of life. Why had he stopped drinking, let alone shav-
ing? Then there was the additional information that Mr. Riccola had suffered a minor head injury in an auto accident a
month before. Conscious of being tired and wanting to go home
(this was the day's last patient), S. determined that, in spite of
his mixed feelings, he would do a thorough neurological examination. To keep himself honest when he might otherwise have
been sloppy with fatigue, he took the precaution of getting the
patient's permission (through his daughter) to call in a medical
student and demonstrate to her the "standard" neurological
exam. Through this side bet he consciously proceeded to increase the odds that he would do a most thorough examination.

The first part of this procedure, the mental-status examination, involved speaking with the patient. With this patient S.
had to have the daughter translate the questions and answers.
Finding Mr. Riccola partially disoriented and exhibiting some
inappropriate judgment, he noticed as well that the daughter
seemed uncomfortable with her father's responses. Upon questioning her he was told that "he's making too many puns." This
S. would not have known, of course, since the puns were in

Italian. S. thought it worth noting that the patient was behaving contrary to the expectations of his daughter, who, after all, knew him well.

Continuing with the neurological exam, S. discovered very slight divergences in the orientation of the right and left eyes and the right and left toes. He could easily have overlooked these findings had he not committed himself to a meticulous exam by calling in the student. By now he was convinced that there was a good probability of a blood clot pressing on the brain (subdural hematoma), which had likely resulted from the auto accident injury but had only reached a critical stage in the past four days. This diagnosis was confirmed by an emergency X-ray test called a CT scan, which showed the pressure on the brain to be increasing to the point where death from massive brain damage was imminent. Mr. Riccola was immediately transferred to the operating room, where surgeons performed a simple procedure to relieve the pressure. A few days later he was his old self and was able to go home.

In this case S. gambled well by recognizing that the results of one gamble, carefully interpreted, could help him choose another gamble. Taking note of the fact that the patient's daughter was betting her time and effort that her father's strange behavior was worth bringing to a doctor's attention, S. gambled that it would be worth his time and effort to look to her as a source of useful information. This gamble produced information that he used in estimating the probable value of doing a careful neurological exam and making the side bet of calling in a medical student, which, since he prided himself on being not only a good doctor but also a good teacher, motivated him that much more. That gamble in turn produced information that led to his doing a CT scan. In this series of successful gambles each gamble changed the odds for the next. Such a series of principled gambles, under the Probabilistic Paradigm, is what scientific experimentation is all about.

Ironically, a CT scan was one of the tests unnecessarily performed on K. This time, however, there were good reasons for choosing to perform the test. In the case of K., where technology was used mindlessly, a life was lost. In the case of Albert Riccola, where technology was used critically, a life was saved. In the one case critical thinking enabled S. to make use of "soft" data (parental neglect) where other doctors looked only for "hard" data (organically based immune deficiency). In the other case critical thinking enabled S. to discover "hard" data (blood clot) where other doctors saw only "soft" data (alcoholism). In the one case S. focused on a kind of causation that could best be observed in the home; in the other he focused on a kind of causation that could best be observed in the hospital. In K.'s case, the hospital setting extinguished critical thinking; in Albert Riccola's case critical thinking put the hospital resources to appropriate use.

15

CAN IT WORK?

S.'s experience in practicing under the two paradigms of medicine had led him to believe that if medicine were to speak the truth in the twentieth century, it would need to speak in probabilistic terms. By facing uncertainty and thinking critically together, patients and doctors could build trust and thereby gamble cooperatively. Out of uncertainty they could create probabilities. S. had seen it happen in his practice; he had felt the excitement of people gaining some control over their lives—some of the time.

He had seen it happen both at the extremes of human experience, as with Mrs. Gormley's death and Roberta and Bob's home birth, and when dealing with mundane and everyday situations. He had seen it happen under difficult circumstances (and with only partial success) in the care that Joe McMillan gave his brother and that Florence Peterson gave her friend Evelyn Dewey. In all of these cases what the patients and families did made a real difference for all concerned, including S. Yet most of the time this wasn't what doctors and patients did. Even S. and his patients weren't applying the new paradigm as much as he would have wished.

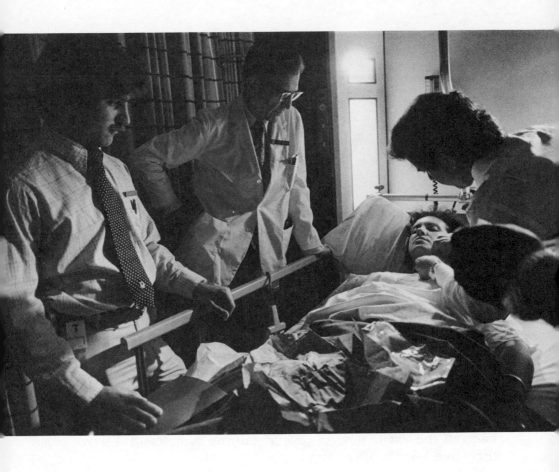

S. realized that his practice was a very imperfect approximation of what he wanted it to be. The same was true of the physicians he recommended when patients asked, "Are there any other doctors who do this?" Why weren't there more physicians and patients who acknowledged uncertainty and made use of probabilities?

It came down to the fact that he, like other doctors, did not practice in a vacuum. He practiced within certain established contexts—the context of widely held beliefs and attitudes, the context of a particular medical system, a particular legal system, the context of limited resources, the context of a way of organizing the production and consumption of goods. In any society a way of thinking supports and is supported by a way of feeling and a way of acting. In our society, as S. was well aware, a way of thinking (the Mechanistic Paradigm), a way of feeling (unconscious fear and denial), and a way of acting (the quest for profit and power) reinforce one another. The barriers to probabilistic thinking that are set up in the workplace and the marketplace make for considerable resistance to the kind of practice S. and his patients were engaged in.

The Limits of Choice

The Probabilistic Paradigm both requires and enables people to make informed choices under conditions of uncertainty. When S. practiced probabilistically, he and his patients made choices together. He viewed much of his work as a process of learning and teaching others how to make informed choices. Yet it seemed that certain choices were almost always closed off. Could people choose to move out of a tenement where their children were subjected to lead-paint poisoning? They might have a choice about whether or not to use the electronic fetal monitor, but they had no choice about whether the monitor was developed, whether their local hospital purchased it, and whether it was overused—all of which decisions would affect their medical bills and insurance rates. Did they have any choice about the stress-related morbidity and mortality fostered by workplaces designed mainly to maximize profits regardless of potential human cost? (Eyer and Sterling, 1977)

S. remembered Mrs. Pinelli, the woman who went through a painful, expensive hypertensive workup that proved to be (and could have been predicted to be) useless. It is not surprising that Mrs. Pinelli failed to make an informed choice. Nothing in her experience as a compliant worker and consumer had prepared her to think critically about the choices she faced concerning her health. She grew up in a society that is not committed to educating people to think critically. At the very most she received "consumer education" in school and from magazines which taught her how to shop intelligently and get the most for her dollar. But this education did not keep her from "buying" the heavily advertised claim that the complete workup was "the best medical care money can buy."

Since probabilistic thinking was strange and foreign to Mrs. Pinelli, Dr. S.'s attempt to introduce her to it was made possible only through a medical student's availability and willingness to donate her time. The exploration of options begun by the student might have led Mrs. Pinelli to forgo the complete workup, thus saving her much pain and her insurance company the cost of both the tests themselves and the days of hospitalization they entailed. But no insurance company was yet willing to invest in the educational process necessary to bring Mrs. Pinelli to the point of making an informed choice. Indeed, in a fee-for-service system the doctor, the hospital, and all their supporting cast stood to profit more by doing *more*, not by doing less. While it is hard to assess the precise impact of this unstated fact on Mrs. Pinelli's decision, it is equally hard to deny that it existed.

It wasn't only Mrs. Pinelli whose choices were limited. S. would have been able to make different choices in treating her if society (through its various reimbursement plans) had placed a higher value on patient education and shared decision-making. As it was, S. was not reimbursed at all for teaching people to think critically and was inadequately reimbursed for many of the things he did in support of people who tried to think critically. He was handsomely remunerated for giving an anesthetic to a woman in labor, but not for working with the woman so that she could handle her uterine contractions without requiring an anesthetic. He could spend an unremunerated hour dissuading a family from transferring an elderly, terminally ill relative from a nursing home to a costly acute-care hospital, while at that same hospital a doctor could make hundreds of dollars in much less time by performing a life-prolonging maneuver such as placing the patient on a respirator. Although the system would pay for Mabel Gormley to be kept breathing by technology, it would not provide as well for her to be given a little "tender loving care" so that she could die in peace and comfort.

Doctors were well aware of the financial advantage to be gained from hospitalizing patients or by performing reimbursable technical procedures in the office. The bias of the legal system also lay in the direction of encouraging the use of expensive, highly profitable technology. A doctor was far more likely to be sued for doing too little than for doing too much. By the same token, practicing "defensive medicine" often meant doing the very things that were profitable to do anyway. So when patients asked S., "Why can't I find other doctors who practice the way you do?" he could have given them more than one reason.

The limitations placed on the choices made by doctors also affected the choices available to patients and families. People could not choose a type of care that no doctors were willing to give. Moreover, people would have to think twice about choosing a type of care for which their doctor would not be reimbursed, since they would have to pay for such care out of pocket. Roberta and Bob's health insurance paid S.'s fee, since S. in "delivering" the baby was thought to be "doing" something. But this insurance policy (which would have paid for a fetal monitor and a team of nurses in the hospital) did not pay for Roberta to be monitored by a birth attendant at home. She and Bob had to make a significant financial sacrifice for a choice that saved their insurance company and its subscribers all the usual costs of a hospital birth (costs that in 1980 averaged $500 per day). Not every family could afford that choice. Mrs. Gormley's family saved their insurance company thousands of dollars by giving the dying woman family care instead of professional and machine care. But not every family could afford to give so much time without compensation.

Finally the hospital itself was not reimbursed for maintaining the backup facilities which patients in Mabel Gormley's or Roberta Johnson's position would occasionally need. If the patient did not *actually use* the facilities, the hospital did not get a cent. It was only natural, then, that hospitals and their personnel were geared toward bringing people into the hospital to be put through the technical procedures for which the reimbursement system was primed to pay.

S. wanted his patients to understand the contexts—economic, political, ethical—in which he and they made decisions, for by understanding, they could perhaps make better decisions. He wanted to tell them about the conditions that constrained their choices—if there was time to tell them, and if it would do any good. Whenever Mrs. Pinelli sat in the office with him during one of her monthly blood pressure checks, he wondered how he could explain it all to her. He wished he could tell her, "You wanted the arteriogram in part because your experience in your bookkeeping job and elsewhere in life has led you to believe that the way to solve problems is by one simple technical operation. On top of that the residents and nurses in the hospital were all telling you that you ought to have the arteriogram 'so you'll be sure.' You see, they face the same kinds of pressures on the job that you do, and they learn the same things. They're afraid *not* to do a procedure that promises to give them certainty. And indeed, the arteriogram does have one outcome that is certain: someone will profit from it; for there is profit in the search for certainty by technical means. And the quest for profit itself reflects a way of thinking in which some single, measurable goal can be exalted over all else. It all fits together in an often jumbled, yet interlocking system, and it's up to us to find a way out of it."

He wanted to tell her these things, but it would have taken his time and her time. They both had other things to do in that time —things that they were being paid to do. Besides, it was all he could do to explain the medication dosages to her so that she wouldn't come in hypotensive (i.e., with her blood pressure abnormally lowered) from taking too much. As S. was learning, there were formidable problems in expecting a patient to use a paradigm in medicine that she wasn't trained or encouraged to use anywhere else.

Sometimes S. did give patients the kind of explanation that he did not attempt with Mrs. Pinelli. For example, when he was treating a so-called hyperactive child, he thought it only responsible to tell the parents, "If you were wealthy, we could do more for your child. We could put him in a school with smaller classes where he would get more personal attention—which certainly won't happen in your public school. But few of us can be wealthy, and so the most we can now do is to give a drug like Ritalin, or experiment with diet or with teaching the child out of school. But these measures do not substitute for the changes in the child's environment that we all too often don't have the power to make. It's the best we can do under the circumstances, but you ought to be aware that under other circumstances we could do something better."

This was what he said when he wasn't too busy or too tired or too overwhelmed, and when he thought that the patient could understand and respond to the information. As a family doctor S. saw patients who differed greatly in their knowledge, intelligence, income, family structure, ethnic background, and ability to speak English. He saw elderly people who had trouble getting to the office, dressing and undressing for examinations, and remembering instructions for taking medication. Some of his patients had no idea what a family doctor was. Some felt a much greater need for certainty than did others. Some were aggressive "consumers" of health care or self-care zealots who acted as if they didn't need a doctor at all, while others were enlightened skeptics who didn't need S. to teach them to think critically. These factors, too, affected people's capacity and willingness to gamble.

The Workplace and the
Marketplace of Medicine

The habits people acquired in the workplace and the marketplace did not magically disappear at the door of S.'s office or the hospital admitting room, for these were also workplaces and marketplaces. Medicine is business—big business. S. had been a hospital corporation employee and was now in business for himself. His patients assumed themselves to be consumers, although S. tried to work with them in such a way that they would come to see themselves as more than that.

Yet S. was part of the system too. He was earning a living, and he was also a consumer. Everything from the clothes he wore to work to the prescription pad given him by the drug salesman were tools of his trade which he consumed as he worked. Practicing one of the most profitable occupations in a profit-seeking society, he could not help but be concerned with the economics of his practice. His work, too, was being done for profit as well as principle. Under the circumstances he sometimes found himself shaking his head and saying to himself, "How can it work when it doesn't pay?"

When S. went into practice, he took on all the responsibilities and details of running a small business that was open twenty-four hours a day. He saw, for example, that although he was paid (either by the patient or a third party) for time spent face to face with patients, much of what he did for patients was done behind the scenes. Driving to and from patients' homes and hospitals, reviewing laboratory results, updating medical records, speaking with patients and their families on the telephone, conferring with specialist consultants, doing the paperwork required to support the visiting nurses in their care of homebound patients—these he considered essential services, but from a business point of view they constituted red tape. He estimated that only about sixty percent of the time he spent on the job was billable. In order to cover his expenses (office space and personnel, answering service, etc.), he had to charge a fee for each of those billable hours that made it difficult for the poor to use his practice. He could not survive in business, for example, if any more than a small proportion of his patients were covered only by Medicaid, the federal-state health insurance for low-income people. For a doctor who went into practice to serve the community, this was a sobering realization.

What made it all worthwhile was that he was his own boss, at least to the extent that such freedom was still possible. Within the constraints of professional standards, relationships with colleagues, and economic necessities, he was free to serve his patients as he and they saw fit. The autonomy and control he gained by being in private practice translated into more choices for patients and families. If there were to be only one type of medical care that a doctor could practice, someone like Mrs. Gormley might not be able to die at home, and couples like Bob and Roberta might not be able to have their baby at home. If there were only one type of medical care available, and if everyone worked for the same corporate bureaucracy, S. could easily envision the existence of "company rules" that would constrain medical choices even further.

When he thought back to the case of K., S. remembered the residents and interns, all of them good, compassionate people, as compliant assembly-line workers tending their single-purpose diagnostic machines. K. was passed down the assembly line, with each machine recording its one result. And if the need for certainty on the part of the institution and the individuals involved weren't enough to ensure that K. would get this mechanistic treatment, the corporation's earnings were directly proportional to the length of time K. remained in the hospital and the number of procedures performed on him.

If the case of K. is any indication, the hospital is much like a factory, where work done by machines (i.e., requiring a large investment of capital) is currently more profitable than work done by people (i.e., requiring a large investment of labor). The hospital worker finds his job to be a routine, attending to machines rather than critically using machines to care for people. Whether in using expensive computer axial tomography in place of a thorough neurological exam to rule out possible life-threatening causes of a prolonged headache, or in treating a patient with a bone infection by giving intravenous antibiotics for six weeks in the hospital instead of giving the medication as a pill at home with comparable effectiveness at a fraction of the cost, the bias generally favors expensive, profitable technology. Thus K. Thus Mrs. Pinelli. Thus Evelyn Dewey.

Even though the profit motive is not always in the foreground, this is not to say that it is not always there. It *was* clearly in the foreground, S. found, in some private community hospitals set up as profit-making businesses. There the staff actually made diagnostic and treatment decisions with an eye toward performing the more profitable procedures. This was not how decisions were made in the academic teaching hospitals where S. worked (the ones where K., Mrs. Pinelli, and Mrs. Dewey were treated). These hospitals, while themselves non-profit organizations, were connected with other institutions (such as drug companies and equipment manufacturers), which profited by their activities. Here the profit motive was served indirectly, through the mechanistic standard of certainty to which the staff was trained to aspire. Engaged in what they saw as the pursuit of truth for humanitarian ends, physicians in the teaching hospitals often ended up performing the same unnecessary procedures which in the private hospitals were motivated by outright greed. Still, "often" is not "always," and misguided idealism is not synonymous with unprincipled self-seeking—which was why S. felt more comfortable in the academic hospital complex (when the services of a hospital were needed at all).

In the medical industry that coexisted with the Mechanistic Paradigm the "need" for certainty insured a "need" for specialized technology, which in turn created a "need" for specialized settings and personnel. (In places where people still got along without these things, an "unmet need" was considered to exist.) If something had to be done with specialized equipment in the hospital, then S. was not the doctor who could do it; somebody else would get the "business." The view that birth, for example, always needed such specialized attention was one with which S., along with couples like Bob and Roberta, disagreed.

S. liked to think of his practice as an alternative to assembly-line medicine—that is, to the anonymity and fragmentation of care that demoralized patients. Yet his practice was tied into the system in a relationship that was in part cooperative, in part antagonistic. S. couldn't do everything himself. He needed the hospital in cases where he did have to call in specialized equipment and highly trained personnel. When he did his neurological examination on the man with the blood clot in the brain, he was thankful that there was such a thing as a CT scan and that surgeons were on call to operate on a few minutes' notice. When a woman about to give birth needed to rest after hours of unproductive labor, he saw how much it meant to be able to bring her to the hospital, sedate her, and keep her under observation while she slept (with the personnel and equipment needed for a possible cesarean section right at hand) in the hope that when she awoke, she would be able to complete a normal vaginal birth. Part of what S. offered his patients, in fact, was the availability of these backup resources and his ability to use them critically and effectively.

Typically, though, patients were pulled into the system as if on a conveyor belt, with neither the patient nor S. having a chance to think critically about the procedures and consultations the patient needed. Mrs. Pinelli was drawn in like a helpless swimmer in an undertow. In her case a specialist physician (S.'s friend, to boot) thought it perfectly natural to assume control of the case from S. and then to relinquish control to the anonymous hospital personnel who ended up having the greatest influence on the patient's decision. Rose Heifetz would be thought of as more sophisticated than Mrs. Pinelli, but sophistication for her meant being acquainted with specialists whom she could see without going through a "middleman" like S. It was hard to win a tug of war with an assembly line.

When Does a Heart Beat Too Slowly?

Patients and their families gave up some control when they went from their homes to the doctor's office; they gave up more control when they went to the hospital. It was with considerable misgivings, therefore, that S. observed yet another level of centralization of medical-care facilities: the regional specialty center, where several institutions joined forces to create a facility or group of facilities gathering together the most prestigious personnel and the most up-to-date equipment for treating a particular condition. This was done with the laudable aim of sharing experience and making the best use of scarce resources for the benefit of patients. However, it also had the effect of limiting the diversity of options and thereby limiting choice for patients, families, and physicians. There was talk, for example, of setting up a regional birth center that would handle all births for people living within a radius of fifty miles. How would Bob and Roberta (let alone S. himself) fit into those plans?

It was in dealing with such medical "conglomerates," sometimes operating unobtrusively within the walls of familiar hospitals, that S. felt most strongly the impotence of the outsider. A case in point was that of a baby born with bradycardia (slow heartbeat) after a normal pregnancy, labor, and delivery (with mild analgesia). S., who was covering for another physician, did not know the family. Called to the hospital to evaluate the baby's condition in the light of the irregularity, S. found nothing abnormal. The baby's heart rate was indeed slow, but it was the same as that of ten percent of all normal babies, and the baby on examination was otherwise healthy and acted normally. Nonetheless unwritten hospital rules (recall Eleanor Perk's "company policy" from Chapter 4) required that the baby be placed on a heart monitor in a special-care nursery, and the nurses indicated that they would not be comfortable deviating from the rules.

S. could read the confusion and anxiety on the faces of the baby's parents. Here he was telling them that nothing was wrong with the baby, yet how could they trust him when they did not know him and the nurses were telling them just the opposite? Whom were they to believe? Just seeing their baby hooked up to a monitor was enough to make the parents worry, and if they worried long enough, they would "want" the baby on the monitor.

In the days that followed, S. tried to have the baby taken off the monitor. By this time the baby's grandmother had mentioned that each of the baby's uncles had been born with the same slow heart rate and none was the worse for it. Meanwhile, though, on the instructions of the chief nurse, the ward nurses had bolstered their position by consulting with a pediatric cardiologist at a nearby hospital. They did this without notifying S., who was at the time the responsible physician. Finally S. contacted the cardiologist directly and, mentioning the baby's normal X ray and electrocardiogram, asked him to look at the baby himself. After being examined and found normal by the cardiologist, the baby was discharged. Through an appeal to machines and institutional authority S. was able to turn off the machine that institutional authority had turned on. "We're glad he called in the cardiologist," said one nurse to another. "We wouldn't have wanted that baby to suddenly die on us."

Who had turned on the machine in the first place? It was not easy to assign responsibility. Several hospitals in the area had merged their neonatal departments with the announced intention of achieving "shared knowledge and coordinated high-level decision-making." What it also achieved, intentionally or not, was absentee authority, remote from and unaccountable to patients, families, and physicians. The lines of communication connecting the various poles of invisible authority ran mainly through the nurses, who were encouraged to "play a greater role in decision-making by consulting with their superiors and freely contacting appropriate personnel at the partner institutions."

It is true that nurses in hospitals generally are not given the chance to think critically and make decisions to the extent that they are capable. Rectifying this discrimination may have been one of the aims of the administrators of the merged program. Whatever their intentions, their actions had the effect of limiting the authority of physicians by implementing policy through highly specialized nurses, who as hospital employees with fewer outside job opportunities were more amenable than physicians to the dictates of the institution. These nurses were a new breed, a breed whose skills were so closely matched to the machines with which they worked that they could not survive outside the temples of high technology. One found many different species of specialists in these temples, all of whom depended for their living on their ability to function smoothly, to follow the rules rather than assume individual responsibility.

A patient or family member or private physician can argue with a staff physician. But how can one argue with a nurse, who, like the minor bureaucrats who appear in Kafka's *The Trial,* has no authority but merely fronts for authority? As in *The Trial* the authority set up by regional medical centers was so diffuse, with no clear chain of command or stated procedures, as to be invulnerable to appeals to reason, principle, or the legitimate authority of experienced and knowledgeable people. Unless, that is, someone put himself out and "made a stink" as S. did. The hospitals were willing to yield in such cases, which were few and far between. After all, they didn't want people to think them authoritarian.

Formula for Consumption

Hospitals and megahospitals were not the only corporate institutions that influenced doctors' and patients' decisions behind the scenes. S. was well aware of the far-reaching power of the drug companies, who subsidized medical journals with their advertisements and who were reaching out with educational programs for doctors on "gaining patient compliance." The drug companies' success in gaining compliance from patients and doctors alike was not lost on other commercial suppliers, for instance the manufacturers of infant feeding formulas.

In 1978 the American Academy of Pediatrics' authoritative Committee on Nutrition issued a set of recommendations concerning infant feeding. Among them were the following: (1) breast-feeding is superior to bottle-feeding both for the mother (in terms of minimizing postpartum bleeding and getting the uterus to contract) and for the baby (in terms of reducing infection and supplying appropriate nutrients); (2) babies should be kept on bottled formula (or, of course, breast milk if it is still being given) up to the age of one year instead of six months as previously recommended, since the formula (which is designed to resemble breast milk) is better for babies than whole (cow's) milk. This recommendation was based on reports that whole milk, with its higher concentration of salt and certain kinds of proteins, may cause allergies and gastrointestinal bleeding in some infants.

For S. the committee's statement was remarkable for what it did not say. Its findings were presented as "scientific data," with no mention of the political or economic context. Actually the committee's first recommendation had already taken place in practice, and the committee was in effect ratifying a shift in society's values. Thirty years earlier breast-feeding had been opposed by most physicians and nurses, who did everything they could to discourage the practice. The La Leche League, a society of breast-feeding mothers, was founded at that time to promote breast-feeding in the face of opposition. For a generation "the data" had dictated bottle-feeding; now suddenly "the data" dictated breast-feeding.

As for the second recommendation, in S.'s view the findings cited did not justify it. The studies of formula versus whole milk between the ages of six months and a year were isolated case histories with no probability factor. S. granted that some babies would show increased sensitivity to some of the ingredients of whole milk. But how many? What were the risks for an otherwise healthy six-month-old? If adverse effects occurred, were they irreversible, or could they be eliminated simply by switching to formula once the baby's inability to tolerate whole milk became evident? It was not even made clear whether the infants studied were over six months old.

The economic implications of the new policy were considerable for both the consumers and producers of commercially prepared formula. Families would be spending more for formula than for whole milk. And their money would be going into different pockets. Formula manufacturers had been suffering a steady loss of their market as a result of the return to breast-feeding. What a fortunate coincidence for them that just when the relevant branch of the medical profession (with whom, it must be added, they had close ties in research and development) officially sanctioned breast-feeding, it also advised

women who did not breast-feed for a full year to continue buying formula for another six months. Now the market that was
being lost in one place could be regained in another.

Because the committee's policy represented a departure
from past recommendations, it embarked upon an educational
program for pediatricians, family-practice physicians, nurse
practitioners, and others in a position to influence people's
decisions concerning infant feeding. The program included direct mailings, announcements in journals, courses for which
physicians received continuing education credit, speaking
tours by prominent physicians and nutritionists, and national
closed-circuit television presentations with telephone hookup
for questions—all underwritten by the formula manufacturers.
A major theme of the presentations was "Problems of Management and Compliance." What, for example, should a doctor do
with a mother who, having started her first two children on
whole milk at six months with no apparent adverse effects,
didn't see why she should treat her third child any differently?
The speakers and brochures advised the doctor to be "supportive," to build an alliance, to use communication skills, to present the new information in a nonthreatening way, to avoid
arousing guilt, and so forth. The goal, however, was to achieve
compliance, not to interpret the data (including the family history of successful feeding with whole milk) with the mother so
that she could make her own choice.

The latter course was the one S. tried to take. Except in cases
where abnormalities in the baby's condition or family history
suggested a greater-than-usual risk of complications from
using whole milk, he told parents, "The advice that's being
officially given now is not to start whole milk until the baby is
a year old. To my mind the evidence on this point is not clear.
I don't know of any harm that would result if you gave the baby
whole milk after six months and then switched back to prepared formula if problems developed. And I ought to tell you
that the companies that make the formulas have a vested interest in pushing the official line. The choice is yours to make."
Although he did not see much likelihood in his being able to
counter such a well-organized, well-financed campaign, he
began writing letters to the American Academy of Pediatrics as

well as to independent research organizations in an effort to clarify the scientific basis for the new recommendations.

The necessity for making the choice, S. reflected, had been created by the omnipresent partnership between big business and institutionalized medicine.

Amending the Mechanistic Constitution

The Mechanistic Paradigm, together with the form that people's relationships tend to take in conjunction with it (power-oriented, profit-oriented, exchange rather than communal), can be thought of as a kind of "constitution" under which doctors and patients practice. Under this constitution doctors and patients avoid feeling uncertain about each other by setting up relationships that have a hierarchical, authoritarian quality, with the doctor and patient playing rigidly defined roles. This kind of relationship fits in well with the rest of mechanistic practice—the assumption that the diagnosis should determine the treatment, the belief that there is one "objectively" right thing to do, and so forth.

It does not fit in well with the needs of our time. Since World War II people have been less and less willing to defer to their doctors. Malpractice suits, outrage over the high cost of medical care, rejection of orthodox medicine in favor of holistic medicine and self-care, and the demand for patients' rights are signs that the mechanistic medical constitution is breaking down. For their part concerned physicians and other health professionals have come up with various "amendments" which introduce some flexibility and responsiveness into the mechanistic constitution. These amendments have made it less likely (though not impossible, as we have seen) for what happened to K. to happen to others. From the perspective of the history of science, however, they represent the same kind of tinkering that physicists did in the late nineteenth and early twentieth centuries in an attempt to save the Mechanistic Paradigm. Such amendments stretch the paradigm so as to enable it to solve particular problems, but they are cumbersome. Although in medicine they have sometimes made it possible for patients' needs to be met and for doctors to practice in a more humane, value-sensitive way, these patchwork devices are themselves undermined by the assumptions of the paradigm onto which they have been grafted. Their significance lies chiefly in that they portend a shift to the Probabilistic Paradigm.

Even the notion of *compliance* (discussed in Chapter 11), chilling as it is, amends the Mechanistic Paradigm by challenging the deterministic assumption that if medicine has been prescribed, it has therefore been taken. It recognizes (albeit grudgingly) that human beings, having a range of feelings, values, and attitudes, are capable of making choices. Nonetheless the compliance model, by failing to recognize that there are sometimes good reasons for disregarding instructions, places a pejorative connotation on the human capacity to choose different courses of action. It has mobilized doctors, backed by drug companies, to work harder at achieving the kind of control allotted to them under the mechanistic constitution.

Other amendments, while not always very effectual, have had the more constructive purpose of legitimizing the exercise of decision-making power by patients and families. The term *informed consent* is used to describe the requirement that a doctor inform the patient (within reason) of the available options and the risks of each. The weakness of this concept lies in the word *consent,* which implies a passive consumer accepting options that the doctor (like a car dealer) presents, rather than participating in creating the options. The words *informed choice* better describe the scientific gambling that patients and doctors under the Probabilistic Paradigm must do together. The *patient advocate* is a new breed of hospital employee who handles complaints and mediates between the patient and the hospital staff. The patient advocate role was created in recognition of the fact that many patients no longer have family doctors or even families to look out for their interests—and in recognition of the fact that medicine has become, like the law, all too often an adversary system. In practice, even with the best of intentions on the part of the hospital, a hospital employee cannot feel fully free to raise issues that may challenge the economic base on which his or her livelihood depends. The *patient's bill of rights,* which is sometimes written into hospital policy or even state law, includes such guarantees as privacy, informed consent, and itemized billing. It is undoubtedly a useful protection as well as a comfort for many people. It might be more useful (and would better reflect a relationship of equality between doctor and patient) if it were accompanied by a bill of responsibilities for patients and a bill of rights for doctors and hospitals. These additions would make clear that patients are participants rather than consumers, and that doctors and hospitals do not retain (as might be assumed under the Mechanistic Paradigm) all rights and powers not specifically given to patients in the patient's bill of rights. The *living will* enables people to specify in writing how they wish to be treated (especially with regard to the use of life-sustaining technology) in the event that they should become terminally ill and unable to communicate. Given the misinterpretations (unintentional and otherwise) that occur routinely with written documents, a living will is most likely to be effective in the context of shared experience, shared expectations, and a shared approach to decision-making among patient, family, and physician. In such a context the written instructions clarify and are clarified by the understanding that exists among the parties (Bursztajn, 1977). What is true of the living will applies as well to all of the "amendments" we have considered. In the context of interpretation supplied by the Mechanistic Paradigm (the context that exists at present) their effectiveness is compromised, their purpose distorted. In a different context—that of the Probabilistic Paradigm—they would be both more useful and less necessary.

S. wanted to help establish that context. Instead of more amendments to the mechanistic constitution, he wanted there to be a new constitution, a new paradigm. His goal, the purpose that gave direction to his work, was the wise use of the Probabilistic Paradigm as a basis for decision-making—first in medicine, and then throughout life. He realized, however, that even the most thoroughgoing attempts to reshape medical relationships and procedures in accordance with the Probabilistic Paradigm might simply produce more amendments to the existing structure of thought, feeling, and action. As long as the Mechanistic Paradigm both governed and was supported by the political and economic relationships by which society functioned, medicine could not stand alone as a place in which people dealt with one another with trust, openness, equality, and a willingness to face the unknown. And though he would have liked to think that there was some prospect of the kind of general social and economic change that would be motivated by the use of the Probabilistic Paradigm, he was pessimistic about the chances of its happening in his lifetime.

Still, it was worth a try, beginning in medicine. He started by sketching out the implications of the paradigm for broader social issues in medicine, such as malpractice judgments and health care funding. What would it be like, he wondered, if the law and the economics of medicine reflected the same principles that guided him and his patients in their daily practice?

Malpractice

Sometimes people misunderstood what S. meant by words like *uncertainty, probability,* and especially *gambling.* They thought that these concepts would give doctors an "out," a way of disclaiming responsibility by attributing bad outcomes to chance. Indeed, in the mistrustful world of the Mechanistic Paradigm, there were some doctors who would try to do this. Some patients wondered whether even S. might not have had that in mind.

Actually nothing could have been further from his mind. Even though S. made it clear that he could not know with certainty, he also made it clear that it was possible to know with some degree of certainty. For example, he could not know precisely what caused Rose Heifetz's cancer or brought about its remission, but he stated with some degree of certainty that Laetrile would not work. In a less than certain world he, like his patients, was responsible for acting on probable knowledge.

Under the Probabilistic Paradigm a doctor would still be responsible for knowing what a doctor should know and doing what it is a doctor's job to do. Malpractice law ought to be able to distinguish between reasonable gambles that just lose and gambles that are unreasonable, whether from incompetence, negligence, or bad faith. When a doctor is held responsible for choice, not chance, malpractice becomes a matter of unprincipled gambling, intentional or unintentional.

This definition, S. realized, would not be so different from the one currently in use. The law as it stands seeks to penalize doctors not for chance outcomes, but for avoidable errors. Deriving the malpractice concept from the Probabilistic Paradigm would have the benefit of clarifying the chance-choice distinction, both in the law itself and, perhaps more important, in people's expectations. Patients who gamble consciously would be less likely to evaluate gambles from hindsight, i.e., to confuse a good outcome with a good gamble, a bad outcome with a bad gamble. Rather they would evaluate gambles as they might have appeared before the fact to a knowledgeable person acting in good faith. Moreover, patients who participated in decision-making would feel less alienated both from the doctor and from the various outcomes. By being able to share the burden of uncertainty from the beginning, they would be less likely to react to disappointment with recriminations. Although malpractice judgments would still be awarded, there probably would be fewer unjustified claims. Without the expectation of certainty doctors would not have such an excessive burden of responsibility.

Under the Probabilistic Paradigm both the doctor and the patient are causes, and as such cannot be completely known or controlled, even by themselves. Acknowledging themselves to be among the causes, patients and families can share responsibility for making and acting upon informed decisions whose consequences they can live with. In this concept of shared (as opposed to diffused) responsibility, in which the patient and family become more responsible without the doctor's becoming any less so, lies the real significance of the Probabilistic Paradigm for medical ethics and malpractice.

Health-Care Funding

If S. had wanted to "sell" the Probabilistic Paradigm, he might have been tempted to claim that its adoption would reduce the costs of medical care. He could not, however, in all honesty make such a broad claim. Quite likely the widespread application of probabilistic thinking in medicine would reduce costs in some areas (e.g., exhaustive, high-technology diagnostic testing) and increase costs in others (e.g., the time doctors spent working out decisions with patients). Less would be spent on machines, more on people.

The costs of medical care depend in part on the kinds of choices people make, individually and collectively. In the present system, however, high costs often result from an absence of choice. The real difference between the present system and the one S. envisioned would be in the way in which the costs would be incurred: who would make the decisions, how consciously and explicitly they would be made, what values they would reflect, how the needs of the individual would be reconciled with the needs of society. An economic solution consistent with the Probabilistic Paradigm would put decisions about the kinds of medical care bought by patients and insurance subscribers (as well as taxpayers) less in the hands of corporate interests and more in those of patients, families, and physicians. People would be choosing what they thought was worth paying for. Even if costs remained as high as they are today, they would not seem so arbitrary and uncontrollable. They would be seen as resulting from considered principles and values.

When the Cavanaugh and O'Farrell families took care of Mrs. Gormley at home, they were made intimately aware of the costs of dying—the costs for the dying person and the costs for the family, the money costs and the costs in time, work, and emotional energy. Without articulating the issue in these terms, they could weigh the costs against the benefits of having

Mrs. Gormley live beyond the point of being able to live a useful or even sentient life. They would have done anything to keep her from becoming terminally ill, but at a certain point they could see that it was time to allow her to die and to go on with their own lives. If Mrs. Gormley had been in the hospital, life-prolonging technology would have been temptingly at hand. In almost any hospital setting today not only she but her family would have been anesthetized from the experience of death and from the costs of caring for a dying person. At home, even if they had been reimbursed for the extra expenses of home care, they still would have experienced the work involved.

S. did not challenge the fairness of the basic insurance principle of averaging out the costs of illness to avoid financial hardship for those who were ill at any given time. As in the case of malpractice claims, he thought it entirely consistent with the Probabilistic Paradigm to say that people should not be penalized for chance events. At the same time, he could not help but observe (as with the Cavanaughs and O'Farrells) that people who participated in making and carrying out decisions concerning their own and their families' health care were in a better position to assume responsibility for the consequences of their choices, both for themselves and for society. Of course, it was not always possible or desirable for patients and families to be so involved in physically carrying out their decisions as Mrs. Gormley's family was. Expensive and remote-seeming technical procedures sometimes were necessary. Still, S. thought, there ought to be some way to bring the consciousness of choice—and along with it the principles of fairness and social responsibility—into everyday medical decision-making.

A system of health-care funding consistent with the Probabilistic Paradigm would give patients and doctors incentives for making principled decisions. By keeping probabilities and values in sight, people could more easily come to principled decisions in a society where limited resources prevent everyone from being reimbursed for everything they might want to do. By how much would a given test reduce the uncertainty of a diagnosis? By how much would a given treatment increase the probability of a good outcome for the patient? These considerations of probability would be weighed against considerations of value and principle. The nature of the illness, for example, would have to be taken into account. A ten percent reduction of uncertainty might be considered worthy of reimbursement in the case of cancer, but not in the case of strep throat. In considering such a reimbursement scheme, however, we also would have to ask whether it is fair for people of greater means to be able to buy the extra ten percent of certainty.

The judgments involved in establishing a health-care reimbursement system cognizant of probabilities and values would be complex and sensitive ones. Who would make them? When he considered this question, S. saw how what he envisioned as an application of the Probabilistic Paradigm could become merely an amendment to the Mechanistic. In a society structured as ours is, guidelines for reimbursement would inevitably be established by a bureaucratic process heavily influenced by profit-seeking interests. Out of such a process would come judgments such as that infants between six months and one year of age should be fed commercial formula rather than whole milk. For a system consistent with the Probabilistic Paradigm such as S. was proposing to work, people would have to be involved not only in their own health-care decisions, but in the political process by which society set up principles for allocating resources. Without such participation patients, families, and doctors would be alienated both from the process and the result.

In attempting to practice the Probabilistic Paradigm in medicine, S. was working to establish trust, both in other people and in the order of a changing universe, so that people could deal effectively with the vicissitudes of reality instead of reacting reflexively out of fear and anxiety. If people could learn trust and critical thinking in the sensitive area of medicine, they would gain, individually and collectively, both the feeling and the actuality of greater control of their lives. They would be less amenable to control by individuals, corporations, or bureaucratic institutions and better able to bring about new ways of thinking, feeling, and acting throughout society. Yet how could people learn to trust in a world that was not now set up to allow for trust? How could people use critical thinking to develop their own rules to live by when the rules they *had* to live by encouraged mindlessness? How could they distinguish between critical thinking and cynicism?

Still, it was a gamble worth taking. They would have to give it a try.

REFERENCES

AINSLIE, G. "A Behavioral Theory of Impulse Control." *Psychological Bulletin,* 82(1975), pp. 463–96.

BERNARD, C. *An Introduction to the Study of Experimental Medicine.* New York: Dover, 1957.

BERNSTEIN, R.J. *The Restructuring of Social and Political Theory.* Philadelphia: University of Pennsylvania Press, 1978.

BOHR, N. "Discussions with Einstein on Epistemological Problems in Atomic Physics," in *Albert Einstein, Philosopher-Scientist,* Third Edition, P. A. Schilpp, ed. LaSalle, Ill.: Open Court (1969), pp. 199–241.

BUNGE, M. *Causality and Modern Science.* New York: Dover, 1979.

BURSZTAJN, H. "The Role of a Training Protocol in Formulating Patient Instructions as to Terminal Care Choices." *Journal of Medical Education,* 52(1977), pp. 347–48.

BURSZTAJN, H., and HAMM, R.M. "Medical Maxims: Two Views of Science." *Yale Journal of Biology and Medicine,* 52 (1979), pp. 483–86.

BURSZTAJN, H., and HAMM, R.M. "On Knowing What Is Good for the Patient: The Uses of Utility Assessment and the Clinician's Intuition of Patient Values." Paper presented at the First Annual Meeting of the Society for Medical Decision Making, Cincinnati, Ohio, September 12, 1979. Unpublished.

CARLSON, R.J., ed. *The Frontiers of Science and Medicine.* Chicago: Henry Regnery, 1976.

CHANDLER, A.D., ed. *Giant Enterprise: Ford, General Motors and the Automobile Industry.* New York: Harcourt, Brace & World, 1964.

CHANOWITZ, B.Z., and LANGER, F. "Premature Cognitive Commitment." Cambridge, Mass.: Harvard University. Unpublished.

CLARK, M., and MILLS, J. "Interpersonal Attraction in Exchange and Communal Relationships." *Journal of Personality and Social Psychology,* 37 (1979), pp. 12–24.

COUSINS, N. "The Holistic Health Explosion." *Saturday Review,* 6 (No. 7, 1979), pp. 17–20.

DREYFUS, H., and DREYFUS, S. "Uses and Abuses of Multi-attribute and Multi-aspect Models of Decision Making." Berkeley: University of California, Department of Philosophy and Department of Industrial Engineering and Operations Research. Unpublished.

EDWARDS, R. *Contested Terrain.* New York: Basic Books, 1979.

EDWARDS, W. "N = 1: Diagnosis in Unique Cases," in *Computer Diagnosis and Diagnostic Methods,* J.A. Jacquez, ed. Springfield, Ill.: Charles C Thomas (1972), pp. 139–51.

ELLSBERG, D. "Risk, Ambiguity, and the Savage Axioms." *Quarterly Journal of Economics,* 75 (1961), pp. 643–49.

EWEN, S. *Captains of Consciousness.* New York: McGraw-Hill, 1976.

EYER, J., and STERLING, P. "Stress Related Mortality and Social Organization." *Review of Radical Political Economics,* 9 (No. 1, 1977), pp. 1–45.

FAISON, J.B.; PISANI, B.J.; DOUGLAS, R.G.; CRANCH, G.S.; and LUBIC, R.W. "The Childbearing Center: An Alternative Birth Setting." *Obstetrics and Gynecology,* 54 (1979), pp. 527–32.

FIORE, N. "Fighting Cancer—One Patient's Perspective." *New England Journal of Medicine,* 300 (1979), pp. 284–89.

FISCHHOFF, B. "Hindsight ≠ Foresight: The Effect of Outcome

Knowledge on Judgment Under Uncertainty." *Journal of Experimental Psychology: Human Perception and Performance,* 1 (1975), pp. 288–99.

FULLER, P. "Introduction," in *The Psychology of Gambling,* J. Halliday and P. Fuller, eds. New York: Harper & Row (1975), pp. 1–114.

GROVES, J. "Taking Care of the Hateful Patient." *New England Journal of Medicine,* 298 (1978), pp. 883–87.

HACKING, I. *The Emergence of Probability.* London: Cambridge University Press, 1975.

HAMPSHIRE, S. "Human Nature." *The New York Review of Books,* 26 (No. 19, 1979), pp. 42c–42d.

HAVENS, L.L. *Participant Observation.* New York: Jason Aronson, 1976.

HEISENBERG, W. *Physics and Philosophy.* New York: Harper & Row, 1958.

HEMPEL, C. "Studies in the Logic of Confirmation," in *Aspects of Scientific Explanation.* New York: Free Press (1965), pp. 3–51.

HOFSTEDE, G. "The Poverty of Management Control Philosophy." *Academy of Management Review,* 3 (1978), pp. 450–61.

KAFKA, F. "The Metamorphosis," in *The Penal Colony,* translated by W. Muir and E. Muir. New York: Schocken Books (1948), pp. 65–132.

KAHNEMAN, D., and TVERSKY, A. "On the Psychology of Prediction." *Psychological Review,* 80 (1973), pp. 237–51.

KELMAN, H.C. "The Role of the Group in the Induction of Therapeutic Change." *International Journal of Group Psychotherapy,* 13 (1963), pp. 399–432.

KITZINGER, S., and DAVIS, J.A., eds. *The Place of Birth.* Oxford: Oxford University Press, 1978.

KOVEL, J. "Rationalization and the Family." *Telos,* 37 (1978), pp. 5–21.

KUHN, T.S. *The Structure of Scientific Revolutions.* Chicago: University of Chicago Press, 1962.

LANGER, E. "The Illusion of Control." *Journal of Personality and Social Psychology,* 32 (1975), pp. 311–28.

LASCH, C. *Haven in a Heartless World.* New York: Basic Books, 1977.

LEE, W. *Decision Theory and Human Behavior.* New York: Wiley, 1971.

LICHTENSTEIN, S., and SLOVIC, P. "Reversals of Preference Between Bids and Choices in Gambling Decisions." *Journal of Experimental Psychology,* 89 (1971), pp. 46–55.

LIFTON, R.J. *The Broken Connection.* New York: Simon & Schuster, 1979.

McCLELLAND, D.C. "Risk-taking in Children with High and Low Need for Achievement," in *Motives in Fantasy, Action, and Society,* J.W. Atkinson, ed. Princeton: Van Nostrand (1958), pp. 306–21.

MOORE, B.R., and STUTTARD, S. "Dr. Guthrie and *Felis domesticus,* Or: Tripping over the Cat." *Science,* 205 (1979), pp. 1031–33.

NEUTRA, R.R.; FIENBERG, S.E.; GREENLAND, S.; and FRIEDMAN, E.A. "Effect of Fetal Monitoring on Neonatal Death Rates." *New England Journal of Medicine,* 299 (1978), pp. 324–26.

NEWTON, I. "Philosophiae Naturalis Principia Mathematica," Book III (1686), in *Newton's Philosophy of Nature,* H.S. Thayer, ed. New York: Hafner (1953), pp. 3–5.

PAUKER, S.G. "Coronary Artery Surgery: The Use of Decision Analysis." *Annals of Internal Medicine,* 85 (1976), pp. 8–18.

PEELE, S., with BRODSKY, A. *Love and Addiction.* New York: New American Library, 1976.

PELLETIER, K.R. *Mind as Healer, Mind as Slayer.* New York: Delacorte Press/Seymour Lawrence, 1977.

PUTNAM, H. *Meaning and the Moral Sciences.* London: Routledge and Kegan Paul, 1978.

———. "A Philosopher Looks at Quantum Physics," in *Mathematics, Matter, and Method,* H. Putnam, ed. Cambridge: Cambridge University Press (1979), pp. 130–58.

RAIFFA, H. *Decision Analysis.* Reading, Mass.: Addison-Wesley, 1968.

ROETHLISBERGER, F.J., and DIXON, W.J. *Management and the Worker.* Cambridge, Mass.: Harvard University Press, 1939.

ROSENTHAL, R. "Interpersonal Expectations: Effects of the Experimenter's Hypothesis," in *Artifact in Behavioral Research,* R. Rosenthal and R. Roshow, eds. New York: Academic Press (1969), pp. 181–277.

ROTHMAN, S.M. "Family Life as Zero-Sum Game." *Dissent,* 25 (1978), pp. 392–97.

SCHRECKER, PAUL. *Work and History.* Princeton: Princeton University Press, 1948.

SENNETT, R. *The Fall of Public Man.* New York: Vintage, 1978.

SHIMONY, A. "Scientific Inference," in *The Nature and Function of Scientific Theories,* R. Colodny, ed. Pittsburgh: University of Pittsburgh Press (1970), pp. 79–172.

SIMONTON, O.C.; MATTHEWS-SIMONTON, S.; and CREIGHTON, J. *Getting Well Again.* Los Angeles: J.P. Tarcher, 1978.

STEPHENS, G.G. "Family Medicine as Counter-Culture." *Family Medicine Teacher,* 11 (No. 5, 1979), pp. 14–18.

THUROW, L.C. "Economics 1977." *Daedalus,* 106 (No. 4, 1977), pp. 79–94.

TOURNEY, G. "A History of Therapeutic Fashions in Psychiatry." *American Journal of Psychiatry,* 124 (1967), pp. 784–96.

TRIBE, L.H. "Trial by Mathematics: Precision and Ritual in the Legal Process." *Harvard Law Review,* 84 (1971), pp. 1329–93.
———. "Policy Science: Analysis or Ideology." *Philosophy and Public Affairs,* 2 (1972), pp. 66–110.

VON NEUMANN, J., and MORGENSTERN, O. *Theory of Games and Economic Behavior.* Princeton: Princeton University Press, 1944.

WEBER, M. *The Protestant Ethic and the Spirit of Capitalism,* translated by T. Parsons. London: G. Allen and Unwin, 1930.

WEINSTEIN, M.C. "Allocation of Subjects in Medical Experiments." *New England Journal of Medicine,* 291 (1974), pp. 1278–85.

WHITE, E. B. "Bedfellows," in *Essays of E. B. White.* New York: Harper & Row, 1977, pp. 80–89.

WITTGENSTEIN, L. *Philosophical Investigations.* New York: Macmillan, 1958.

INDEX

THE AUTHORS

HAROLD BURSZTAJN, M.D., is a resident in psychiatry at the Massachusetts Mental Health Center and a clinical fellow in medicine at the Massachusetts General Hospital. He is the author of several articles on the philosophy of medicine. Born in Poland, Dr. Bursztajn graduated from Princeton and in 1977 from the Harvard Medical School, where his honors thesis concerned the relationship between scientific paradigms and clinical decision-making in primary care. His work as a University Scholar at Princeton, the Harvard Medical School honors thesis, and his ongoing research with Dr. Hamm form the conceptual framework for *Medical Choices, Medical Chances.*

RICHARD I. FEINBLOOM, M.D., is director of the Family Health Care Program of the Harvard Medical School and a partner in the Family Practice Group of Cambridge, Massachusetts. He is author, with the Boston Children's Medical Center, of the *Child Health Encyclopedia* and the major contributor to their *Pregnancy, Birth and the Newborn Baby.* Dr. Feinbloom is also an outspoken advocate of car safety for children and of improved television programs for children. He has testified before the U.S. Senate on these and similar issues.

ROBERT M. HAMM, PH.D., is an experimental psychologist at Harvard University and author of several studies of decision-making behavior. He has taught psychology at Harvard and conducted research at the Massachusetts Mental Health Center. Dr. Hamm is also currently a research fellow in the Division of Primary Care at the Harvard Medical School.

ARCHIE BRODSKY, a writer, is co-author of several books, including *Love and Addiction, Burnout: Stages of Disillusionment in the Helping Professions,* and *The Active Patient's Guide to Better Medical Care.* A graduate of the University of Pennsylvania, Mr. Brodsky has done editorial consulting and written articles and reviews in the fields of medicine, psychology, and human services.